Language, Mind and Brain

To the memory of Mieczysław Dąbrowski

Language, Mind and Brain

Some Psychological and Neurological Constraints on Theories of Grammar

EWA DĄBROWSKA

EDINBURGH UNIVERSITY PRESS

Edinburgh University Press Ltd
22 George Square, Edinburgh

Typeset in 10/12 Times New Roman
by Servis Filmsetting Ltd, Manchester, and
printed and bound in Great Britain by
The Cromwell Press, Trowbridge, Wilts

A CIP record for this book is available from the British Library

ISBN 0 7486 1474 5 (hardback)
ISBN 0 7486 1475 3 (paperback)

The research for this book was supported by

A · H · R · B

arts and humanities research board

Contents

List of figures

List of tables

Acknowledgements

I would like to thank my teachers, Roman Kalisz and Tomasz Krzeszowski, who first introduced me to cognitive approaches to language, and thus started me on the long way that led to this book. I am very grateful to Magdalena Smoczyńska for encouraging me to take up work on child language, and generously providing me with a coded version of the Kraków corpus to get me going. The research on the acquisition of Polish case inflections reported in Chapter 8 is based on this data.

I began working on the book while I was visiting the Max Planck Institute for Evolutionary Anthropology in Leipzig. During the visit, and on many subsequent occasions, I had many interesting and fruitful discussions with Elena Lieven, Mike Tomasello, Holger Diessel and Heike Behrens. Many of the ideas in this book emerged and developed during these discussions, and I am extremely grateful to all of them for their generosity and encouragement. Special thanks are due to Mike Tomasello and Elena Lieven, who have read and commented on parts of the manuscript and provided many valuable and insightful comments. I am also indebted to Wojciech Kubiński, Ola Kubińska, Agata Kochańska, Anna Tymińska and Beata Williamson for help with the data collection.

Most of the book was written during a period of leave funded by the University of Sheffield and the Arts and Humanities Research Board (grant number AN5597/APN15868). The research on case inflections reported in Chapter 8 was supported by a British Academy Small Research Grant (grant number RB 100556).

I would like to thank Mouton de Gruyter for permission to reproduce figures 7.4, 7.5, and 7.6, which originally appeared as figures 1, 2, and 3, respectively, in P. Brown, 'The INs and ONs of Tzeltal locative expressions: the semantics of static descriptions of location', *Linguistics*, 32, 743–90.

Most of all, I would like to thank my husband, Michael Pincombe, for acting as linguistic consultant and voice of reason on topics related to the book and many others. Michael read the entire manuscript and identified many issues that needed clarification or correction; he produced the artwork in Chapter 7; and his humour, good cheer and paprikás have helped to keep me happy and sane (well, almost) during the duration of the project.

1 Introduction

Linguistics is often defined as 'the branch of cognitive science dealing with language' – but, most linguists hasten to add, it is an 'independent branch', by which they mean that language can, and should, be studied in its own terms, without reference to psychological or neurological concepts and theories. On this view, the role of linguistics is to provide hypotheses for other disciplines to test. Some linguists are even more 'separatist': all too often, when research on language acquisition or processing contradicts hypotheses developed on the basis of purely linguistic data, they succumb to the temptation to ignore it, justifying this decision by appealing to notions such as 'performance' as opposed to 'competence'. This approach has resulted in a proliferation of linguistic theories, many of which appeal to constructs which are extremely implausible both psychologically and biologically, and an estrangement from other disciplines studying the human capacity for language. It is becoming increasingly clear to many linguists that in order to make further progress in the study of language, we need to constrain linguistic theorising in some way. Since human language resides in the human mind, the most promising source of constraints on theories of language is properties of the human mind/brain.

This book is an attempt to show how linguistics can benefit by incorporating insights from other disciplines. Part I, 'The Basic Specifications', draws on the relevant research in language processing, acquisition, and impairment, comparative psychology, and genetics to develop a set of 'design specifications' for language which should be the starting point of any linguistic theory that purports to be psychologically realistic. The purpose here is not to engage in debate or evaluate the research in these disciplines, but to concentrate on those findings which are relatively uncontroversial and which are of special importance to linguistic theory. For readers with little prior knowledge of these disciplines, this will be a useful introduction to the relevant psychological and neurological issues.

These general specifications are further developed in Part II, 'The Building Blocks of Language', where they are applied to three central aspects of linguistic organisation: lexical semantics, inflectional morphology, and syntax. Knowing how a system emerged often provides valuable clues about its organisation, so each of these areas is explored from a developmental perspective as well as from the point of view of the adult end state. Part II also addresses several issues of central importance to linguistic theory: the status of rules, the relationship between grammar and the lexicon, and the relationship between innate structure and acquired knowledge. The final chapter is devoted to approaches to language which meet the specifications developed earlier, with particular prominence given to cognitive and construction grammar.

Another recurrent theme throughout the book is the need to make linguistics an empirical science. This means, above all, that linguistic theories should be assessed on how well they explain the data and the empirical predictions they make – not on their formal elegance. It also means that, in order to reach reliable conclusions, linguists need to make use of a wider range of data sources.

Particularly important among these are examples of real usage collected in large corpora of texts, both written and spoken. During the first three decades following the 'Chomskyan revolution', it was fashionable in certain circles to assert that corpus data provides an inadequate foundation for linguistic theory, for two main reasons. First, even the largest corpora necessarily contain only an infinitesimally small part of the possible sentences of any given language, and may not contain any instances of the structures that are of interest to the analyst. Worse still, corpus data is 'noisy', in that it often contains ungrammatical sentences. Due to these limitations, it was proposed that linguists should rely on grammaticality judgements rather than on collections of actual texts.

As a matter of fact, grammaticality judgement data can also be very noisy. Naïve informants often reject grammatically well-formed sentences which are semantically or pragmatically odd, or merely difficult to process, and accept ungrammatical sentences in certain contexts. Because of this, many linguists do not even bother to collect grammaticality judgements, preferring instead to rely on their own intuitions, or those of a few colleagues. Such an approach, however, is completely unacceptable if linguistics is to be regarded as a scientific enterprise. A researcher's own intuitions may be blunted after repeated experience with ungrammatical sentences, or, worse still, contaminated by his or her theoretical commitments. Therefore, while they are an excellent source of hypotheses, they should, except in the clearest cases, be confirmed by a systematic survey of native speakers' judgements. This will also allow the researcher to establish how much variation there is among speakers of the same language, which could have far-reaching theoretical implications.

However, useful as they are, grammaticality judgements cannot replace corpus data. Only the latter provides information about structures which people actually use – about language in its natural habitat, as it were – and, crucially, their relative frequencies, which often offers valuable clues about how languages work. Furthermore, corpora sometimes yield unexpected information about systematic exceptions to generalisations proposed by linguists – a kind of data which we cannot afford to ignore. So, while the concerns about corpus data enumerated earlier are valid, they do not entail that linguists should not rely on this information source, but merely that they should use other sources as well. Elicitation and grammaticality judgement studies, for example, are a useful way of getting around the problem of accidental gaps in corpora; and experiments in which the researcher manipulates the language (e.g. by presenting speakers with a nonce word and asking them to use it in a particular construction) yield valuable information about productivity. In the following pages, we will use all of these data sources, since it is only by combining information from a number of different sources that we can hope to begin to understand the astonishingly complex phenomenon we call language.

Part I

The Basic Specifications

2 Language processing: speed and flexibility

1. The complexity of the task

Most people – including many language professionals – take language for granted. We produce and interpret utterances so quickly and effortlessly that it's easy to overlook the enormous complexity of the task. It will be useful, therefore, to begin our discussion by examining some of the difficulties involved in processing perfectly ordinary language. I will illustrate these problems using one simple sentence, picked more or less at random from a book that happens to be lying on my desk as I am writing this – David Lodge's *Paradise News*:

(1)   *Tess blew her nose on a paper tissue.*

If you were to hear this sentence instead of reading it, what would reach your ears would be a series of air vibrations; yet almost instantaneously you would be able to work out its meaning: a woman picks up a piece of tissue, covers her nostrils with it, and clears her nose by vigorously expelling air through it. To arrive at this interpretation, you must have performed a number of operations: identified the words; accessed their relevant senses; determined the grammatical relationships between them; and integrated lexical, syntactic, and contextual information with real-world knowledge to construct an interpretation of the sentence in context. Each of these operations involves the integration of multiple and only partially reliable cues.

Let us begin with the first stage: word recognition. The major problems here are variability of the speech signal and segmentation. The acoustic properties of speech segments vary according to the context in which they occur: the /b/ sounds in *blew, bet, bear* and *rob*, for example, are phonetically quite distinct. Furthermore, since the acoustic properties of speech depend on the shape of the vocal tract and everybody's vocal tract is shaped slightly differently, what we perceive as 'the same' sound is actually quite different when produced by different speakers, or even by the same speaker on different occasions. The segmentation problem is a consequence of the fact that speech is continuous (speakers don't normally pause between words), and hence word boundaries are not 'given' in the acoustic input but must be inferred by the listener.

Because of the lack of invariance and the segmentation problem, even this 'low-level' processing poses a considerable challenge, which is perhaps best appreciated in the context of current developments in automatic speech recognition. Despite decades of intensive research, we are only beginning to see computer applications that are reasonably accurate at identifying words in continuous speech. Most of the existing programs are trained to recognise the voice of a particular speaker in a particular acoustic environment, with little background noise; and although their performance is good enough to make them commercially viable, they still make many errors.

Once the listener has segmented the speech signal and identified the words, he or she must access the relevant sense of each word and determine how they combine to form constituents. Both of these operations are fraught with difficulty, since most words are ambiguous, and there is often more than one way of constructing a well-formed syntactic structure from a given string of words.

Let us begin with lexical ambiguity. The first word in our sentence, *Tess*, is a proper name, and hence has no conventional linguistic meaning apart from specifying that the referent is female and probably human. However, the next word, *blew*, is multiply ambiguous. As the past tense form of the verb *blow*, *blew* could have any of the following meanings:

1. moved (of air particles), as in *The wind blew in my face*;
2. caused to move by blowing, as in *The wind blew snow in my face*;
3. sent out a stream of air from the mouth or nose, as in *He blew (air) into the balloon*;
4. produced (e.g. smoke rings or bubbles) by blowing air out of one's mouth;
5. blew air into a wind instrument, as in *She blew the trumpet*;
6. (of a musical instrument) produced a sound: *The trumpet blew outside*;
7. burst, as in *His tyre blew*;
8. experienced a burst tyre while driving, as in *He blew a tyre*;
9. spent (money etc.), as in *He blew his inheritance on a sports car*;
10. wasted (an opportunity), as in *She blew her chance*;
11. burned out, as in *The fuse blew*;
12. exhaled vigorously through the nose in order to clear it.

(This is a selection of some of the most frequent meanings; any sizeable dictionary will list many more.) The same phonological form, when spelt *blue*, is also associated with the following meanings:

13. having a particular colour;
14. sad, as in *Why are you feeling blue?*;
15. pornographic, as in *a blue movie*.

The next content word, the noun *nose*, can designate any of the following:

1. a part of the body;
2. the sense of smell, as in *a dog with a good nose*;
3. intuition, as in *a reporter with a nose for a story*;
4. the most forward part of an aircraft;
5. the open end of a pipe.

It can also have a range of verbal meanings:

6. (of an aircraft) to come down steeply;
7. to go forward carefully;
8. smell for;
9. search for;
10. pry into, as in *nose into other people's affairs*.

The word *paper* also has several different senses:

1. substance manufactured from wood fibre used for writing, drawing etc.;
2. newspaper;
3. a set of examination questions;
4. essay;
5. to cover with paper;

and the same is true of *tissue*, which can refer to any of the following:

1. woven fabric;
2. a mass of cells, as in *muscular tissue*;
3. a small piece of thin soft absorbent paper;
4. web, as in *a tissue of lies*.

In addition to these multiply ambiguous open-class words, our sentence also has three function words, *her*, *on*, and *a*. These, too, can signal a variety of meanings. *Her* can be either a possessive determiner (as in *her nose*) or the objective form of the pronoun *she* (as in *I gave her a pen*). The preposition/particle *on* is one of the most highly polysemous words in English. Instead of listing all the possible senses, which run into the hundreds, I will simply list a few representative usages:

(2) a. *All the books on politics are on this shelf.*
     b. *She hung the picture on the wall.*
     c. *She had a dog on a lead.*
     d. *I wrote it on a piece of paper.*
     e. *Have you ever worked on a farm?*

f. *The house is on the river.*
g. *We watched the boats on the river.*
h. *There weren't many people on the train.*
i. *I've never seen a smile on her face.*
j. *The meeting is on Thursday.*
k. *Does your car run on unleaded?*
l. *I heard it on Radio Four.*
m. *She's on the phone.*
n. *The book was on special offer.*
o. *He read on.*
p. *Turn the lights on.*
q. *He is working on a new book.*
r. *That's just not on!*

Finally, the determiner *a*, in addition to various specialised uses which will not be discussed here (but see Quirk et al. 1985: 265–97), can be used to indicate that the speaker wishes:

1. to refer to a specific member of the class designated by the following noun; thus, one possible interpretation of *Sally wishes to marry a millionaire* is that she wants to marry a particular millionaire;
2. to refer to any member of the class designated by the noun; thus *Sally wants to marry a millionaire* could also mean that she is willing to marry anyone with a seven-figure account (in other words, any old millionaire will do);
3. to refer to all the members of the class designated by the noun; thus *A girl should be realistic* means that all girls should be realistic;
4. to quantify the number of objects referred to by the noun; for example, *in a day or two* means 'in one or two days'.

To resolve these ambiguities, the listener must use grammatical, lexical, collocational, and pragmatic information. Let me illustrate this process using the second word in our example, the phonological form /bluː/. In the context of our sentence, /bluː/ is the past tense of the verb *blow* rather than the adjective *blue*, since (1) there is no noun for it to modify and (2) it comes immediately after the subject, and hence is likely to be the first element of the verb phrase, which is usually a verb or an auxiliary. The fact that the subject NP is animate effectively eliminates senses (1), (6), (7) and (11), which normally co-occur with subjects designating wind, a wind instrument, a tyre, and a fuse, respectively. Senses (4), (5), (8), (9) and (10) are also ruled out for collocational reasons: they normally take direct objects which designate a gaseous formation such as smoke rings (sense 4), a wind instrument (5), a tyre (8), money or equivalent (9), or an opportunity (10). Our sentence could mean that she blew into a nose-shaped piece of plastic, or that she sold her nose in order to buy a paper tissue – but such interpretations are extremely unlikely. Since noses usually come attached to faces, sense (2) is ruled out on the basis of our knowledge of the world (although the sentence could, in theory, mean that she propelled a plastic mould of a nose, or a real nose which had been severed from someone's face, by blowing until it landed on a paper tissue – either by exhaling air from the lungs or by using a device such as a bellows). The direct object *her nose* is incompatible with sense (3), which is used in intransitive constructions or with an NP designating the substance that comes out of the lungs such as air or smoke. This leaves (12), the nose-clearing sense, as the preferred interpretation of the phonological form /bluː/ in the context of our example.

Let us now briefly look at syntactic processing. English is a fairly rigid SVO language, so the listener can safely assume that the preverbal NP (*Tess*) is the subject. If we consider just lexical category information, the sequence *blew her nose* could be interpreted either as a verb followed by a direct object, where *her* is a possessive determiner in the object NP (analogous to *ate his lunch*) or a verb with two objects (analogous to *gave him lunch*). However, *her* cannot be the object of the verb, for two reasons. First, *blow* is monotransitive (it only allows one object), so if *her* were its object, there would be no way of attaching the NP *nose* to the verb phrase. Secondly, since *nose* is a singular count noun, it must be preceded by a determiner. Therefore, the entire expression *her nose* must be the object of *blew*.

The next four words, *on a paper tissue*, clearly constitute a prepositional phrase. To interpret the sentence, the listener must determine how it combines with the preceding words. There are three possibilities here: the PP could be a complement to the verb, an adjunct, or a modifier of the noun. In the first case, the sentence would have the same structure as *Tess put the milk in the fridge*. This possibility is ruled out by the fact that *blew* is monotransitive, and hence takes only one complement, the direct object. In the second case, *on a paper tissue* would specify either the location or the direction of Tess's doings, and the syntactic structure would parallel that for *Tess read the book on the train*. Finally, the PP could postmodify the noun *nose*. Imagine that Tess has two noses, and has put one of them on a paper tissue. In this context the sentence could mean that she blew the nose which was on the paper tissue, and would be similar in structure to *Tess sold the house in Canada*.

Our example is a very simple sentence, and hence the amount of syntactic ambiguity that the reader or listener must cope with is fairly modest.[1] However, syntactic ambiguity becomes a major problem when the processor is confronted with longer, more complex sentences characteristic of written discourse. It is well known from the natural language processing literature that the number of candidate parses increases exponentially with sentence length. Consider the following example, borrowed from Martin et al. (1987). Their grammar assigns three structural analyses to the sentence *List the sales of products in 1973* (the prepositional phrase *in 1973* can modify the verb *list*, the expression *sales of products*, or just the noun *products*). If we add a single word to the sentence, making it *List the sales of products produced in 1973*, the number of analyses increases to 10; and if we add *with the products produced in 1972* at the end of the last sentence, the number of alternative structural descriptions (assuming the grammar developed by Martin et al.) is exactly 455.

Returning to Tess and her nose: to determine which of the two grammatically acceptable readings identified above is the one that the speaker intended, the listener must again use pragmatic information. Since noses are usually attached to their owners and people don't normally have more than one, the easiest way to specify which nose you mean is by identifying the owner by means of a possessive modifier; hence, a prepositional phrase after *nose* is unlikely to be a postmodifier. It must therefore be an adjunct specifying either where Tess was when she blew her nose or where what she blew out of her nose ended up. Stating that Tess was *on a paper tissue* is not a very good way of locating her in space, since tissues are rather small in relation to a person, and do not have a fixed location. On the other hand, paper tissues are excellent for blowing your nose on, so by far the most likely interpretation of the sentence is that Tess used the tissue to clear her nose.

The listener must also decide whether *her* refers to Tess or to another female not mentioned in the sentence. English grammar allows both possibilities, so again, the correct interpretation depends on pragmatic knowledge. Since it is impossible to clear another person's nose by exhaling air on a paper tissue,[2] we must conclude that *her* refers to Tess.

I have deliberately chosen to illustrate the complexity of the processing task with a very simple (if somewhat insalubrious) sentence: one with no embedding, no dislocated constituents, no long-distance dependencies. The example illustrates rather nicely the amount of ambiguity that listeners must cope with, as well as the fact that successful comprehension requires the integration of lexical, syntactic and real-world knowledge. The discussion so far, however, has completely ignored another important feature of ordinary language use which introduces a whole new dimension of complexity: the fact that much of the linguistic input that reaches our ears is degraded.

First, the acoustic signal itself is often distorted or partially inaudible – because of either background noise, or various modifications that speakers make in rapid speech, or both. In a now-classic study, Pollack and Pickett (1964) spliced words out of a recorded conversation and asked speakers to identify them. Only about 50 per cent of the words presented in isolation were intelligible, but performance improved dramatically when the same words were heard in a short phrase. By varying how the linguistic context was presented (visually or visually and auditorily), Pollack and Pickett were able to show that the improvement was partially attributable to listeners adjusting to the specific quality of the speaker's voice and partially to the lexical and syntactic constraints introduced by the additional material, a conclusion which was corroborated by later research (see Massaro 1994; Samuel 1986). Thus, in addition to all the complexities already discussed, listeners are also frequently forced to guess what the speaker actually said.

Casual speech is also 'noisy' in a metaphorical sense, in that it contains a fair number of sentence fragments and false starts as well as some sentences which are outright ungrammatical. This means that some of the grammatical cues that language users can exploit when processing more carefully edited discourse (e.g. written texts) are unavailable or even misleading. We know very little about how people process ill-formed sentences, although existing studies suggest that morphosyntactic anomalies present surprisingly little difficulty (Braze et al. 2002; Jou and Harris 1991).

2. Speed

In spite of this complexity, humans process language extremely fast. In informal conversation people produce, on average, about 150 words per minute. Furthermore, most conversations are reasonably contingent (people respond to each other's points) and proceed quite smoothly, with the next speaker taking the floor within about 500 milliseconds (i.e. half a second) of the first speaker finishing his turn (Bull and Aylett 1998). Within this interval, the new speaker must finish decoding the preceding utterance, decide on a relevant response, construct her own message (or at least its beginning) and launch the appropriate articulatory sequence. In fact, people often do this much faster. It is not unusual for successive turns to overlap slightly (by about a syllable or so). In such cases the second speaker has to do all her planning while her predecessor is still executing his turn.

These observations about the speed of ordinary language processing are confirmed by more controlled studies in laboratory conditions. One early demonstration was a series of experiments by Marslen-Wilson and colleagues (e.g. Marslen-Wilson 1973) in which participants were asked to 'shadow' a model, that is to say, repeat everything the model said as quickly as possible. Some people are able to do this with only a quarter second latency – in other words, they are only about a syllable behind the model. Analysis of the performance of such close shadowers suggests that they are not merely parroting a string of sounds, but processing the message at higher levels. For example, they often correct errors (*His knife tut the bread neatly* is repeated as *His knife cut the bread neatly*), and their own errors tend to be semantically and syntactically appropriate (e.g. *It was beginning to be light enough so I could see . . .* was shadowed as *It was beginning to be light enough so that I could see . . .*; *He had heard at the fire brigade . . .* became *He had heard that the fire brigade . . .*).

We can obtain more detailed information about the precise timing of the various subprocesses from work on language comprehension. Studies of spoken word recognition suggest that people can reliably identify words in isolation after hearing the first 300–30 ms; and when presented in a sentential context, many words can be identified after as little as the first 200 ms

(Grosjean 1980; Marslen-Wilson 1987) – well before the speaker has finished articulating them!

Lexical ambiguity is also resolved very quickly. In fact, one of the most hotly debated issues in psycholinguistics is whether the contextually irrelevant meanings of ambiguous words are accessed at all, or whether access is selective from the very beginning. This is a question of considerable theoretical significance. If comprehenders are able to use context to access only the relevant sense, we would have to conclude that language processing is highly interactive. On the other hand, initial activation of all senses is usually taken as supporting modular accounts of processing, according to which language comprehension and production is performed by a series of relatively autonomous components – one specialising in word recognition, another in syntactic analysis, and so on. Unfortunately, the large number of studies investigating the processing of ambiguous words have produced mixed results: some studies support the selective access account, and others do not (see Simpson 1994 for a review). There is an emerging consensus that the reason for these conflicting findings is that lexical access is not an 'all-or-nothing' phenomenon: the different senses of an ambiguous word are probably activated to varying degrees, depending on their relative frequencies (with frequent meanings being inherently easier to activate) and the strength of the contextual constraints. Thus, highly entrenched senses are difficult to suppress regardless of how inappropriate they may be in a given context; but contextual factors seem to have a considerable effect on the activation of less frequent senses.

However this debate is eventually resolved, the important point is that even when several meanings are initially accessed, the contextually irrelevant ones are deactivated very quickly. Tanenhaus et al. (1979) and Seidenberg et al. (1982), for example, found that if an ambiguous word was presented immediately after a word which was semantically related to one of its senses, both senses were primed – that is to say, people were able to make lexical decisions faster. If, however, the target word was presented after a short delay (about 200 ms), the facilitatory effect was found only when the prime was related to the relevant sense of the target word, which suggests that the irrelevant sense had already been eliminated at that point. This was true for noun/verb ambiguities (*He bought a watch/They decided to watch*), which can be resolved using morphosyntactic information, as well as noun/noun ambiguities (*You should have played the spade/Go to the store and buy a spade*), which require the integration of linguistic and real-world knowledge.

These early studies have shown that semantic and pragmatic knowledge are integrated with the incoming acoustic information extremely quickly. This was confirmed by more recent studies which attempted to determine the point at which participants establish reference by monitoring their eye movements as they examined a visual display accompanying a linguistic stimulus. When people are presented with a visual context for a spoken sentence, their eye movements are closely synchronised with the unfolding spoken sentence. For example, if they hear an instruction such as *Put the apple on the towel* while viewing an array consisting of an apple, a towel and a few distractor objects, they look at the apple on hearing *apple*; then, on hearing *towel*, they shift their gaze to the towel. Thus, tracking a person's eye movements gives us a window onto the mental processes underlying comprehension.

Using this methodology, Eberhard et al. (1995) were able to demonstrate that when the visual array does not contain a distractor object with a similar-sounding name, people are able to integrate acoustic, linguistic and visual information and pick out the intended referent on average 55 ms before the speaker has finished articulating the word. Altmann and Kamide (1999) went one better and showed that in a sufficiently constraining context, listeners can identify the probable referent before the speaker even *begins* the corresponding word. In their experiment, people listened to sentences which contained verbs with fairly specific selectional restrictions (e.g. *The boy will eat the cake*) as well as more general verbs (e.g. *The boy will move the cake*). Both types of stimulus were accompanied by a visual scene containing the objects mentioned in the sentence (in this case, a boy and a cake) as well as some distractors (e.g. a train set, a ball and a toy car). In this context, the verb *eat* is highly predictive, since there is only one edible object in the scene, whereas *move* is not. Listeners were able to use this information online and, in the *eat* condition, looked at the cake shortly after the offset of the verb.

Syntactic analysis and the integration of grammatical, semantic and contextual information also proceed at lightning pace – so fast, in fact, that it is very difficult to determine whether these are distinct processing stages, or whether the processor immediately integrates all the information available. Evidence for the former position comes from the so-called 'garden-path effects'. When confronted with structurally ambiguous input, readers and listeners often have a strong preference for one analysis over the other (Ferreira and Clifton 1986; Frazier 1987; Rayner et al. 1983). For example, on encountering the sentence fragment *put the book on the shelf*, people have a strong tendency to interpret the prepositional phrase as a complement of the verb (a phrase specifying where the book was put) rather than a modifier of the noun (specifying where the book was located before it was moved). Sentences in which this expectation is violated (e.g. *She put the book on the shelf in the box*) are more difficult to process, and the difficulty manifests itself in longer reading times in the disambiguating region (i.e. the second prepositional phrase). The traditional interpretation of this finding is that the processor has been led 'up the garden path' to an incorrect analysis, and additional processing time is needed to reject it and compute a new one.[3] Crucially, such effects sometimes arise even when context or pragmatic considerations favour the dispreferred reading (Ferreira and Clifton 1986; Rayner et al. 1983). This has been taken as supporting a modular view of language processing in which syntactic analysis is 'informationally encapsulated' and precedes semantic and pragmatic processing. This conclusion, however, is controversial, since many studies have found that semantic and pragmatic processing operate on the same time scale as parsing, and, if the contextual bias is strong enough, can even guide syntactic analysis (Altmann et al. 1998; Marslen-Wilson and Tyler 1987; Ni et al. 1996; Spivey et al. 2002; Trueswell et al. 1994). Moreover, regardless of whether there is a purely syntactic stage, it is clear that other types of processing are also performed very rapidly: the processing cost of a garden path (the time required to reject the initial analysis and compute a new one) is usually quite short: 100 ms or thereabouts.

The view that semantic and pragmatic processing begins immediately and proceeds as quickly as parsing appears to be corroborated by research on event-related brain potentials (ERPs). This involves measuring electrical activity at the scalp while a person is engaged in some linguistic activity – often listening to sentences containing some kind of anomaly, since anomalies elicit distinctive ERPs which can be linked to a specific point in the sentence. There are three main ERP profiles associated with language processing:

1. The *left-anterior negativity (LAN)* is a negative-amplitude wave in the left anterior region which begins about 200 milliseconds after the onset of the critical word and lasts for about 300 ms. Some researchers (e.g. Friederici 1995) argue it is associated with initial phrase-structure analysis based on word category information; others (Kutas and King 1995) claim that it is a reflection of verbal working memory processes.
2. The *N400* is a widely distributed bilateral negativity observed from about 200 ms until about 600 ms post-onset, with a peak at around 400 ms. It is thought to be related to semantic processing.
3. The *syntactic positive shift (P600)* is a widely distributed positive wave observed in the posterior parts of both hemispheres from about 500 to 800 ms post-onset, with a peak at around 600 ms. It is associated with a variety of grammatical anomalies, including violations of phrase structure and verb subcategorisation, subject–verb agreement, and reflexive–antecedent agreement.

Thus, ERP responses to semantic anomalies are observed at the same time as (and possibly earlier than) responses to syntactic anomalies (Brown et al. 2000; Osterhout and Nicol 1999). Both begin while the word is still being heard and are completed at the end of the word or shortly afterwards. In fact, a latency of 200 ms post-onset suggests that the brain begins to react to the anomaly even before there is enough acoustic information to identify the word uniquely. This is confirmed by a study by Van Petten et al. (1999), who timed the beginning of the N400 effect with respect to the isolation point – the point in the word at which most people are able to recognise it. Van Petten and colleagues identified the isolation point for a number of English words using the gating technique. (This involves presenting people with very short initial fragments of a word: e.g. the first 50 ms, 100 ms, 150 ms and so on, until they have identified the word correctly.) They then presented another group of participants with sentences which ended in a word which was either fairly predictable from the context (e.g. *He spilled some of the oil onto the engine because he didn't have a funnel*) or incongruous (*He spilled some of the oil onto the engine because he didn't have a tunnel*) and measured ERPs for the final word. They found, in line with previous research, that the incongruous completions elicited a much larger N400 than the congruous completions. The profiles for the two conditions began to diverge about 200 ms before the isolation point. This shows that the participants in the experiment must have either anticipated likely completions for the sentences and matched them against the incoming signal, or used the first phonemes of the word to activate a cohort of candidate words and compared their semantic representations with the semantic representation of the sentence being processed. Whatever they did, the experiment shows that the incoming acoustic information is immediately integrated with the representation of the sentence at multiple levels.

3. Processing shortcuts

Thus, the enormously complex processing required to interpret an utterance is carried out extremely quickly. To appreciate the significance of this fact, it is important to realise that human brains are fairly slow processors. Neurons in the human brain typically fire about 200 times per second. The clock speed of most modern desktop computers is between 100 million and 1,000 million cycles per second – about a million times faster. Yet, while humans process ordinary conversation quickly and effortlessly, computers run into serious difficulties at just about every level of processing.

So how do we do it? How is it possible for listeners to convert an acoustic wave into a contextually interpreted utterance in a matter of seconds – often even before the speaker has finished articulating it? Or, looking at the issue from the perspective of language production, how is it possible for speakers to decide on the message, retrieve the appropriate lexical items, integrate them into a grammatically coherent whole, and articulate the utterance in the same time span?

The answer to this question comes in two parts. First, while individual neurons are relatively slow, we have quite a lot of them – somewhere in the region of 100 billion, each connected to between 1,000 and 10,000 other neurons. Consequently, a large number of computations are carried out in parallel by different neurons – or more realistically, by different assemblies of neurons. This has profound (and as yet largely unexplored) implications for theories of language processing.

Secondly, humans (and animals generally) are very good at using processing shortcuts: simple heuristics, which, though not 100 per cent reliable, are good enough for most situations (in contrast to algorithms, which are guaranteed to provide the correct solution but are very demanding computationally). In the following three subsections, we will explore some of these in relation to language processing.

3.1 Prefabricated units

The simplest way of avoiding having to carry out complex computations is to memorise the result and simply retrieve it from memory when required. In linguistic terms, this means accumulating a large store of 'prefabricated' chunks: ready-made sentences and smaller units (phrases, inflected words) which can be combined into sentences with minimum effort.

It is incontrovertible that language users store *some* prefabricated units – for example, idioms such as *spill the beans* and social formulas such as *How are you?* But to what extent does ordinary language use depend on such ready-made chunks? To answer this question, we need to consider some basic facts about human memory, the statistical structure of texts, and our daily experience of language.

3.1.1 We are able to store vast amounts of information

Our brains are superb information storage devices. There is a general consensus among cognitive psychologists that, for all practical purposes, our long-term memories can be considered to have infinite storage capacity (Barsalou 1992: 148; Schneider and Bjorklund 1998: 469), and some researchers have argued that encoding into memory is 'an obligatory, unavoidable consequence of attention' (Logan 1988: 493). We are also good at retrieving information from memory when we need it, particularly if we have been repeatedly exposed to it. What makes this possible is the fact that our memory is content addressable: we can access memory representations virtually instantaneously on the basis of just about any attribute. For example, on hearing a word we can retrieve information about its meaning, grammatical properties, and the words it typically collocates with. We are often able to do this on hearing just part of a word: our brains immediately complete the pattern by filling in the missing details. Similarly, we can activate a concept and retrieve the phonological and grammatical properties of the corresponding word or words. If we can do this for words, we can also do it for phrases and other complex units: in fact, retrieval of complex units may be easier than retrieval of individual words of comparable frequency, since the component units can act as retrieval cues (provided that the complex unit has been analysed into its components and that both are parts of the same associative network). For example, let us assume that a speaker has stored the units *open*, *door* and *open the door*. The last is considerably less entrenched than the former two (because it is less frequent); however, it may still be relatively easy to retrieve because the speaker can access the component units (*open*, *door*) which in turn will activate the whole phrase.

3.1.2 The language we hear is full of recurrent word combinations

Erman and Warren (2000) examined a sample of spoken passages from the London–Lund corpus and written passages from the LOB corpus. They found that 59 per cent of the words in spoken discourse were parts of prefabs; in the written sample, the proportion was slightly lower – 52 per cent. This figure probably underestimates the number of prefabs, since Erman and Warren counted only word combinations which were in some way idiomatic. However, there is no reason to assume that people don't also memorize fully compositional units such as *read a book*, *I am trying to . . .*, or *brothers and sisters.*

To arrive at an upper bound for the frequency of prefabs in discourse, we could simply count all the recurrent word combinations in a particular data set. Such an analysis was undertaken by Altenberg (1998), who identified all word combinations which occur at least twice in exactly the same form in the London–Lund corpus. He found that the corpus, which comprises just under half a million words, contained over 201,000 such combinations representing over 68,000 different types. Together, these recurrent word combinations made up over 80 per cent of the words in the corpus. Even this figure might be an underestimate, however, since Altenberg counted only continuous combinations, while many prefabs may contain slots (e.g. *for ___ years*, where the slot can be filled by any numeral greater than 1, or *I haven't the ___ idea*, where the slot has a more restricted set of fillers: *slightest, faintest, least, foggiest, remotest*: see Eeg-Olofsson and Altenberg 1993; Moon 1998).

3.1.3 People experience vast amounts of language in their daily lives

A frequency of two in a corpus of half a million words may not seem very much. To put this figure in perspective, it will be useful to have an estimate of how much language people experience in their daily lives. In normal adult conversation, about 150 words are spoken every minute (Huggins 1964; Maclay and Osgood 1959). Much of what we hear on television and the radio – news reports, weather forecasts, commercials – is considerably faster than this; and skilled readers read 200–400 words per minute. A rate of 150 words per minute is equivalent to 9,000 words per hour. Assuming an eight-hour 'language day' – that is to say, that most people spend about eight hours a day engaged in some kind of linguistic activity (talking, reading, watching television, listening to the radio, browsing the Internet etc.) – they will hear or read about 72,000 words in a typical day. This adds up to 504,000 words, or more than the entire London–Lund corpus, in just a week. Thus, assuming the London–Lund corpus to be representative, a frequency of two in the corpus equals about two every week of one's life.[4]

3.1.4 People memorise prefabricated chunks

There are reasons for believing that people memorise multi-word chunks which are much less frequent than this. Conventional multi-word units such as idioms, proverbs, institutionalised metaphors, sayings and so on must be learned precisely because they are conventional ways of expressing a particular idea. Yet corpus research suggests that most of them are fairly rare. In her study of such 'phrasal lexemes' Moon (1998) found that 70 per cent had a frequency of less than 1 per million, and 40 per cent did not occur at all in her 18-million-word corpus. Most of the expressions that Moon studied were drawn from the *Collins COBUILD* dictionary, which is intended for learners of English as a second language, and hence is quite selective in its coverage: it is meant to be 'a guide to ordinary everyday English' (Sinclair 1987: xix) and specifically avoids any specialised or unusual expressions. Thus, we can plausibly assume that most native speakers of English are familiar with the vast majority of the phrasal lexemes that Moon studied – including expressions such as *hang fire, kick the bucket, one man's meat is another man's poison, speak for yourself*, which are among the 40 per cent that did not occur at all in the corpus. It seems, therefore, that people have no trouble learning large numbers of idiomatic multi-word units even if these are relatively infrequent. It doesn't follow from this that people also memorise fully compositional units – but it is not an unreasonable conjecture, given that they have both the capacity and the opportunity. Note that in order to claim the opposite – that people *do not* memorise expressions which they are in principle capable of assembling themselves – one must assume that in addition to our memory and processing mechanisms we are equipped with a screening device which either deletes redundant information from memory or prevents it from being encoded in the first place.

Nevertheless, most linguists (and many psycholinguists as well) take it for granted that linguistic expressions are either computed or stored, and that if a form can be computed, it is not stored. This is only an assumption, not supported by any evidence – but it is a powerful one nevertheless, and as a result, there has been relatively little work devoted to the storage of complex expressions which are fully compositional. The one exception to this is work on regularly inflected forms such as *kissed* or *cats*, much of it conducted in the context of the debate on the dual mechanism theory of morphological processing (see Chapter 8).

One of the tell-tale signs of memory storage is sensitivity to frequency: memory representations of high-frequency items are more entrenched, and hence are accessed more quickly and more reliably than low-frequency items. Several studies have demonstrated frequency effects for regularly inflected forms, which suggests that at least some regular forms are stored. Stemberger and MacWhinney (1986, 1988), for example, presented English-speaking adults with regular verb stems and asked them to supply the past tense form as quickly as possible. They found that their subjects made fewer errors on high-frequency verbs, a result which is difficult to explain if one assumes that all regular forms are constructed by applying a rule. Other studies suggest that high-frequency regular forms are processed more quickly. In lexical decision experiments, where participants have to decide as quickly as possible whether a particular stimulus is a word or not, reaction times are shorter for high-frequency forms, even when the frequency of the root is controlled for. This finding has been reported for the Dutch third person singular (Schreuder et al. 1999), the Dutch plural (Baayen et al. 1997), and English noun morphology (Sereno and Jongman 1997).[5]

Bod (2001) used a similar method to show people may also store simple sentences. He presented people with high-frequency sentences (e.g. *I like it*), low-frequency sentences (e.g. *I keep it*), and ill-formed strings consisting of the same words (e.g. *It I like*). The high- and low-frequency sentences were identical in syntactic structure, were equally plausible and contained lexical items of similar frequencies. The participants' task was to decide as quickly as possible whether the word string was an English sentence or not; and they made this decision faster for the high-frequency sentences.

Additional evidence suggesting that people store regularly inflected forms comes from studies which examined pronunciation. Word-final stops in certain consonant clusters are usually shorter and articulated less clearly than in other positions, or they may be deleted altogether, particularly in rapid speech: for example, *band* and *guest* may be pronounced [bæn] and [gɛs] respectively. Such simplifications are usually restricted to consonant clusters which are part of the same morpheme: the final clusters in *banned* and *guessed* tend not to be simplified, in spite of the fact that these words are homophonous with *band* and *guest* (New 1972). However, the final [t] and [d] in high-frequency past-tense forms behave like the corresponding segments in monomorphemic words: they are often omitted in rapid speech, and, when present, they tend to be pronounced less clearly (Bybee 1995, 2000), which suggests that, like the monomorphemic forms, they are stored.

As indicated earlier, there is very little work investigating whether adults store regular (i.e. non-idiomatic) combinations of words, although we do know that children do, and that such units play an important role in language acquisition (see Chapter 9). Bybee and Scheibman (1999) have demonstrated that similar reductions occur in high-frequency word combinations: the form *don't* in the expressions *I don't know, I don't think, why don't you* is phonetically very different from the *don't* we find in novel combinations, which, by the logic outlined above, suggests that it is part of a stored chunk. There is also some less direct evidence from language change. It is well known that frequently occurring word combinations often fuse into single words. For example, in English, *going to, want to, have to* are often pronounced *gonna, wanna, hafta* (note, too, the conventionalised spelling); auxiliaries are often contracted when they follow pronominal subjects (*I'm, we've, she'll*) and the negative particle *not* may attach to the preceding auxiliary (*haven't, doesn't*, etc.). It is also quite common for prepositions to fuse with the following article, as in the German *am* (*an + dem*), *zur* (*zu + der*), *aufs* (*auf + das*) etc. For such phonological reductions to occur, the participating words must have become single chunks of structure in speakers' minds, since they are not systematic but restricted to specific combinations of words.

3.1.5 *Prefabricated chunks facilitate language processing*

We have seen that people store 'ready-made' chunks of language – probably very large numbers of them.[6] There is also evidence that the availability of such stored units facilitates processing. I have already noted that high-frequency regularly inflected forms and sentences appear to be processed more quickly and more accurately than low-frequency forms. Further relevant evidence comes from research on idioms. People take longer to process the literal meanings of conventional idiomatic expressions than the non-literal meanings (Gibbs 1980; Mueller and Gibbs 1987); and idioms are processed faster than comparable novel word combinations (Gibbs and Gonzales 1985; Peterson and Burgess 1993). This explains why most people would never even consider the various bizarre interpretations of *Tess blew her nose on a paper tissue* discussed at the beginning of this chapter: the availability of the semi-idiomatic prefab *X blow XPOSS-DET nose* pre-empts the more compositional interpretations.

There is also plenty of more informal – and more ecologically valid – evidence. Bilinguals who use different languages in different situations – for example, one language at home and the other at work – often avoid using a language in the wrong setting (the 'home' language at work or vice versa); and, when forced to do so, can become surprisingly dysfluent. All speakers, whether bilingual or monolingual, tend to be more fluent when discussing a familiar topic. This is without doubt partly attributable to non-linguistic cognitive demands, but also to the fact that they cannot rely on preconstructed phrases. For similar reasons, as shown by Goldman-Eisler (1968), when people are asked to retell the same story, they become more and more fluent with each retelling. They also tend to use the same expressions in the subsequent versions, which indicates that the increase in fluency is not due simply to speakers' having already decided which aspects to narrate and in what order. (In real life, you can sometimes observe this phenomenon at dinner parties. It is usually fairly easy to identify a fellow guest's 'party piece', even if you have never heard it before, because it is delivered much more fluently than other anecdotes.)

Some particularly interesting evidence of the effect of using prefabricated chunks on fluency is presented by Kuiper (1996), who studied fast sport commentators, auctioneers, and other individuals who can speak abnormally quickly in certain situations. Their secret, Kuiper shows, is a large repertoire of ready-made phrases, which they string together in a more or less linear fashion. However, when not required to speak abnormally fast, these 'smooth talkers' switch to a different speech mode ('colour commentary mode') which is characterised by less stereotypical language and normal dysfluencies.

3.2 Shallow processing

Since most prefabricated chunks are sentence fragments, in order to form a complete utterance, speakers must usually piece together several prefabs or combine prefabs with words. For example, in order to form an utterance such as *Why don't you stay at home tonight?*, the speaker might integrate two pre-constructed units (*why don't you VP*, *stay at home*) and the adverb *tonight*; in order to construct our original example, *Tess blew her nose on a paper tissue*, the speaker will need three chunks, *X blow XPOSS-DET nose*, *on a N* and *paper tissue*, as well as the pronoun *her* and the proper noun *Tess*. Such piecing together requires grammatical knowledge, since the component chunks must be combined in a specific way if the result is to be grammatical. For example, only units of a particular kind (viz. VPs with a bare infinitive) can be inserted into the slot after *why don't you*; the possessive determiner in the second sentence must be coreferential with the subject; and so on. However, the processing required to accomplish this is relatively shallow: the speaker must attend to the relationships between units and the underspecified parts of other units, but not to every detail of their internal structure.

There is growing evidence that the processing involved in ordinary language comprehension is, in fact, fairly shallow: that is to say, people may integrate the meanings of the most salient lexical items, some easily accessible grammatical cues, and contextual information to arrive at a semantic interpretation without fully parsing the sentence.

One of the earliest studies demonstrating this was conducted by Fillenbaum (1974), who asked a group of students to paraphrase some sentences as accurately as possible. Although they were specifically instructed not to improve the sentences or make them more sensible, the participants in the study often 'normalised' pragmatically anomalous sentences. For example, perverse threats such as *Clean up the mess or I won't report you* were given a more plausible paraphrase (e.g. *If you don't clean up the mess I will report you*) 54 per cent of the time. The participants were then asked to reread each sentence and its paraphrase in the presence of the experimenter and asked whether they could 'see some shred of difference' between the two – and even then, they failed to spot the discrepancies 34 per cent of the time.

We cannot be sure what caused Fillenbaum's subjects to give inaccurate paraphrases. They may have taken a 'pragmatic shortcut' – that is to say, arrived at an interpretation without fully analysing the sentence; but it is also possible that they interpreted the sentence correctly, but, since the interpretation didn't make much sense, rejected it in favour of something more plausible. However, the fact that some participants appeared to be unable to spot the discrepancy between the meanings of the original sentences and their paraphrases of them when they were specifically invited to do so in the second phase of the experiment does suggest that they took the 'pragmatic shortcut' route.

Further support for this interpretation of Fillenbaum's results is provided by Ferreira (2003), who found that people often misinterpreted passive sentences describing unlikely events: for example, when asked to name the affected participant in *The dog was bitten by a man*, the participants said 'man' in over 20 per cent of all trials. However, they practically never made this mistake with active sentences: *The man bit the dog* was virtually always interpreted correctly. So it is not the case that people have a tendency to 'correct' pragmatically odd sentences: normalisation seems to occur primarily with sentences which are non-canonical, and hence fairly difficult to process.

In my own work (Dąbrowska 1997), I have shown that shallow processing can also occur in the absence of a pragmatic bias towards an incorrect interpretation and is inversely correlated with educational achievement: that is to say, the more formal schooling a person has had, the more likely they are to make full use of the grammatical information available. The least educated participants in the study were usually able to extract locally encoded information, but had difficulty in processing long-distance dependencies. For example, when confronted with parasitic gap[7] sentences such as *It was her boss that Louise persuaded that Margaret will interview*, they were much better at identifying the interviewer (Margaret) than the interviewee (the boss). They were also sometimes unable to establish hierarchical relationships between clauses in multiply embedded sentences. Thus, the sentence *Paul noticed that the fact that the room was tidy surprised Shona* was frequently interpreted to mean 'Paul noticed that the room was tidy and this surprised Shona' – in other words, the respondents appeared to extract simple clauses from the input (Paul noticed something, the room was tidy, something surprised Shona) and then attempted to integrate their meanings without making use of the grammatical information available. Similar results have been reported by Chipere (2001, 2003).

Let us conclude the discussion with a particularly tricky example. Wason and Reich (1979) found that nearly all the people they tested misinterpreted the sentence *No head injury is too trivial to ignore* to mean 'No head injury should be ignored, however trivial it may be'. But according to the rules of English grammar, the sentence cannot possibly mean this: it can only mean the exact opposite. Consider the following:

(3)   a. *No child is too obnoxious to look after.*
           'Every child should be looked after, no matter how obnoxious.'
        b. *No question is too stupid to answer.*
           'Every question should be answered, no matter how stupid.'
        c. *No mistake is too trivial to correct.*
           'Every mistake should be corrected, no matter how trivial.'

Therefore:

(4)   *No head injury is too trivial to ignore.*
        'Every head injury should be ignored, no matter how trivial.'

Why is it that people systematically misunderstand the last sentence, but not the other three? The problematic sentence is quite complex, both syntactically and semantically. The noun phrase *no head injury*, which functions as the theme of *ignore*, does not appear in its usual direct object position (as in *We ignored the head injury*) but at the beginning of the sentence, as the subject of the main verb, which makes it difficult to establish the relationship between them. The sentence also contains three negatives: the particle *no* and two logically negative expressions, *too trivial* (i.e. 'not serious enough') and *ignore* ('take no notice'). Furthermore, it is very odd from a pragmatic point of view, since it presupposes that serious matters should be ignored and trivial things attended to (cf. *This is too trivial to ignore*), as well as enjoining the addressee to ignore head injuries, which are widely known to be potentially dangerous. It is not particularly surprising, then, that many people misinterpret the sentence. What is interesting, however, is that they are so confident about their erroneous interpretation and find it extremely difficult to 'see' the correct one, even when they are told what it is.

3.3 Frequency

Fluent language users are remarkably sensitive to the statistical properties of their language. This sensitivity manifests itself at all levels of linguistic organisation, from phonemes and combinations of phonemes through to words and grammatical constructions (Ellis 2000), and appears to be quite detailed. People seem to know not just the relative frequencies of individual words and word senses, but also how often they appear in specific constructions: for example, that some transitive verbs (e.g. *accuse*) are much more likely to occur in the passive construction than others (e.g. *watch*: see Trueswell 1996). Similarly, when a verb allows more than one type of complement, people know which kind of complement it typically takes: e.g. while both *push* and *move* can occur in either a transitive or an intransitive construction, *push* 'prefers' the former and *move* the latter (MacDonald 1994); *accept* takes NP complements more often than sentential complements, while *suggest* has the opposite preference (Garnsey et al. 1997); *imply* is more likely than *hope* to take an overt complementizer when it occurs with a sentential complement (Trueswell et al. 1993); and so on (see MacDonald 1999 for further examples).

People are also sensitive to frequency information at more abstract levels. For example, when confronted with an ambiguous expression such as *Someone stabbed the wife of the football star who was outside the house*, where the relative clause (*who was outside the house*) can modify either the 'upstairs' or the 'downstairs' NP (*the wife* or *the football star*, respectively), English speakers usually prefer the latter interpretation – that is to say, in the absence of contextual information supporting the other reading, they interpret the sentence to mean that it was the football star, not the wife, who was outside the house. However, speakers of many other languages, including Spanish, normally choose the other interpretation when they hear or read the corresponding sentence in their own language.[8] This reflects the statistics of the language: corpus counts show that in English, a sequence consisting of a noun followed by a prepositional phrase and a relative clause is usually associated with the 'downstairs' interpretation, whereas the opposite is true in Spanish (Mitchell 1994: 398). A compelling piece of evidence demonstrating speakers' sensitivity to such factors is provided by an intervention study by Mitchell, Cuetos and Corley (see Mitchell 1994: 398), who got two groups of Spanish-speaking 7-year-olds to read stories which contained sentences with this kind of ambiguity. In one set of stories, the relative clause modified the higher noun, and in the other set, the lower noun. The children were matched in their initial preference for one or the other interpretation; but when they were tested two weeks later, their preferences had diverged.

Knowledge about the relative frequency of words and constructions manifests itself primarily in ease of activation and processing times: at all levels of linguistic organisation, high-frequency forms are inherently easier to activate and hence are processed faster. Thus, when the input is ambiguous, people consistently prefer the higher-frequency interpretation. By its very nature, probabilistic information is not 100 per cent reliable. However, reliability improves considerably when several different sources of probabilistic information are combined (Redington and Chater 1998). The main advantages of using probabilistic information is that it speeds up the processing of typical cases – that is to say, it speeds up processing most of the time – and it also helps to narrow down the search space when there are a vast number of alternative analyses, which is often the case with complex sentences found in written texts (such as this one!). For this reason, there is a growing tendency to incorporate probabilistic information into automatic parsers (cf. Bod 1998; Briscoe 1994).

4. Implications for linguistic theory

Some linguistic expressions (e.g. irregular forms) are retrieved from the memory and others (e.g. all novel expressions) must be computed. Still others, such as frequently occurring word combinations and inflected forms of common words, can be either retrieved or computed. However, there is a trade-off between storage and computation: a set of general, highly compact rules does not require a large storage capacity, but poses severe demands on the processing system; and conversely, the retrieval of prefabricated chunks is computationally less demanding, but requires a large and efficient memory.

Linguists like general rules and principles. When choosing between competing accounts of the same phenomena, they have traditionally relied on the principle of economy. General solutions are always preferred to more specific ones, and it is assumed that any regularities that can be captured by means of general rules and principles should be so captured. It is also held as a matter of course that anything that is computable need not be, and hence is not, stored.

However, it is doubtful that the principle of economy is an appropriate standard by which to evaluate linguistic theories, if these are intended to be psychologically realistic. Human brains are relatively slow processors, but have enormous storage capacity. From a psychological point of view, therefore, retrieval from memory is the preferred strategy. People store vast numbers of prefabricated units, and rely on them whenever possible – even when they are fully compositional and could also be assembled using rules. It follows that linguistic knowledge is represented in a highly redundant manner, and that the same expression may be processed in different ways on different occasions.

It is important to bear in mind that most prefabricated units are fairly small: between two and three words. Thus, in order to construct a complete utterance, speakers must usually combine several prefabs, or a prefab and one or more word-sized units. This requires linguistic knowledge since, if the resulting structure is to be well-formed, units of a particular kind must be combined in a strictly defined way. Thus, a psychologically realistic grammar must contain combinatorial mechanisms which can accommodate complex units as well as simple units.

We have also seen that humans have very detailed knowledge about the frequency of linguistic units, and are able to use this knowledge in resolving ambiguities. In principle, it is possible that information about frequency is stored separately from linguistic knowledge proper, as a kind of vast appendix to the grammar. However, it is much more likely that our sensitivity to frequency is simply a direct effect of the amount of experience we have with various structures: frequent constructions are processed faster and with less effort because people have had more opportunity to practise them. This would suggest that our mental representation of language is shaped by language use, and hence, it is counterproductive to draw a sharp distinction between competence and performance.

Notes

1. Note, however, that there are a number of local ambiguities. As indicated in the main text, *her* could be either a determiner introducing the noun phrase functioning as the object of *blow* or the object itself: the ambiguity is resolved when the processor encounters the next word, *nose.* Likewise, *on* could be a preposition or an adverbial particle modifying *blow* (as in *She blew her nose on and on*, meaning 'She continued blowing her nose'). Finally, on encountering *paper,* the processor could construe it as the object of the proposition *on* rather than a modifier of the following noun. Notice that in each case the ambiguity is resolved at the very next word.
2. Not in the usual way, anyway. There are some rather disgusting possibilities, but I will leave these to the reader to explore.

3. An alternative view is that the processor constructs several analyses in parallel, but the dispreferred ones take longer to assemble.

4. Of course, we have no way of knowing whether a particular expression which occurred twice in the London–Lund corpus really has a frequency of four per million. It is possible that it was only ever produced twice in the entire history of the English language. Likewise, it is possible that many fairly frequent expressions are not represented in the corpus at all – after all, compared to the whole body of texts in the language we call English, or even the linguistic experience of a single native speaker, the corpus is laughably small. However, assuming that the corpus contains a representative sample of spoken texts, we can be reasonably confident that the *mean* frequency of the expressions that occur twice in the corpus is about four per million.

5. Some studies (Pinker and Prince 1992; Ullman 1999) have failed to find frequency effects for regulars in English. This is probably a ceiling effect: English past tense and plural inflections are very simple, and hence comparatively easy to compute.

6. Pawley and Syder (1983: 192) estimate that speakers have 'hundreds of thousands' of such ready-made units in their repertoire.

7. A parasitic gap is a gap which has the same antecedent as another gap in the sentence, and which could not occur if the sentence did not contain the other gap: therefore, its presence is 'parasitic' on that of the other gap. In the example given in the text, the ordinary gap occurs after *persuaded* and the parasitic gap after *interview*; the noun phrase *the boss* is the antecedent for both.

8. I first became aware of this ambiguity, and the fact that there may be language-specific preferences in interpretation, when I was doing a Spanish language course as an undergraduate. One day, during a discussion about whether there was such a thing as true love, my teacher declared that *El único amor verdadero es el amor del dinero, y el amor del perro, que se compra* ('The only true love is the love of money, and the love of the dog, which one buys'). I interpreted the relative clause as modifying the word *dog*, and dismissed the argument as completely irrelevant ('It doesn't matter whether you buy it or not, the important thing is that the dog loves you'), whereas my teacher obviously intended the other interpretation and insisted that you can't talk about true love if it (love, not the dog) is bought. It wasn't until after I left the class that I realised what he meant.

3 Language acquisition: robustness

Language acquisition, it is sometimes claimed, is 'highly sensitive to maturational factors' and 'surprisingly insensitive to environmental factors' (Fodor 1983: 100; see also Crain and Lillo-Martin 1999; Gleitman 1981; Stromswold 2000). To be sure, language develops in all normal children exposed to language, even in highly adverse circumstances: in neglected and abused children, in cognitively impaired children, and in children who have limited access to information from the external world due to sensory deprivation, i.e. deafness or blindness. Furthermore, many researchers have been impressed by the fact that children often go through similar developmental stages. In Stromswold's words:

> Within a given language, the course of language acquisition is remarkably uniform . . . Most children say their first referential words at 9 to 15 months . . . and for the next 6–8 months, children typically acquire single words fairly slowly until they have acquired approximately 50 words . . . Once children have acquired 50 words, their vocabularies often increase rapidly . . . At around 18 to 24 months, children learning morphologically impoverished languages such as English begin combining words to form two-word utterances . . . Children acquiring such morphologically impoverished languages gradually begin to use sentences longer than two words; but for several months their speech often lacks phonetically unstressed functional category morphemes such as determiners, auxiliary verbs, and verbal and nominal inflectional endings . . . Gradually, omissions become rarer until children are between three and four years old, at which point the vast majority of English-speaking children's utterances are completely grammatical. (Stromswold 2000: 910)

Stromswold also notes some more specific commonalities. For example, English-speaking children acquire the grammatical morphemes of their language in roughly the same order: first the progressive -*ing*, closely followed by the locative prepositions *on* and *in*, then the plural -*s*, irregular past-tense forms such as *ate*, *slept* and *drunk*, the possessive -*'s*, the uncontractible copula (as in *Yes, she is*), the articles, and regular past-tense inflections. Still later come the third-person -*s* and uncontractible auxiliary forms, and, finally, the contractible copula and auxiliary (e.g. *She's tired, He's coming*) (see Brown 1973; de Villiers and de Villiers 1973). Auxiliaries and various complex constructions such as questions, Stromswold (1995) maintains, are also acquired in the same order by nearly all children.

The universality and alleged uniformity of language acquisition are sometimes taken as evidence for an innate universal grammar which develops according to a biologically determined timetable and does not depend on other cognitive subsystems. As we shall see in this chapter, there are some serious problems with this argument.

1. Individual differences

First, we might observe that the 'remarkable uniformities' that Stromswold speaks of are not all that remarkable. We don't need to postulate a universal grammar to explain why children produce single-word utterances before two-word combinations, why the latter precede longer utterances, or why early word combinations are generally telegraphic. What is more, even this rather uninteresting progression is only a tendency: some children's earliest utterances are short phrases and sentences such as *Look-a-that!* or *Whassat?* which are only later analysed into their component morphemes.

Second, many of the observed similarities can be easily explained by appealing to factors such as conceptual complexity, salience and frequency. For example, the concepts of plurality and possession are more accessible to young children than the purely grammatical concept of agreement; hence, the plural and possessive suffixes are learned earlier than the third-person -*s*; past-tense forms of irregular verbs are generally acquired earlier than past-tense forms of regular verbs because irregular verbs tend to be much more frequent (nine of the ten most frequent English verbs are irregular); uncontractible copula and auxiliary forms are acquired earlier than contractible forms of the same items because they are phonetically more salient; the progressive inflection and the prepositions *in* and *on* are acquired early because they designate relatively simple concepts and are syllabic (and hence acoustically salient); and so on.

Third, although there are many similarities between children acquiring the same language, there are also vast individual differences. Such differences are perhaps most obvious, and easiest to quantify, in lexical development. The comprehension vocabularies of normally developing children of the same age can differ tenfold or more (Bates, Dale and Thal 1995; Benedict 1979; Goldfield and Reznick 1990), and there are also enormous differences with regard to what proportion of their expressive vocabularies children are able to use in production: some children's expressive vocabularies are nearly as large as their receptive vocabularies (i.e. they are able to produce almost all the words they understand), while others may be able to understand more than 200 words, but still not produce any (Bates, Dale and Thal 1995). Children also differ with regard to the kinds of words they learn in the initial stages of lexical development. So-called 'referential' children initially focus primarily on object labels (that is to say, concrete nouns), while 'expressive' children have more varied vocabularies with more verbs and adjectives and a significant proportion of social routines and formulas such as *stop it*, *I want it*, *don't do it* (Nelson 1973, 1981). Finally, there are differences in the pattern of growth. While many children do go through the 'vocabulary spurt' that Stromswold alludes to at some point between 14 and 22 months, a significant minority – about a quarter – show a more gradual growth pattern with no spurt (Goldfield and Reznick 1990).

Grammatical development is also anything but uniform. Children may begin to combine words as early as 14 months or as late as 25 months, and show correspondingly large differences in MLU (mean length of utterance) and other global measures of grammatical development a year later (Bates, Dale and Thal 1995). At 42 months, the differences between the most and least advanced 'normal' children are equivalent to 30–36 months (Wells 1985). Some children learn to inflect words before they combine them into larger structures, while others begin to combine words before they are able to use morphological rules productively (Smoczyńska 1985: 618; Thal et al. 1996). Some children are extremely cautious learners, while others are happy to generalise on the basis of fairly sparse evidence, which results in large differences in error rates (Maratsos 2000). Marked individual differences have also been found in almost every area of grammatical development where researchers have looked for them, including word order, negation, case marking, the order of emergence of grammatical morphemes – and, yes, in the development of English auxiliaries (Jones 1996; Richards 1990; Wells 1979), questions (de Villiers and de Villiers 1985; Gullo 1981; Kuczaj and Maratsos 1983) and multi-clause sentences (Huttenlocher et al. 2002; see also Lieven 1997 for a review).

Children also differ in acquisition styles, or the strategies they use to learn to speak (Nelson 1981; Peters 1977; Peters and Menn 1993). 'Analytic' or 'referential' children begin with single words, which they articulate reasonably clearly and consistently. 'Holistic' or 'expressive' children, on the other hand, begin with larger units which have characteristic stress and intonation patterns, but which are often 'mush-mouthed' and may consist partly or even entirely of filler syllables such as [dadada]. Peters (1977) argues that holistic children attempt to approximate the overall 'shape' of the target utterance while analytic children isolate and produce single words. These different starting points have a profound influence on the course of language development, since they determine how the child 'breaks into' grammar. Analytic children must learn how to put words together to form more complex units. They typically do this by first learning how to combine content words, whereby they produce telegraphic utterances such as *Put ball sofa.* Later on in development they discover that different classes of content words require specific function words and inflections (nouns take determiners, verbs take auxiliaries and tense inflections etc.), and learn to supply these. Holistic children, in contrast, must segment their rote-learned phrases and determine what role each unit plays in the larger whole. Unlike analytic children, they sometimes produce grammatical morphemes very early in acquisition, usually embedded in larger unanalysed or only partially analysed units. In other creative utterances, they may use nonsense 'filler syllables' – often a schwa or a nasal consonant – as placeholders for grammatical morphemes. As the child's linguistic system develops, these fillers gradually acquire more phonetic substance and an adult-like distribution, and eventually evolve into function words of the target language (Peters 2001; Peters and Menn 1993; see also Chapter 9). Thus, while both groups of children may eventually converge on similar grammars, they get there by following very different routes.[1]

There is evidence suggesting that the choice of language-learning strategy is at least partially dependent on the child's environment (Hampson and Nelson 1993; Lieven 1994, 1997; Pine 1994). The analytic style is typical for first-born children of middle-class parents, whose linguistic experience consists mostly of one-on-one interactions with a parent. The expressive style, on the other hand, is found more often in later-born children and children who grow up in extended families, who engage more in polyadic interactions with various family members. Occasionally, the same child may develop different strategies when acquiring different languages. Elizabeth Bates's daughter Julia, for example, adopted a fairly analytic style in English, which she learned mostly in dyadic contexts, and a more expressive style in Italian, learned primarily in the context of large family gatherings (Bates et al. 1988).

It should be stressed that the existence of individual differences is not necessarily incompatible with a nativist view of language development. Differences in the rate of acquisition could be a result of different rates of maturation of the language faculty; and many developmental asynchronies could be attributed to individual modules maturing at different times. Nativist theories can also accommodate differences in acquisition style, as long as they allow for individual differences in the genetic endowment for language, although this is problematic to the extent that acquisition styles are linked to specific environmental influences and/or non-linguistic cognitive and affective factors. Two points, however, should be clear from the above discussion. First, we cannot argue for innateness on the basis of the alleged uniformity of language acquisition, because language acquisition is *not* uniform. Secondly, large individual differences suggest that there is considerable flexibility in the way that the genetic program unfolds – that is to say, the genetic program appears to be relatively 'open'.

2. The role of input

Language can develop in very inauspicious circumstances: in blind children, who have limited access to contextual information that helps sighted children guess the meanings of the adult utterances they hear; in cognitively impaired children, who may be unable to make use of much of this information; and in neglected children, who have limited access to linguistic data from which to construct their mental grammars. Since all normal children develop language except in situations of extreme deprivation, the argument goes, language acquisition must be driven by internal processes, and does not depend on input except as a trigger. In this section, we will critically examine the above argument.

It is undeniable that there are vast differences in how much input children get, and the quality of that input. In a study of child–mother interaction, Huttenlocher et al. (1991) found that the most talkative mothers in their sample spoke up to 10 times as much per unit of time as the least talkative mothers. Since parents also differ in the amount of time they spend with their children, the actual differences in the sheer quantity of language children hear are probably even greater (see also Hart and Risley 1995, 1999). The usual nativist take on such findings is that they show that only a minimal amount of input is necessary to trigger language development, since all normal children, including those of taciturn or neglectful parents, do develop language.

Once again, however, the conclusion is premature. First, the amount of input does matter, since children who hear less language develop language more slowly (Hart and Risley 1995, 1999; Huttenlocher 1998). A recent study of the linguistic abilities of children from socio-economically deprived backgrounds found that half had moderate-to-severe language delays (Locke and Ginsborg submitted; Locke et al. 2002). Since the children scored at age-appropriate levels on a test of cognitive development, their poor performance on linguistic tasks cannot be attributed to unfamiliarity with the testing situation or a general cognitive delay. The authors argue that the language delay found in these children is a direct consequence of the simple fact that their parents do not speak to them as much as middle-class parents do. Not surprisingly, even more severe language delays are found in neglected children, children of depressed and substance-abusing mothers, and institutionalised children – but, significantly, not in abused children (Culp et al. 1991): the latter presumably do get a good deal of language input, even if it does not occur in a loving environment.

Quality matters, too. Certain maternal speech styles are associated with faster language growth (Hampson and Nelson 1993; Murray et al. 1990). The children of more directive mothers learn language more slowly (Della Corte et al. 1983; Tomasello and Todd 1983), while children whose utterances are frequently recast by their parents tend to make faster progress (Baker and Nelson 1984; Farrar 1990). There are robust correlations between children's ability to produce and understand multi-clausal sentences on the one hand and the frequency of such sentences in the speech of their parents and, and, more importantly, their teachers on the other hand (Huttenlocher et al. 2002). The latter is theoretically more significant, since, unlike the former, it cannot be attributed to genetic factors. Many studies of twins have found that they are often substantially delayed relative to other children (see Mogford 1993), presumably because they get less 'personalised' input than singletons. But perhaps the most convincing evidence for the relevance of input tailored to the child's needs comes from studies of spoken language development in hearing children of deaf parents. While such children are rarely completely cut off from spoken language, they clearly get less of it than children born to hearing parents. Even more importantly, they often get little personalised input from adults, which has a profound influence on their language development.

Consider, for example, Jim, a boy studied by Sachs et al. (1981). Jim's parents had very little oral language and communicated with each other in sign, but they did not sign to him. He was exposed to English primarily through television, which he watched frequently, but he also occasionally played with hearing children. Sachs et al. began to study Jim's linguistic development when he was aged 3;9, just as he was beginning speech therapy. It was immediately clear that Jim's language was not just delayed, but qualitatively different from that of normally developing children. Although he had a reasonably good vocabulary (only slightly smaller than an average child of his age), his comprehension was quite poor, and he also had severe articulation problems. Perhaps as a result of these, he only produced very short utterances: his mean length of utterance (MLU) at the beginning of the study was 2.2, which would be appropriate for a child just over two. Unlike ordinary children learning English, Jim made many word order errors, and often produced decidedly 'un-English' sentences such as those in (1).

(1)   a. *Not window two window.*
        b. *My mommy my house a@sc play ball.*
           '(?) I play ball at home with my mommy.'
        c. *House a@sc chimney my house a@sc my chimney.*
           '(?) My house has got a chimney.'
        d. *This is how a@sc plane.*

He also had particular difficulty with inflectional morphology and function words, which he omitted 63 per cent of the time – about twice as often as normally developing children with a comparable MLU.[2]

There are two important lessons to be learned from Jim's case. First, 'mere exposure' to language does not automatically lead to acquisition, since he was unable to learn English from the television.[3] It seems that, in addition to simply hearing a lot of language in context, children also need at least occasional interaction with a competent language user who does the sorts of things that parents do: repeat and rephrase utterances that the child did not understand, and provide some sort of feedback on the child's production. This could be in the form of expansion of the child's incomplete utterances, puzzlement at incomprehensible utterances, or simply a continuation of the topic introduced by the child or compliance with a request, both of which would indicate that the child's communicative intentions have been understood. Secondly, Jim's language shows that restricted input affects morphosyntactic development as well as lexical development – in fact, in his case the former was clearly much more seriously affected than the latter. It is worth pointing out that Jim's case is not isolated: Todd and Aitchison (1980) report similar deviant constructions in the speech of another hearing child of deaf parents.

So both the quality and the sheer quantity of input do matter. On the other hand, they do not seem to matter as much as one might expect, since children who get only a tenth of the input addressed to the most priveleged children do not take ten times longer to achieve the same level of competence. How can we explain this apparent discrepancy?

It is important to bear in mind that most children get vast amounts of input. Cameron-Faulkner et al. (2003) estimate that a typical toddler hears between 5,000 and 7,000 utterances per day. This means that between the ages of 1, when language acquisition may be said to begin in earnest, and 4, when most children achieve productivity in the basic structures of their language, they will have heard something of the order of 6,570,000 utterances, including about a million WH questions, a million Y/N questions, 660,000 instances of the full transitive construction (a subject followed by a verb followed by an object), about 40,000 relative clauses, and almost 7,000 passives.[4] So halving the amount of input may have little effect on language learning simply because most children get more input then they actually need: half of 6.6 million is still a very large number.

The second point to bear in mind is that while reducing the amount of language experience may have little effect on the linguistic development of some children, it does affect others – namely, children with low IQs, small short-term phonological memory capacity, and sensory deficits – who appear to be far more vulnerable to the effects of suboptimal input (Snow 1995). Thus, quality and amount of input may help to explain an apparent paradox. There are reports in the literature of children who developed language normally in spite of very low IQ, small short-term phonological memory capacity, or other impairments, which have led some researchers to conclude that language development does not depend on such cognitive abilities. On the other hand, speech therapy clinics are full of disabled children with severe language problems, which suggests that there are close links between linguistic and non-linguistic development. We can reconcile these conflicting facts by recognising that non-linguistic cognition does matter – but good input can compensate for cognitive impairments (within limits); and, conversely, good language learners may be able to compensate for suboptimal input. However, when several inauspicious circumstances conspire, language will suffer.

This suggests that language may develop differently in different circumstances. To investigate this possibility, we will consider one special population – blind children – in more detail.

3. Language development in blind children

The linguistic development of blind children can be potentially very informative in the context of the debate on the role of innate factors in language acquisition. If language acquisition involved merely setting the parameters in an innate program, we would not expect to find many differences between sighted and blind children: after all, both groups hear language, and both are equipped with the same universal grammar, so both should follow the same course of development. On the other hand, if language acquisition were heavily dependent on experience, we might expect that blindness will have a profound effect on the course of development, since much information that is normally available to the child – information about the visual properties of objects and events in the environment, about what their interlocutors are doing, what they are looking at, their gestures and facial expressions – is inaccessible to blind learners.

How, then, does language develop in blind children? The short answer is that it depends on the child. According to one study, about 40 per cent have speech abnormalities of some kind (Elstner 1983). But most blind children have no speech abnormalities, just a small delay; and some develop completely normally (Gleitman 1981; Pérez-Pereira and Conti-Ramsden 1999).

An additional factor which may account for these large differences is the fact that many blind children also suffer from other handicaps. Deviant language development seems to be the rule when the child has other disabilities in addition to blindness or is growing up in an unfavourable social milieu. According to Graham (1968, cited in Elstner 1983), almost half of all blind children who are multiply handicapped are completely without language. The incidence of language disorders in the group studied by Elstner, which included a number of children who had other problems, was 76 per cent. Furthermore, while most of the abnormalities in sighted children are phonetic or phonological, the blind children's problems tended to be lexical-semantic and morphosyntactic; and there were more morphosyntactic abnormalities in the speech of completely blind children than in children with partial vision.

The conclusion, then, is that blindness by itself does not cause language difficulties, although it often results in a small delay. However, when combined with other problems, such as low IQ or an impoverished home environment, it can lead to serious language problems.

But why are impairments which do not necessarily cause problems in other children so disastrous in the blind, and why should blind children be more likely to produce deviant language? The answer, I suggest, comes down to the fact that blind children develop language somewhat differently from seeing children. Because many aspects of contextual information are not accessible to them, blind children must make very good use of whatever information they have got, and cognitive impairment may preclude them from doing so. Furthermore, blind children have to be more 'proactive' in obtaining information about meaning. There are two ways in which learners can determine what a new linguistic expression means: they can either observe competent speakers use it and note as much as possible about the context, or they can experiment – that is to say, produce it and see what happens. Since blind children cannot observe as much as sighted children, they must experiment more. The result is that they often produce utterances which they clearly do not understand. This 'meaningless language' or 'verbalism' of the blind is sometimes regarded as an indication of deviant development, or even cognitive impairment. However, it seems more illuminating to view it as a very good way of obtaining clues about what linguistic expressions might mean.[5]

There is considerable evidence that blind children make more use of imitation, repetition and verbal routines than seeing children, and tend to adopt a holistic learning strategy (Dunlea 1989; Mulford 1988; Pérez-Pereira 1994; Urwin 1984). This suggests that they rely more heavily on distributional information, presumably in order to compensate for the lack of visual information (Pérez-Pereira and Castro 1997). This language learning strategy, of course, makes greater demands on the child's phonological memory. Thus, a short phonological memory span, or poor auditory processing skills, will affect blind children more than seeing children, and may be another reason for the large individual differences in the linguistic accomplishments of blind children.

A particularly striking example of how a blind child's heavy reliance on verbal routines may result in the production of very unusual structures is given by Wilson and Peters (1988). Between the ages of 3;2 and 3;6, the child they studied, Seth, produced a number of questions such as those given in (2) below (Wilson and Peters 1988: 251–3).

(2) a. *What are we gonna go at* [=to] *Auntie and?* [answer: Auntie and Priya]
  b. *What did I get lost at the, Dad?* [answer: at the store]
  c. *What are you cooking pan?* [answer: pancakes]

Such utterances are peculiar by any standards; but they are particularly problematic for Principles and Parameters theory, since they apparently violate universal constraints on movement. Sentence (2a) violates the coordinate structure constraint, which states that items cannot be moved out of a coordinate structure (or a more general constraint, subjacency, which states that constituents cannot be moved across more than one bounding node: in this case, NP and S). Sentences (2b) and (2c) are violations of the maximal projection property of movement rules (the requirement that only maximal projections can be moved to the specifier position). In (2b), only the noun has been moved, not the entire noun phrase, and in (2c), only the second part of the compound noun.

This anomalous usage had its origins in an information-eliciting game that Seth's father used to play with him, in which the father produced an affirmative sentence with a 'blank' and Seth had to fill in the blank, like that:

(3)   a. [Getting ready for breakfast]
              F: *Put your . . .*
              S: *Bib on.*
         b. [After breakfast]
              F: *What did you eat? Eggs and . . .*
              S: *Mbacon.* (Wilson and Peters 1988: 262–3)

It seems that in the anomalous utterances in (2), Seth put such a 'sentence with a blank' in an interrogative structure.

These anomalous constructions in Seth's speech were not, of course, a direct result of blindness, but rather a consequence of his unusual linguistic experience. They do, however, offer particularly compelling evidence that unusual experience can result in unusual language production.

4. The robustness of language

We have seen that there are considerable individual differences in the way that children learn to use language. Some children first produce single words (mostly nouns) and later learn to combine them to form more complex expressions; others begin with short phrases or sentences and extract words from them; and still others – probably the majority – use both strategies. Some children are rapid piecemeal learners and use a variety of grammatical constructions in very early stages of development, before they have fully analysed them; others look for more general patterns and consequently may appear to be less advanced. Some children jump to conclusions on the basis of relatively little data – a risky strategy which results in high error rates; others are more cautious and consequently make relatively few errors.

We have also seen that it is not true that language acquisition is *in*sensitive to environmental and non-linguistic cognitive factors. Environmental deprivation, sensory impairments and, as we shall see, cognitive deficits all have an effect on language development. However, unless several different factors conspire, children are usually able to overcome these adverse circumstances and develop normal language. As we will see in the next two chapters, children with very low IQs and children who have suffered damage to the areas of the brain which normally specialise in linguistic processing may also develop relatively normal language, although the actual course of development may be quite different from that found in normal children. And, of course, if a child is exposed to two, three or even four languages, she will learn all of them, provided she gets enough input in every language.

The most striking feature of human language acquisition, then, is its robustness. The language learning system is able to adapt flexibly to a wide range of very different circumstances. Clearly, this flexibility is not infinite; but within limits, the language learning system applies whatever mental resources are available to the (sometimes impoverished) input data to construct a functional (though perhaps imperfect) system. This kind of flexibility is incompatible with an acquisition sequence whose exact course is predetermined genetically. A rigid genetic program cannot make allowances for such diverse contingencies of language development as exposure to more than one language, extremely limited exposure to language, early brain damage, or lack of supporting input from other modalities. The flexibility of language development, then, and the existence of a great deal of individual variation suggest that languages are learned, not acquired.

Notes

1. This is a somewhat idealised picture. Most children use a mixture of both strategies.
2. It should be stressed that Jim's problems are not be attributable to a linguistic impairment, since he made excellent progress after intervention. His MLU rose to 2.9 in just a month, and by age 6;11, he was performing above age level on most measures of linguistic ability.
3. Note, too, that at the time that Sachs et al. began observing Jim, he had not acquired sign language, in spite of the fact that he could observe his parents signing on a regular basis. He did, however, make considerable progress in sign later.
4. These estimates are based on frequency data given in Cameron-Faulkner et al. (2003) for questions and transitives, Gordon and Chafetz (1990) for passives, and Diessel and Tomasello (2000) for relatives.
5. I am not suggesting that blind children consciously adopt this strategy. On most occasions, their goal is simply to get adult attention – but they end up getting a variety of clues about the meaning of their utterances.

4 Language in the brain

It has been known for well over a century that damage to the 'language areas' of the brain often has catastrophic effects on an individual's ability to produce and understand language. Lesions in the third frontal convolution of the left hemisphere, the so-called Broca's area, often lead to Broca's aphasia, which is characterised by slow, effortful speech and difficulties with function words and inflections (cf. example (1) below). Patients suffering from this type of aphasia are usually able to understand ordinary spoken language, although they may struggle on formal tests of comprehension where they are deprived of contextual information and must rely on grammatical cues alone. For example, they may be unable to work out who chased whom given a semantically reversible passive sentence such as *The boy was chased by the girl*, but will have no problems with *The soup was eaten by the girl*, where they can use a non-syntactic strategy. Lesions to Wernicke's area, i.e. the upper posterior part of the left temporal lobe, in contrast, tend to lead to severe comprehension difficulties in the presence of fluent but often deviant speech (cf. example (2)). Such patients make frequent lexical errors, substituting semantically related but inappropriate words (e.g. *table* for *chair*) or incorrect sounds (e.g. *bekan* for *began*), or, in more severe cases, unidentifiable phonological forms such as *taenz*.

(1)   [Retelling the story of the fox and the crow] *King . . . Singing . . . Singing loud . . . Meat. Perfect!* (Goodglass 2001: 64)

(2)   [Response to a therapist's question about why he is in hospital] *What's wrong with me because I . . . was myself until the taenz took something about the time between me and my regular time in that time and they took the time in that time here and that's when the the time took around here and saw me around in it it's started with me no time and then I bekan work of nothing else that's the way the doctor find me that way.* (Obler and Gjerlow 1999: 43)

The frequent occurrence of such impairments following damage to Broca's and Wernicke's areas indicates that these regions are crucially involved in language processing. It has also led some researchers to speculate that linguistic knowledge is actually embodied in the wiring of these areas of the brain: specifically, that Broca's area is the seat of grammatical knowledge while lexical knowledge is at least partially represented in Wernicke's area. As we shall see, however, such claims are rather problematic for a number of reasons.

1. The localisation issue

The first problem with the strict localisation view is the fact that the relationship between the lesion site and the nature of the resulting impairment is far from straightforward. Language impairment sometimes occurs after brain damage outside the classical language areas (Dronkers et al. 2000), even in right-handed monolingual patients with no known prior neurological condition which might have caused a reorganisation of language function in the brain. If fact, aphasic-like symptoms may occur after damage to subcortical areas like the basal ganglia and the thalamus (Basso et al. 1987; Brown 1975; Crosson et al. 1986; Démonet et al. 1991; Lieberman 2002). This suggests that many regions of the brain outside the classical language areas are involved in language processing – a supposition confirmed by a growing number of brain imaging studies (Démonet et al. 1992, 1993; Mazziotta and Metter 1988; Posner et al. 1988; Warburton et al. 1996; Wise et al. 1991; Zatorre et al. 1992).

Conversely, damage to the 'language areas' does not always lead to language impairment, or to the predicted type of impairment. Dronkers et al. (2000) describe patients with damage to Broca's area who are not agrammatic, and patients with lesions to Wernicke's area who do not have Wernicke's aphasia. Furthermore, persistent full-blown aphasias are rarely found in patients with damage to Broca's or Wernicke's area alone: when the lesion is confined to just the classical language areas, patients usually recover (Dronkers et al. 2000; Lieberman 2002).

Recovery after damage to the language areas of the brain is particularly good in children. As a rule, children recover quite quickly from the effects of the lesion, and, if it occurs before the onset of language, the expectation is that they will make a more or less full recovery – that is to say, within a few years, their language abilities will be within the normal range, though usually slightly below normal controls (Aram 1998; Bates 1999; Bates et al. 1997). Lesions sustained in middle and late childhood typically do leave some deficits, although these are more likely to be apparent in the children's writing and schoolwork than in ordinary conversation (Bishop 1993; Martins and Ferro 1992, 1993; van Hout 1991).

It is also worth noting that the aphasic symptoms observed in children who have suffered brain damage are very different from those found in adults. Wernicke's (fluent) aphasia is extremely rare in children, even after damage to Wernicke's area, as is the telegraphic speech characteristic of Broca's aphasia. Child aphasics typically don't talk very much, and when they do, they use simpler structures – but they rarely make errors. Furthermore, children are likely to have a mild aphasia after just about any kind of brain damage, including damage to the right hemisphere and the non-linguistic parts of the left hemisphere (Aram 1998; Gardner 1974). This suggests that the localisation of linguistic functions is much more widely distributed in children than in adults, which doesn't fit in very well with the idea that the basic blueprint for grammar is genetically prespecified and embodied in the wiring of Broca's area.

But the most dramatic illustration of the plasticity of linguistic organisation comes from studies of individuals who lack the left hemisphere altogether. Some cases of catastrophic childhood epilepsy can be cured or at least alleviated either by removing the entire hemisphere in which epileptic attacks begin (hemispherectomy) or, more commonly, by stripping it of its cortex (hemidecortication). Not surprisingly, children who have undergone such drastic surgery suffer from a variety of deficits, including linguistic deficits. However, the nature of their impairment is often very different from what one might expect, given what happens in brain-damaged adults.

It is important to bear in mind that the hemispherectomised population is very heterogeneous: patients differ in the actual condition which led to the operation, the age at which it appeared, the age at which they were operated on, the success of the operation in controlling seizures, and the state of the remaining hemisphere. All of these factors, and probably many more, have an effect on how well language develops after surgery. Consequently, the final outcome after hemispherectomy is extremely variable. However, given the special status of the left hemisphere in language processing, we would expect its removal to have a dramatic and devastating effect on an individual's language abilities, while removal of the right hemisphere should normally spare language (although it might impair the ability to use prosody and to interpret figurative language, both of which are known to require right-hemisphere involvement). This expectation, however, is not corroborated by the available evidence.

A recent survey of 49 post-hemispherectomy patients (Curtiss and de Bode 1998) found no significant relationship between side of lesion and language outcome. In fact, nearly a third of the *right* hemispherectomised patients had no productive language at all, compared to 16.7 per cent of the left hemispherectomies, which suggests that the right hemisphere plays an important role in language acquisition. Even more surprisingly, seven of the thirty left-hemispherectomised patients – that is to say, over 23 per cent – had normal or nearly normal language.

Curtiss and de Bode acknowledge that their measure of linguistic ability, the 'Spoken Language Rank', is fairly crude, so it is possible that a more sensitive test of morphosyntactic abilities would reveal subtle deficits in the left-hemispherectomised group. Such deficits were found by several researchers, including Dennis and Kohn (1975), Dennis and Whitaker (1976), Dennis (1980), and Vargha-Khadem and Polkey (1992). Dennis and Kohn (1975), for example, used the Active-Passive-Negative test, in which the patient is presented with two pictures (e.g. a picture of a girl pushing a boy and a boy pushing a girl) and a sentence (e.g. *The boy is being pushed by the girl*) and asked to point to the picture that matches the sentence. The sentences vary in voice (active v. passive) and polarity (affirmative v. negative). Dennis and Kohn found that both groups performed well on active sentences, but the left-hemidecorticate group had more problems with passive and especially negative passive sentences, from which they conclude that the right hemisphere is not as proficient at linguistic processing as the left hemisphere. This conclusion, however, has not gone unchallenged. Bishop (1983) argues that performance on passive negatives is low in children and in individuals with low IQ, and that the left-hemidecorticates' performance was not in fact significantly different from that of age- and IQ-matched controls; and Ogden (1988) found that the deficits in left-hemidecorticates' performance on passive-negative sentences disappeared when the test sentences were presented in writing rather than orally.

Thus, both left- and right-hemidecorticates typically have language problems, although it may be the case that the left-hemidecorticates are less proficient in the more complex aspects of morphosyntax. It must be stressed that the deficits are detectable only through specialised tests: the spontaneous speech of the more proficient left-hemidecorticated patients is fluent and grammatical. It is clear, then, that the isolated right hemisphere is capable of sustaining a great deal of syntactic processing.

2. Preservation of grammatical knowledge in Broca's aphasia

There is also growing evidence that agrammatics, and aphasic patients in general, may not have lost their linguistic knowledge. Aphasic patients' linguistic performance is often highly variable, and may improve or deteriorate considerably from day to day, or at certain times of the day (Goodglass and Kaplan 1972: 12; Linebarger 1989: 199). It is also very dependent on the nature of the task: patients often perform better on more structured tasks. For example, they might be able to complete a passive sentence begun by a therapist even if they are unable to construct one themselves. Furthermore, agrammatic production does not necessarily co-occur with agrammatic comprehension: some patients can understand grammatical distinctions conveyed by word order and function words but are unable to use the same constructions in their own speech, while others have relatively normal speech but cannot use grammatical information in comprehension (Blackwell and Bates 1995; Linebarger et al. 1983). To make things even more complicated, some cases of agrammatism are modality-specific: the symptoms may be manifest only in the patient's speech, or only in writing. All these facts suggest that agrammatic patients (or at least those agrammatic patients who show such uneven profiles) have not lost their grammatical knowledge, but have difficulty accessing it – in other words, that their deficit is not one of competence, but of performance.

There is also evidence that even 'truly' agrammatic patients show some sensitivity to grammatical structure. In one study (Wayland et al. 1996) patients were asked to listen to sentences and press a button when they heard a particular word. The researchers found that agrammatic participants' reaction times were slower when the sentence was ungrammatical (e.g. when a verb occurred in a syntactic context appropriate for a noun or vice versa). These results suggest that the agrammatics were sensitive to the morphological cues signalling grammatical category even though they did not produce the relevant morphemes in their own speech. Even more intriguingly, there is now a whole raft of studies showing that agrammatic patients often perform surprisingly well on grammaticality judgement tasks (see Linebarger 1989, 1990; Linebarger et al. 1983; Wulfeck and Bates 1991; Wulfeck et al. 1991). Linebarger et al. (1983), for example, asked agrammatics to evaluate the acceptability of sentences such as those in (3)–(5) below, and found that they gave the correct response about 80 per cent of the time – a level of performance which is far from perfect, but nevertheless well above chance.

(3)   a. *Did the old man enjoy the show?*
        b. **Did the old man enjoying the show?*

(4)   a. *I want you to go to the store now.*
        b. *I hope you will go to the store now.*
        c. **I want you will go to the store now.*
        d. **I hope you to go to the store now.*

(5)   a. *Frank was expected to get the job.*
        b. *Which job did you expect Frank to get?*
        c. **This job was expected Frank to get.*

It is worth noting that many of the ungrammatical sentences used in the study were *locally* grammatical, so the relatively high level of performance could not have been achieved if participants carried out only a superficial analysis. As the authors point out:

> At least the following kinds of syntactic ability are required by our task: an awareness of strict subcategorisation frames, considerable sensitivity to the function vocabulary, the ability to compute hierarchical phrase structure, and the ability to handle discontinuous syntactic dependencies. It appears that the task could not be performed successfully by using general semantic knowledge or an appreciation of transitional probabilities and/or prosodic patterns associated with particular lexical items. In general, any appeal to 'template matching' as an alternative strategy for performing this task seems to us to require templates which

are in fact generalizations over structures of considerable syntactic spec-
ification. (Linebarger et al. 1983: 386ff)

Yet another source of evidence suggesting that aphasic disorders may
involve lack of access to grammatical knowledge, rather than lack of knowledge as such, comes from studies of bilingual aphasics. Most bilingual speakers suffering from aphasia are impaired in both of their languages, but in a
significant minority of cases, the speaker's languages may be differentially
affected. In some patients, one language is severely impaired while performance in the other remains relatively good. Others show unexpected patterns
of recovery: for example, the two languages may recover in succession, or the
patient may improve in one language but not in the other, or one language may
recover while the other deteriorates (see Paradis 1977, 1998). Occasionally
patients may show different symptoms in different languages: for example, a
patient may behave like a Broca's aphasic in one language and like a
Wernicke's in another (Albert and Obler 1978; Silverberg and Gordon 1979).
But perhaps the most exotic case of linguistic impairment following brain
damage is a condition known as 'alternate antagonism with paradoxical translation' described by Paradis et al. (1982). Their two bilingual patients could
use both of their languages spontaneously, but not at the same time (alternate
antagonism). Moreover, they were able to translate *into* the language that was
not available for spontaneous production, but not into the other language
(paradoxical translation). For example, one of their patients, a French/Arabic
bilingual referred to as AD, was on some occasions able to speak French but
not Arabic and to translate into Arabic but not into French; on other occasions, she showed the opposite pattern. Clearly, AD could not have lost either
of her languages, although she was not able to access them at will.

The findings reviewed above suggest that the linguistic impairments experienced by many aphasic patients are attributable to processing difficulties, not
to loss of linguistic knowledge (although global aphasia probably does involve
loss of knowledge). This interpretation appears to be supported by several
studies which showed that aphasic-like symptoms can be induced in *normal*
people under cognitive overload or when the stimuli are partially masked by
noise (Blackwell and Bates 1995; Dick et al. 2001; Miyake et al. 1994; Tesak
1994). Miyake et al., for example, got their subjects to read sentences presented to them word by word at a very fast rate. This method of presentation
significantly reduced the subjects' ability to use grammatical cues in interpret-
ing relatively complex grammatical structures such as relatives, but had little
effect on simpler sentences. In the Blackwell and Bates study, a group of
undergraduates had to keep a series of digits in memory while performing a
grammaticality judgement task. Their performance, though superior to that
of aphasics, was clearly impaired relative to no-digit controls. Interestingly,
agreement errors were especially difficult to detect in such conditions. Since
aphasics also have particular difficulty with agreement morphology, the study

offers strong evidence in favour of the claim that the selective vulnerability of grammatical morphemes in aphasia may be at least partly attributable to global diminution in cognitive resources.

Most of the work reviewed so far is based on aphasia in speakers of English and other typologically similar languages. In recent years, however, it has become increasingly clear that brain damage may affect speakers of different languages in different ways and consequently, that some of the conclusions about the organisation of language in the brain arrived at on the basis of data from the familiar European languages may be in need of revision. Two main findings are relevant in this connection. First, it appears that users of typologically very different languages may suffer aphasia after lesions which do not cause linguistic problems in speakers of English. The traditional literature on aphasia, for example, is virtually unanimous in asserting that in the vast majority of cases, language impairment occurs after damage to the dominant hemisphere – i.e. the left hemisphere in right-handers and the right hemisphere in most left-handers. Damage to the non-dominant hemisphere may affect a patient's pragmatic skills, but it rarely results in serious deficits in the core linguistic areas of lexis and grammar. However, this does not appear to be the case in Chinese. Hu et al. (1990) reported that in their sample of Chinese right-handed aphasics, about 30 per cent had suffered damage to the *right* (i.e. non-dominant) hemisphere. This suggests that Chinese speakers, or at least a large proportion of Chinese speakers, make much greater use of the right hemisphere when speaking than do speakers of Indo-European languages. Researchers working on sign language have also found that linguistic deficits in signers can occur following damage to the right hemisphere and some 'non-linguistic' regions of the left hemisphere as well as Broca's and Wernicke's areas, suggesting that the areas of the brain involved in processing sign language only partly overlap with those used by spoken languages (Corina 1998). These findings have been confirmed by imaging studies (Corina 1996; Neville and Bavelier 2000). Thus, it appears that experience with different languages might cause speakers to recruit additional regions of the brain in addition to the classical language areas.

Secondly, it has been shown that the 'traditional' aphasias, and Broca's (non-fluent) aphasia in particular, look very different in typologically different languages. One of the hallmarks of Broca's aphasia in English-speaking patients, apart from dysfluency and other problems with articulation, is agrammatism, which is often manifested as 'telegraphic' speech: the patient is able to produce nouns and some other content words, but has severe difficulty with function words and grammatical endings, resulting in speech output reminiscent of the style we find in telegrams. However, non-fluent aphasics in highly inflected languages such as Polish, Serbo-Croatian, German and Italian, and agglutinative languages such as Turkish, Finnish and Hungarian, are not agrammatic – that is to say, they do not omit inflections, though they often use them inappropriately (Bates et al. 1991; Menn and Obler 1990;

Slobin 1991). Slobin (1991), for example, found that inflectional morphology in Turkish Broca's aphasics was 'remarkably well preserved . . . with hardly a trace of telegraphic speech' (1991: 150). His subjects tended to provide the right grammatical morphemes where required, although compared to normal controls, the range of affixes in their speech was quite restricted – similar to the range of forms available to Turkish 3-year-olds. Slobin also notes that in cases of word-finding difficulty, patients often used pronouns instead of nouns, and these were correctly inflected. Even the most non-fluent patient, whose speech consisted mostly of single word utterances, provided the appropriate case inflections on nouns.

Thus, the results from highly inflected languages are at odds with those obtained from English-speaking patients. The 'agrammatic' patients described by Slobin and Bates et al. had suffered similar lesions to 'agrammatic' English-speaking aphasics, yet they had clearly not lost all grammatical knowledge. It seems safe to conclude, then, that grammatical knowledge does not reside in the pattern of connections in Broca's area.

3. The co-occurrence of lexical and grammatical deficits

In popular treatments of language disorders, particularly those intended for consumption by linguistics students, Broca's aphasia is often treated as a primarily grammatical impairment, while Wernicke's aphasia is presented as a lexical deficit. Such a characterisation, though it fits in very well with the traditional division of a speaker's linguistic knowledge into a 'grammatical' and a 'lexical' component, is very misleading.

First, it is now well known that Wernicke's aphasics, in addition to their obvious lexical problems, also have grammatical deficits. Although they do not omit function words and grammatical inflections in production, they tend to use them inappropriately and often produce ill-formed structures. This is particularly obvious in highly inflected languages such as Polish, Czech or German, where substitution of an inappropriate grammatical morpheme is likely to result in a sentence which is ungrammatical rather than merely semantically anomalous (Pick 1973 [1913]; Ulatowska et al. 2001). They also perform poorly on grammatical comprehension tasks (Kertesz and Osmán-Sági 2001; MacWhinney et al. 1991) and grammaticality judgement tasks (Grodzinsky and Finkel 1998).

Conversely, the agrammatic performance of Broca's aphasics is virtually always accompanied by word-finding difficulties (particularly with verbs and other relational words) and other disturbances of lexical processing such as reduced semantic priming (Dick et al. 2001). Indeed, it appears that lexical deficits of some description accompany *all* forms of aphasia (Dick et al. 2001; Marshall 1986), although their severity does not necessarily correlate with the severity of the patient's other deficits. Furthermore, as pointed out by

Elizabeth Bates and her collaborators (Bates and Goodman 1997, 1999; Dick et al. 2001), there are some rather striking parallels between a person's lexical and grammatical difficulties, which can be observed in a wide range of deficits, including developmental disorders, aphasia, and the linguistic impairments which accompany Alzheimer's dementia and normal ageing. Thus, individuals who omit function words also tend to omit lexical items rather than substitute inappropriate ones. This pattern is found in Broca's aphasia as well as in other 'non-fluent' deficits such as Down's syndrome and some forms of specific language impairment. In contrast, lexical substitution errors (semantic paraphasias) and the substitution of inappropriate grammatical functors (paragrammatism) are the hallmarks of Wernicke's aphasia, and are also quite characteristic of the speech of individuals suffering from another 'fluent' disorder, Williams's syndrome. Finally, the excessive use of pronouns and semantically 'light' forms such as *thing*, *make* and *do* in anomia and Alzheimer's disease (and, to a lesser extent, in normal ageing) is accompanied by a similar reduction of the grammatical repertoire: individuals belonging to these groups tend to avoid complex syntactic structures such as passives (Bates, Harris et al. 1995). The co-occurrence of lexical and grammatical deficits in all these groups and the similarity in the symptoms that they demonstrate across linguistic domains strongly suggest a common underlying mechanism.

4. The resilience of language

It is undeniable that some regions of the brain are more involved in linguistic, and specifically grammatical, processing than others. However, the strongest version of the anatomical specialisation hypothesis – that grammar resides in the pattern of connections in Broca's area – is clearly false. As we have seen, there is considerable evidence that individuals who have suffered lesions to Broca's area do not lose their grammatical knowledge, but are simply unable to access it at will. Furthermore, the most entrenched grammatical patterns, such as basic word order or case inflections in morphologically rich languages, generally do remain accessible. This suggests that linguistic knowledge is represented in a redundant manner in various regions of the brain, with the language areas acting as a kind of central switchboard. There is also evidence of close links between grammatical and lexical deficits, which in turn suggests that these two aspects of a speaker's linguistic competence are closely intertwined.

   Another important lesson to be learned from the research on aphasia is that our capacity to use language is extremely resilient. In immature individuals, language can survive the loss of the 'language areas' or even of the entire left hemisphere. In adults, such large-scale reorganisation is not possible, perhaps because the regions which take over language processing in brain-damaged children are already committed to other functions. However, there is evidence that even adults are able to recruit new areas or make new connections to some extent. Furthermore, adults are certainly able to compensate for the damage suffered by developing new language processing strategies. Both of these facts lend further support to the claim that the architecture supporting the human language faculty is very flexible.

5 Language and other cognitive processes

1. The modularity hypothesis

One of the most controversial issues in contemporary psycholinguistics is the extent to which our linguistic abilities depend on 'general purpose' cognition. In the 1980s and 1990s, many researchers (e.g. Ferreira and Clifton 1986; Fodor 1983; Smith and Tsimpli 1995; Yamada 1990) proposed that language is relatively independent from other cognitive capacities and is subserved by a specialised cognitive 'module'. This controversial hypothesis is based on two types of arguments. First, it has been proposed that the specialised language processor is faster, and therefore **informationally encapsulated**: the early stages of language processing rely exclusively on lexical and syntactic knowledge, and other kinds of knowledge can only be accessed after a preliminary syntactic analysis has been completed. As we saw in Chapter 2, language processing is indeed very fast; however, there is no strong evidence that the 'purely linguistic' processes – i.e. lexical access and parsing – outpace processes which depend on non-linguistic real-world knowledge. A second, much more powerful argument for the modularity hypothesis is the existence of apparent **dissociations** between language (especially grammar) and other cognitive processes: it seems that language can be seriously disrupted while other processes remain relatively unaffected, and, conversely, severe cognitive impairment may be accompanied by little or no grammatical deficit.

As observed in the introductory chapter, linguistics has developed in relative isolation from research on human psychology. The apparent dissociation of language from other cognitive processes supports the status quo: it appears to justify the separation of linguistic theory from other disciplines. We shall see in this chapter, however, that the case for modularity has been overstated. We begin with a brief summary of the evidence for the autonomy of language, and then proceed to a discussion of some of the problems with the argument.

The textbook example of a relatively 'pure' language impairment is Broca's (non-fluent) aphasia. Broca's aphasics have problems with just about every aspect of language. They find it difficult to access the words they need, and in extreme cases, may be able to retrieve little more than concrete nouns. Their

speech is slow, poorly articulated and agrammatic (they often leave out obligatory function words and inflections, at least in English and typologically
similar languages). They are also unable to use grammatical cues in comprehension: for example, they have problems with reversible passives such as *The
boy is being chased by the girl*, where it is impossible to tell from the meaning
of the words alone who does the chasing and who is being pursued. However,
the general cognitive abilities of Broca's aphasics are good: they are able to
solve complex problems (as long as these don't require the use of language),
they behave in socially appropriate ways, and they can make excellent use of
contextual information to infer the meaning of an utterance. In fact, their
pragmatic skills often allow them to compensate very successfully for their
grammatical deficit, and for this reason Broca's aphasia was for a long time
regarded as a purely productive deficit.

Deficits which seem to affect language and language alone have also been
observed in acquisition. While the majority of developmental language disorders can be attributed to hearing loss, general learning difficulties or emotional
problems, some children develop language late and with considerable difficulty in spite of the fact that they appear to be completely normal in every
other respect. Such children, diagnosed as suffering from specific language
impairment, or SLI, usually have problems with several aspects of language
use, including articulation, vocabulary and grammar. Their utterances are
shorter and less fluent than those of normal children; they frequently omit
function words and affixes, and tend to avoid more complex grammatical
structures. They also make more errors of commission than other children,
and perform below age norms on comprehension tests. Most SLI children do
eventually learn to speak normally, although some residual problems often
remain; consequently, they are at risk for reading disorders, and tend to
perform less well than unimpaired children at school.

More surprisingly, language can apparently develop more or less normally
even in the face of severe cognitive impairment. Williams' syndrome (WS) is
a case in point. WS is a rare neurodevelopmental disorder characterised by a
complex of physical abnormalities (including heart and circulatory defects
and a characteristic 'pixie-like' face) and mental retardation. Individuals with
WS typically have performance IQs of about 50–60 and have difficulty finding
their way around or performing simple everyday tasks such as tying their shoe-
laces. Their linguistic skills, however, appear to be remarkably well preserved.
WS adolescents are fluent and articulate – quite loquacious, in fact. Their
utterances are generally well-formed and contain a variety of complex grammatical structures, including full passives, relative clauses and multiple embedding. Here, for example, is how a 17-year-old WS girl with an IQ of 50
described the experience of having an MRI scan:

(1)   *There is a huge magnetic machine. It took a picture inside the brain.*
        You could talk but not move your head because that would ruin the

whole thing and they would have to start all over again. After it's done they show you your brain on a computer and they see how large it is. And the machine on the other side of the room takes pictures from the computer. They can take pictures instantly. Oh, it was very exciting! (Bellugi et al. 1993: 183)

Individuals with WS also perform well on some formal tests of language development. They tend to achieve high scores (sometimes above their mental age) on vocabulary tests, both receptive and expressive. They also perform relatively well on tasks tapping various grammatical abilities, including comprehension of passives, negatives, conditionals, and anaphoric and reflexive pronouns (Bellugi et al. 1994; Clahsen and Almazan 1998). Finally, they have good metalinguistic skills: for example, they are able to define familiar words and to identify (and often correct) ungrammatical sentences (Bellugi et al. 1993, 1994). Thus, it is clear that their linguistic skills far outstrip their non-verbal abilities.

We find another striking example of the selective sparing of linguistic abilities in Christopher, a 'linguistic savant' studied by Smith and Tsimpli (1991, 1995). Although Christopher appears to have a normal verbal intelligence, his non-verbal IQ scores are extremely low (from 40 to 76, depending on the test); at age 30, he fails a theory-of-mind test which poses no problem for normal 4-year-olds and conservation tasks which normal children solve at the age of 5; and he must be institutionalised because he is unable to look after himself. However, Christopher has an unusual talent for learning languages: in addition to his native English, he is able to read, write and communicate in some fifteen other languages.

Thus, language, and in particular grammar, can be significantly impaired in the absence of other cognitive problems, and, conversely, language can be disrupted while other cognitive processes remain relatively unaffected. Many researchers argue that such a 'double dissociation' shows that language is mediated by dedicated neural circuits, and hence independent from other cognitive processes and 'hardwired' – that is to say, genetically predetermined (see, for example, Pinker 1999; Smith and Tsimpli 1995).

2. Problems with the double dissociation argument

Such far-reaching conclusions, however, are rather premature, for several reasons. First, saying that some individuals have 'intelligence without language' while others have 'language without intelligence' (cf. Pinker 1995) is a vast oversimplification, as the observed dissociations between language and other cognitive processes are partial. Global aphasia – the total loss of the ability to communicate by means of language – is comparatively rare and is apparently always accompanied by cognitive deficits (van Mourik et al. 1992).

In most aphasic patients, some linguistic abilities are preserved (see Chapter 4), so it is inaccurate to say that they lack language; and while they usually perform well on cognitive tests, their non-linguistic cognition is rarely, if ever, completely unaffected. A number of studies, for example, have reported that aphasics obtained lower scores than other brain-damaged patients on non-verbal intelligence tests (see Baldo et al. 2001; Hamsher 1998; Keil and Kaszniak 2002; Lebrun and Hoops 1974), although it is not clear whether this is a result of aphasia as such or of constructional apraxia (inability to copy or construct complex figures), which often accompanies aphasia. Many aphasics also have problems with relatively simple tasks which do not involve language, such as using the right colours to fill in outline drawings, associating non-linguistic sounds with pictures, showing what one does with various objects (e.g. a toothbrush), and sorting. The co-occurrence of the linguistic problems with such non-linguistic deficits does not entail that there is a functional link – it is possible, for example, that these non-linguistic tasks are subserved by adjacent areas of the brain which are damaged at the same time as the language areas – but it should make us careful in drawing conclusions about the presumed independence of language from other cognitive processes.

The same point can be made even more forcefully with regard to language-impaired children. Individuals with SLI have problems with language, but they are certainly not 'languageless'; and although, by definition, they have normal or above-normal intelligence, there is ample evidence that various sub-populations of children diagnosed with SLI suffer from associated non-linguistic deficits. The most often reported impairments involve auditory processing and short-term memory, but a variety of other problems have been observed as well (Bishop 1992; Curtiss and Tallal 1991; Curtis et al. 1992; Gathercole and Baddeley 1990; Hill 2001; Johnston 1997; Jones et al. 1994; Merzenich et al. 1996; Montgomery 1995; Vargha-Khadem et al. 1995). Again, the co-occurrence of language disorders with such non-linguistic defi-cits does not prove that the former are a consequence of the latter: it is pos-sible that the children had been misdiagnosed, or that their non-linguistic problems are a result of the language impairment (cf. Stromswold 1996). However, the existence of such associated deficits suggests that the term '*spe-cific* language impairment' is a misnomer.

The case for 'language without intelligence' is equally problematic. It is true that the 'hyperlinguistic' individuals mentioned earlier have low intelligence. The WS subjects described in the literature usually have IQs of about 50–60, and Christopher's full-scale IQ is probably between 70 and 80. However, this does not mean that they are cognitive vegetables. As Tomasello (1995) points out, IQ is a number derived by dividing a person's mental age by their chron-ological age (and multiplying the result by 100). Thus, the IQ of 50 obtained by the girl quoted in the preceding section means that, at 17, her performance on an intelligence test was equivalent to that of an average 8-and-a-half-year-old. The studies documenting the good performance of WS subjects on linguistic tasks involved adolescents and young adults with mental ages between 5 and 9. Since normal children in this age range speak fluently and understand passives, negatives, conditionals etc., we should not be surprised by the fact that WS adolescents are also able to understand such structures. The same argument also applies to Christopher, of course – and in his case, one might also add that his verbal IQ scores were within the normal range, that he performed extremely well on a test of pragmatic inference, and that he was able to teach himself foreign languages by reading grammar books. Thus, describing people like Christopher or the WS patients studied by Bellugi and her colleagues as lacking intelligence is simply preposterous.

Furthermore, it is important to note that none of these 'hyperlinguistic' individuals actually has normal language. People with WS show considerable language delay in infancy (Bellugi et al. 1994; Paterson et al. 1999; Thal et al. 1989). They tend to make good progress in middle and late childhood, and by adolescence, their linguistic skills are comparable to those of normally developing 6–7-year-old children (Karmiloff-Smith et al. 1997; Volterra et al. 1996) – that is to say, about right for their mental age, although even adolescents have difficulties with complex syntactic structures (Grant et al. 2002). In other words, the linguistic skills of individuals with WS are good only in comparison with their non-verbal abilities. This was demonstrated particularly dramatically by Stojanovik et al. (in press), who, unlike other researchers, directly compared WS and SLI individuals on the same tests. In line with previous research, they found dissociations. The SLI participants performed at age-appropriate levels on standardised tests of non-linguistic cognition, and below age levels on language tests. The WS participants, on the other hand, performed well on language tests *relative to their non-verbal cognition scores.* Crucially, however, they were *no better than the SLI participants on the language tasks* (in fact, they were slightly worse on some measures). Given that SLI is supposed to be a selective impairment of language, it makes no sense to say that language skills in WS are 'intact'.

Similar observations can be made about Christopher. We do not know much about his early linguistic development (he was already 29 when Smith and Tsimpli began their investigation), although we do know that he was a late talker. His command of foreign languages, while impressive, is far from perfect: in fact, he seems to have internalised very little syntactic knowledge, although his vocabulary and morphology are very good. He tends to follow English word order in spontaneous production and translation, and his grammaticality judgements are strongly influenced by English. Smith and Tsimpli conclude that 'Christopher's syntax is basically English with a range of alternative veneers' (1995: 122) and observe that 'it is possible that despite speaking many languages, Christopher really has only one grammar' (129).

On the other hand, argue Smith and Tsimpli, Christopher's command of his native English is virtually perfect. He performed at ceiling on TROG (Test of Reception of Grammar), which shows grammatical knowledge equivalent to at least that of a normal 11-year-old. Furthermore, he was able to make very subtle distinctions, as well as correct ungrammatical sentences, on a grammaticality judgement task. For example, he correctly identified the (a) sentences below as ungrammatical, and offered the grammatical versions given in (b):

(2)   a. *This is the girl that I saw her with John at the cinema.*
        b. *This is the girl that I saw with John at the cinema.*

(3)   a. *Mary believes the claim which John is a very intelligent man.*
        b. *Mary believes the claim that John is a very intelligent man.*

(4)   a. *Which student do you think that could solve the problem?*
        b. *Which student do you think could solve the problem?*

Such subtle judgements clearly require sophisticated syntactic knowledge. However, Christopher makes very little use of this knowledge in production. His spontaneous conversation is generally monosyllabic. On the rare occasions when he does produce longer stretches of discourse, his speech is 'mildly repetitive and full of snatches that appear to have been memorised from textbooks' (Smith and Tsimpli 1991: 327) – and, one might add, not very native-like (cf. example (5) below). Furthermore, he often produces ungrammatical sentences when translating into English.

(5)   IT *How did you learn Hindi?*
        C   *From book.*
        IT *Like Greek.*
        C   *Yes. Shall we try a bit of um exercises where, where the where you want to go to a girl who doesn't speak Hindi and her mother says: Are you are you permitted to go here because there's a film on and there and mother says* a:j, a:j ek film – *you* – a:p – tu um kiya: baza:r kya: zaba:r *um now – how do I write 'Hindi'? Is it, is it this way to write 'Hindi'?*

   Smith and Tsimpli attribute these difficulties to his non-linguistic cognitive impairment. While this may account for the mistakes in translation (which is without doubt a very demanding task), it does not seem like a plausible explanation for his difficulty with normal everyday conversation – after all, WS adolescents are fluent conversationalists in spite of the fact that their cognitive impairment is even more severe than Christopher's.
   In summary: it is true that in some people language is seriously impaired in the absence of equally obvious problems with non-verbal cognition, while others develop relatively good language in spite of severe cognitive deficits. However, such dissociations are partial. 'Hyperlinguistic' individuals have unusually good language, relative to their non-verbal abilities, while language-impaired

individuals have poor language skills, again relative to other cognitive domains. In both groups, however, the deficit is a matter of degree.

We now turn to a more important question: what exactly do these dissociations show? They do indicate that language is not merely an outgrowth of 'general cognition'. But then there is no such thing as 'general cognition': what we have is a varied repertoire of cognitive skills and abilities. Some of these (e.g. auditory short-term memory) are clearly implicated in language acquisition and processing, while others (e.g. the ability to find one's way around in an unfamiliar neighbourhood) are not. It is to be expected, then, that some cognitive deficits will have a profound effect on language performance, while others will be of little or no consequence.

On the other hand, the dissociations do not show that grammar is an innate, domain-specific and informationally encapsulated module – indeed, the very fact that they are partial entails that there are important links between verbal and non-verbal cognition. Specifically, the fact that both lexical and grammatical development is significantly delayed in virtually all mentally impaired children – including those who are described as 'hyperlinguistic' – suggests that certain 'cognitive infrastructures', to borrow Elizabeth Bates's (1994) term, must be in place before grammatical development can begin. One should stress, however, that these are fairly modest: equivalent, perhaps, to the mental abilities of a normal 2-year-old (cf. Bates 1997). Furthermore, the fact that the language of the mentally handicapped – again including those who are 'hyperlinguistic' – is also impaired, albeit sometimes to a lesser degree than other aspects of their cognitive functioning, suggests that some grammatical abilities require more elaborate cognitive infrastructures.

This brings us to the final point: it is not accurate to say that language processing in 'hyperlinguistic' individuals is simply 'not quite as good' as in normals: there is evidence that it may also be *qualitatively* different. Several researchers have noted that the spontaneous speech of people with WS often includes strange word choices. For example, one of the young people studied by Bellugi observed that *The bees abort the beehive* (that is to say, leave it); another indicated that she would have to *evacuate the glass* (empty it) (Bellugi et al. 1994: 32). Individuals with WS also tend to use more low-frequency words than normals on word fluency tasks, which prompted some researchers to conclude that their mental lexicons are organised in an unusual (Bellugi et al. 1994) or even deviant (Pinker 1991) fashion.

The language of children and adolescents with WS also shows some grammatical peculiarities. In contrast to normal children and adults, for example, they perform better on high-frequency than on low-frequency regular verbs, but show no frequency effects on irregulars (Thomas et al. 2001). Karmiloff-Smith and colleagues (1997) found that their French-speaking WS subjects made significantly more gender-agreement errors than controls, especially when the experimental stimuli were nonce words rather than real words. Particular difficulties with agreement were also observed in the speech of an

Italian WS girl studied by Capirci et al. (1996). Capirci et al. also note that the girl made syntactic errors that do not occur in the speech of normal children at comparable stages of linguistic development. Finally, Karmiloff-Smith et al. (1998), using an online language task, found that their WS subjects showed normal sensitivity to phrase structure violations and restrictions imposed by an auxiliary on the form of the following verb, but not to lexical verb subcategorisation frames.

Such findings suggest that people with WS may acquire and process language in a qualitatively different way (cf. Bellugi et al. 2000; Karmiloff-Smith 1998; Karmiloff-Smith et al. 1998). There is some support for this conclusion from brain imaging studies, which have shown that WS individuals show distinctive ERP patterns which are not found in any other group (Bellugi et al. 1994; Neville et al. 1993). Furthermore, they show no left-hemisphere dominance for language – that is to say, unlike normal adults and older children, they process language bilaterally.

As we saw earlier, Christopher's language is also deviant, though apparently in different ways. The difference is most readily seen when we compare his spontaneous speech with that of WS subjects. People with WS speak fluently and generally correctly and use a variety of complex syntactic structures. Christopher's conversation, in contrast, is monosyllabic and non-native-like. On the other hand, Christopher performs much better than WS subjects on formal tests of language development and on grammaticality judgement tasks.

At the moment we know too little about the language abilities of 'hyperlinguistic' individuals to draw any definite conclusions. It is possible, however, that they learn and process language in qualitatively different ways from normal people. If this is the case, their abilities offer further evidence of the human brain's ability to wire itself for language – in different ways, according to the mental resources available – rather than of the existence of an innate, informationally encapsulated language module.

6 Biological underpinnings

1. A genetically specified language module?

All normal humans, and no other species, have language. Many animals, of course, have quite elaborate communication systems, but human language is very different from animal 'languages' – they are not just simpler, but qualitatively different. Unlike other species, humans are able to refer to objects in their environment (as well as to absent or imaginary entities) and combine words and phrases to form novel messages. Furthermore, human languages, even if they require some innate knowledge, are largely learned, since children growing up in different linguistic communities end up speaking different languages. Last but not least, human languages, unlike the vocalisations of our closest ape relatives – the chimpanzees – are under cortical control, and hence conscious and deliberate. Chimpanzee vocalisations, in contrast, are 'bound': they are triggered by a particular emotional state, are very difficult to suppress in its presence, and cannot be produced in its absence (Goodall 1986).

Virtually all language researchers agree that language acquisition would be impossible without some kind of innate structure: a flatworm cannot learn Flemish, or a chicken Chinese, however hard they and their teachers might try. What is much less clear is what kind of innate structure is necessary for this task, and the extent to which it is task-specific (devoted exclusively to language learning). According to the generative tradition, which dominated linguistic research for much of the latter half of the twentieth century, all humans are endowed with 'Universal Grammar', a mental module specifying the universal properties of human languages and the parameters along which they can vary, without which language acquisition would be impossible. Universal Grammar is believed to have evolved after we separated from the apes and to contain knowledge which is applicable exclusively to language learning – in other words, it is regarded as an adaptation which is both species- and task-specific.

However, the idea of a language module or 'organ' (cf. Anderson and Lightfoot 2002; Chomsky 1975, 2000), though it may initially seem attractive, becomes considerably less appealing when we consider the neuroanatomical evidence. One reason for this is that so far, despite intensive research, no one has been able to find this module. Anatomically, the human brain is not very different from that of the great apes. It is considerably larger (about three times the size of that of a chimpanzee), and it differs in the relative proportions in that humans have more association cortex and a larger cerebellum. However, there is no evidence that humans evolved new cortical areas or structures not present in the apes (Elman et al. 1996; Müller 1992, 1996; Preuss 2000). The so-called 'language areas' (Broca's and Wernicke's areas) have homologues in ape brains (Preuss 2000) and are involved in other cognitive operations as well (Fiez et al. 1995; Fox et al. 1988; Mazziotta et al. 1982).

One might object that the presence of homologous areas in ape brains does not entail that the details of the microcircuitry are the same: it is possible that in the course of human evolution, our brains have been 'rewired' to encode linguistic knowledge (and presumably knowledge underlying other uniquely human abilities). However, there are several reasons for doubting that the genome specifies the details of cortical connections, as opposed to the general pattern.

First, there is an arithmetical problem which Müller (1996: 626) has dubbed the problem of the 'poverty of the genetic code'. The human brain contains approximately 100 billion neurons. Assuming that each neuron is connected to 1,000 other neurons (a rather conservative estimate), we have 10^{14} (i.e., 100,000,000,000,000) synapses. The human genome, however – which encodes information necessary for building the rest of the body as well – contains only about 24,000 genes ('How many genes' 2003), about 99 per cent of which are shared with chimpanzees (Ebersberger et al. 2002). The disparity between these two figures suggests that the details of cortical microcircuitry are probably not fully specified in the genome, but rather emerge through complex interactions of genetic and environmental factors (cf. Elman et al. 1996).

Secondly, there is considerable evidence that cortical tissue is quite plastic in that it can support a variety of different representations, depending on the input it receives (Deacon 1997, 2000; Elman et al. 1996; Johnson 1998). We have already seen in Chapter 4 that if the regions which are normally responsible for linguistic processing are damaged early in infancy, language usually develops in other parts of the brain. Similar reorganisations have also been observed for other cognitive functions in many species. When a particular area is deprived of its usual input, it may assume another function. For example, if a monkey's finger is amputated, the area which would normally receive input from it will be 'colonised' by input from adjacent fingers; or parts of the auditory cortex may take over visual processing if they do not receive input from the ears. Such reassignment of function is most pronounced if the damage takes place early in infancy, but also occurs to some degree in mature individuals. Furthermore, when a living brain is surgically 'rewired' so that a particular region receives input from a different source – so that the auditory cortex receives information from the eyes, for example – the new recipient region develops some characteristics of the normal recipient region (in our example, the auditory cortex takes on visual representations). But perhaps the most dramatic evidence for plasticity has come from experiments involving transplantation of fetal neural tissue to a different area of the brain in another animal of the same species, or even a different species. Amazingly, the transplanted neurons grow appropriate connections and become functionally integrated with the host neurons (Deacon 1997, 2000), demonstrating that the genetic program for growing the brain is not only flexible, but also quite similar across species. For obvious ethical reasons, such experiments have not been performed on humans, but research on brain reorganisation in amputees and congenitally deaf or blind individuals is generally consistent with the animal data. Moreover, there have been several apparently successful attempts to transplant fetal pig neural cells into the brains of human patients suffering from Parkinson's disease in an effort to improve their motor control. A postmortem carried out after one such patient died revealed that the pig cells had survived and had grown appropriate connections in the host brain (Deacon et al. 1997).

It must be stressed that there are limits to this plasticity (cf. Johnson 1993, 1998). While it is possible for a lesioned brain to reorganise itself, particularly if the lesion occurred early, this is by no means always the case: the results of brain damage can be catastrophic. Similarly, while it is possible to transplant fetal neural tissue to a different site in another brain, it is certainly not possible to transplant anything anywhere. Furthermore, we do not know how well the transplanted tissue or rewired brains work. Although they do seem to take on representations appropriate to the input they receive, they may not do so as efficiently as an intact brain would. Thus, the fact that brain tissue is fairly plastic in the sense that it can take on a variety of representations does not rule out a certain degree of specialisation: it is perfectly possible that some regions are better suited for certain tasks than others. Even a fairly modest degree of plasticity, however, is incompatible with the view that specific regions are predestined to support a particular function because they encode the information necessary for that function.

Thus, it seems that the genetic 'wiring diagrams' for the brain are fairly crude: fetal axons 'know' the general area where they should terminate, but not the specific cell. Patterns of connectivity which can support complex computations such as language processing emerge later, largely as a result of experience (cf. Elman et al. 1996; Johnson 1998). In what sense, then, can language be said to be innate? To answer this question, it will be useful to appeal to a taxonomy of 'ways to be innate' offered by Elman et al. (1996; see also Elman 1999). Elman et al. distinguish between three types of innateness:

1. Representational: the genome prespecifies the neural microcircuitry required for the activity, thus in effect endowing the organism with innate knowledge.

2. Architectural: the genome specifies the general characteristics of the processing system such as the types of neurons and their properties, the types
of neurotransmitters, the degree of interconnectivity in various regions of
the brain, and the overall patterns of connectivity (i.e. which brain regions
are connected and their characteristic sources of input and output).
3. Chronotopic: the genome controls the timing of the developmental processes which build the brain, such as the number of cell divisions at particular stages of development and the patterns of synaptic growth and
pruning in various regions.

The evidence for cortical plasticity reviewed above argues against innately
specified cortical representations.[1] This suggests that the innate biases that
construct a brain capable of acquiring language operate at the other two levels.
Architectural and chronotopic constraints require less genetically specified
information, so the small number of genes in the genome (relative to the
number of synapses in the brain) is not a problem. They operate indirectly, by
enabling certain processes and making certain outcomes highly probable, but
they also allow for variations after injury or when environmental conditions
are different. However, architectural and chronotopic constraints are not specific enough to encode details of linguistic knowledge: instead, they build a
brain that can perform certain types of computations and support certain
types of learning.

It follows that human adaptations to language involve innate information-
processing and learning biases rather than innate knowledge. We now turn to
the question of what these adaptations might be, and how they might have
evolved.

2. Human adaptations to language

2.1 Preadaptations

Our evolutionary history saw two periods of relatively rapid increase in brain
size. During the first of these, which occurred between 2 million and 1.5
million years ago, the brains of our ancestors doubled in size from approximately 450 to 900 cubic centimetres, and during the second, which began
about half a million years ago and lasted until about 300,000 years ago, they
reached their present size of approximately 1350 cc. Both of these periods of
brain expansion appear to have coincided with changes in the upper respira-
tory tract which would have enabled our ancestors to produce a wider range
of sounds (Lock and Peters 1996), so it is likely that they correspond to major
developments in the evolution of language, perhaps the emergence of symbolic communication and combinatorial syntax respectively.

However we interpret the fossil record, it is clear that language is a relatively recent innovation. Since evolution is a highly conservative process which works by modifying or combining existing systems rather than creating new ones from scratch, the recent origin of language makes it virtually certain that it builds on pre-existing abilities which evolved for other purposes. These would have included, among others:

1. proto-phonological capacities, i.e. the ability to produce and recognise sounds and to coordinate complex motor routines involving the articulators;
2. proto-semantic capacities such as the ability to categorise percepts and to construct complex concepts (as well as some elementary concepts and/or feature detectors);
3. the capacity to form cross-modal associations (necessary to learn form–meaning pairings);
4. the ability to store and retrieve such pairings when required.

All of these abilities are particularly well developed in humans, but they are also found in apes (Lock and Colombo 1996; Premack 1980), so they can be regarded as preadaptations for language. Since they are clearly useful for language, it is reasonable to assume that, once humans acquired a rudimentary linguistic system, they were selected for, and refined as a result: the vocal tract became increasingly suitable for speech production, we became better at co-ordinating motor routines, acquired more sophisticated conceptual abilities and a better memory (especially for cross-modal associations), and so on. However, before any of this could happen, our ancestors had to acquire an ability without which it is impossible to have language as we know it: the capacity for cultural learning.

2.2 Cultural learning and mind-reading

The capacity for cultural learning made possible the transmission of cultural innovations, which in turn cleared the path for cumulative cultural evolution: a process in which later generations do not have to reinvent everything from scratch, but can build on the accomplishments of preceding generations.

Cumulative cultural evolution is a necessary condition for language: without it, language would never get off the ground. One person, or even a small group of people, cannot create a language: it takes a whole community – or, to be more exact, several cohorts of learner-inventors in a community. We know this from research on the development of gestural communication in the deaf. Deaf children deprived of sign language input develop a rudimentary form of communication ('homesign'), but not a full language. The emergence of a true language requires a critical mass of individuals who interact on a regular basis (Kegl et al. 1999). It also requires time, as demonstrated by Senghas and Coppola (2001), who documented how Nicaraguan Sign

Language emerged after a number of deaf children were brought together in special schools and was grammaticalised by successive cohorts of learners who built on the conventions established earlier.[2]

Cumulative cultural evolution (whether linguistic or non-linguistic) appears to be a uniquely human trait, and relies on a characteristically human form of learning: imitation (Tomasello 1999). Our ape relatives do develop certain 'cultural' practices such as eating termites in a particular way or using two stones to crack nuts. They also can, and do, learn to use gestures communicatively. However, neither of these behaviours is acquired in the same way as human cultural practices and gestural signs. To appreciate the difference, it will be useful to begin with a quick look at learning in chimpanzees and other non-human primates.

Chimpanzee communicative gestures are learned through a process known as ontogenetic ritualisation. They originate from a non-communicative behaviour intended to accomplish a particular goal; in the course of ritualisation, the behaviour gets abbreviated and comes to be used as a means of getting another individual to do so something. For example, an infant chimpanzee might pull the mother's arm to reach her nipple, and the mother will typically respond by allowing him to suck. After the behaviour has been repeated a number of times, the mother anticipates the infant's actions and begins to respond as soon as he has touched her arm. The baby in turn discovers that he doesn't actually need to pull the mother's arm: all he needs to do is touch it. Thus, the gesture becames abbreviated and acquires a meaning: 'Let me suck'.

An important characteristic of ritualised gestures is that they are idiosyncratic: they are used only by the two individuals who participated in the ritualisation process. In fact, neither of the two individuals can be said to know the gesture fully in the way humans know linguistic signs, because each knows only half of it: in our example, the baby knows how to produce it, and the mother how to interpret it, and they never reverse roles. Of course, in this case, it would be inappropriate for the mother to ask to be allowed to suck; but such one-sidedness is characteristic of gestures learned by ritualisation (Tomasello 2003).

Another form of social learning which is typical for chimpanzees is emulation. In emulation, an animal observes another animal produce an effect, and later learns to reproduce the effect. Emulation is thus similar to imitation, in that both involve learning from a model. The crucial difference is that in imitation, the learner learns that a particular effect can be achieved by using a particular method; in emulation, the learner learns that a particular effect can be achieved, but not the method – the latter is learned later, typically by trial and error. A good example of emulation is the acquisition of the nut-cracking technique by chimpanzees living in the Tai forest, which involves placing a nut on a hard stone and hitting it with another stone. The behaviour is peculiar to the group living in Tai and is learned (other populations of chimps do not crack nuts in this manner). Nuts are an important source of food for Tai chimps, and hence juveniles have plenty of opportunity to observe adults cracking nuts. In spite of this, they require years of practice before they master the technique: young chimps spend a great deal of time hitting hammers against anvils without putting a nut in between, striking nuts with a hammer without first placing them on an anvil, or striking nuts on an anvil with the hand rather than a hammer (Boesch 1993; Boesch and Boesch-Acherman 2000). Thus, each learner basically rediscovers the invention for himself. Such learning is slower, and not faithful enough to achieve cumulative cultural evolution.

Learning by ritualisation and emulation also occurs in humans, but the most characteristic form of social learning in our species is imitation. In imitation, both the method and the result it produces are learned by observation. Curiously, non-human primates are either unable to learn in this way, or their abilities to do so are severely limited. Tomasello and colleagues demonstrate this by means of a simple experiment (see Tomasello 1999: 32). They removed one chimpanzee from the group and taught her to produce a particular gesture, for which she was rewarded with food. They then returned the animal to the group, where other individuals could observe her perform the gesture and get her reward; but although they clearly wanted the food, none imitated the gesture. Other researchers (e.g. Whiten et al. 1996; Celli et al. 2001) have argued that some non-human primates, notably chimpanzees, are capable of some learning by imitation. Crucially, however, none of the studies that attribute imitative abilities to chimpanzees involved imitation of communicative signs.

Tomasello (1999) concludes that there are two critical differences between social learning in humans and other primates. First, humans appear to be much more tuned to the details of the model's behaviour, and aim to reproduce them faithfully (even irrelevant details which are not necessary for the successful execution of the action: Nagell et al. 1993). Secondly, while other primates seem to focus on the environmental effects of the actions they observe, human learners focus on the model's *goals*. This is because we perceive other humans as intentional agents, and naturally attribute intentions to them: on seeing someone struggling with a lid on a box, a human observer cannot help but perceive that person as a *trying to open the box*. Human infants as young as 18 months imitate actions that the model tried to perform but failed (in other words, they can work out what the model's goals were even if they had not seen the action succeed: Meltzoff 1995), but they tend not to imitate unintentional actions (Carpener et al. 1998). This, Tomasello argues, is because humans have a theory of mind: we know that other humans are intentional agents like ourselves, and we can put ourselves 'in their shoes'. Because of this, we perceive other people as having intentions (including communicative intentions) and are very good at working out what those intentions might be.

These two characteristics of human cultural learning are highly relevant to the development of language, both in the individual and in the wider historical sense. The propensity for *faithful* imitation ensures that all individuals in a community acquire (more or less) the same signs. Our mind-reading skills, on the other hand, ensure that we attach roughly the same meanings to these signs.[3] Both of these abilities are a necessary prerequisite for language.

2.3 Cortical control over vocalisations and coordinating action sequences

The vocalisations of chimpanzees and other non-human primates are innate responses triggered by a particular emotional state, rather like laughter or sobbing in humans. They are controlled by the viscero-motor system, an automatic response system connected with arousal states. Human speech, in contrast, is under voluntary control: we can decide what to say in a particular situation – or whether to say anything at all (although the latter ability may be severely impaired in some individuals). This means that in the course of hominid evolution, control over the oral musculature has shifted to the cortex.[4]

Cortical control, apart from enabling us to say what we want when we want, had two further consequences. First, it gave us the ability to learn new vocalisations, thus vastly increasing our vocal repertoire and, concomitantly, the number of distinct messages that could be conveyed. Secondly, it made it possible to harness other cortical systems – notably those for coordinating complex motor routines – for use in communication, thus enabling our ancestors to combine simple vocalisations to form more complex ones and establishing the foundations for syntax.

This suggests that syntax (or at least some aspects of syntax) might be a specialisation of the more general ability to coordinate complex motor routines and combine units hierarchically (cf. Lieberman 1991, 1998, 2002). Several lines of evidence seem to support this conclusion. First, imaging studies show that the same regions of the brain – notably, Broca's area – play a vital role in syntax, speech motor control, and programming sequences of manual movements (Fox et al. 1988; Kimura 1993). This is corroborated by research on deficits resulting from brain injury. As noted in Chapter 4, Broca's aphasia is frequently (though not always) accompanied by constructional apraxia, which suggests that the regions responsible for coordinating language use and purposive manual movements partly overlap.[5] Moreover, Grossman (1980) noted that even in the absence of apraxia, Broca's aphasics have a selective deficit in reconstructing the hierarchical organisation of an abstract diagram from memory. Motor deficits are also very common in children suffering from SLI (Bishop 2002; Hill 2001). Conversely, syntactic deficits have been observed in patients suffering from motor diseases such as Parkinson's (Lieberman et al. 1990, 1992). While such associations are not perfect (not all syntactic deficits are accompanied by a motor deficit, and not all people with impaired motor control also have language problems), their coincidence is high enough to suggest a common underlying problem.

Additional evidence for a possible link between motor planning and language comes from comparative studies of humans and other primates. All primates are able to learn sequences of actions or stimuli, which suggests that it is an ability that we inherited from our common ancestors. However, a more detailed analysis of the performance of humans and modern-day non-human primates reveals that there are some subtle differences in how they approach the task: specifically, humans plan the whole complex sequence before executing it, whereas non-human primates appear to program each stage independently (although chimpanzees show some ability to plan ahead; see Conway and Christiansen 2001 for a discussion).

The ability to program and execute a whole sequence of actions as one unit may have developed in humans as an adaptation to throwing (Calvin 1983, 1993). Accurate throwing is useful for chasing away predators and for hunting. However, it is quite a demanding task, in that it requires the coordination of the action of many muscles and very precise timing. Furthermore, because it is a very brief action, there isn't enough time for the brain to respond to feedback from the moving arm; therefore, unlike slower actions such as climbing a tree to reach a piece of fruit, the whole motor sequence for throwing must be planned before the launching phase is initiated. As Calvin put it:

> your arm is an unguided missile shortly after the throw has begun. You must plan perfectly as you 'get set' to throw, create a chain of muscle commands, all ready to be executed in exactly the right order . . . You need something like a serial buffer memory in which to load up all the muscle commands in the right order and with the right timing relative to one another. (1993: 234)

Calvin also notes that because neurons are rather inaccurate time-keepers, in order to achieve the precise timing necessary to hit the target at any distance, the planning mechanism must average the output of a very large number of neurons, and hence it is possible that the advantages of accurate throwing might have driven the selection for a bigger brain in our ancestors.

Whatever its evolutionary origins, the ability to package a series of actions as a single unit allows more elaborate planning, since the complex unit itself can be incorporated into a larger action plan. It could also be 'exapted' for linguistic use: a sequence of words functioning as a single unit – that is to say, a phrase – can be incorporated into a larger unit, thus giving rise to hierarchical syntax. It is interesting to note, then, that while the giant apes are able to learn hierarchically structured action sequences, their ability to do so is quite limited – similar to that of a 2-year-old human child (Conway and Christiansen 2001).[6] This appears to parallel the upper limit of their linguistic abilities. Attempts to teach language-like systems to captive apes have shown that they can learn simple ordering rules, but they do not seem to be able to combine phrases hierarchically.

3. Language adaptations to humans

While it is undeniable that in the course of human evolution our brains and vocal apparatus adapted to the exigencies of linguistic communication, we should not lose sight of the fact that languages, too, are products of evolution. The emergence of language is a process in which individual speakers make innovations which either do or do not spread through the community. Whether or not a particular variant will spread depends at least in part on its 'communicative fitness'. Other things being equal, speakers naturally prefer structures which are easier to produce; and through failure to communicate, they learn to avoid structures which are difficult to understand.[7] This means that when there is more than one structure expressing a particular function, the structure which is more difficult to process will be used less frequently. The next generation of speakers will have the same processing biases, but also fewer opportunities to learn the more difficult structure. This will result in a further drop in frequency of the more difficult variant, until it eventually disappears.

In other words, the story of the emergence of language is one of co-evolution: humans adapted to language, but language (or rather languages) also adapted to humans. Indeed, there are reasons to think that languages did most of the evolving. As Deacon (1997) points out, languages need humans more than humans need languages (if it came to the crunch, we could probably survive without them; but they need our brains to survive and reproduce) – so the selectional pressures on languages were stronger. Furthermore, cultural change is several orders of magnitude faster than biological change. Any substantial restructuring of the brain requires hundreds of thousands or even millions of years. Grammars, on the other hand, can change radically in a few centuries, and lexical innovations spread in a matter of years – and, in this era of mass media, sometimes in a matter of months or even weeks.

One particularly good example of language adjusting to humans is the phenomenon of categorical perception of speech sounds. When presented with a range of stimuli which differ along some continuous parameter, such as voice-onset time (VOT), people tend to perceive sounds up to a certain point on the continuum as belonging to one category and sounds that fall beyond that point as belonging to another category. For example, stops with a VOT of less than 35 ms are perceived as voiced, while those with a greater VOT are perceived as voiceless. Thus, an artificially produced sound that is intermediate between a prototypical /t/ and a prototypical /d/ is not perceived as something 'in between' the two phonemes, but as either one or the other, depending on whether the VOT is less than or more than 35 ms. We know that at least some such perceptual biases are innate because they are present in very young infants, even when the contrast is not phonemic in the ambient language.

Our tendency to perceive speech sounds categorically is useful from a communicative point of view, since it allows efficient coding of phonemic distinctions, and used to be regarded as a prime example of an innate special-isation for language – or, to be more precise, for speech. However, categorical perception is not 'for' language, or speech. Some non-speech sounds are also perceived categorically (Premack 1980). More importantly, categorical percep-tion of human speech sounds is found in a number of other species, including chinchillas and Japanese quail (Kluender et al. 1987; Kuhl 1981; Miller and Jusczyk 1989; Springer 1979). In other words, the existence of categorical per-ception of speech sounds in humans is not evidence that our species adapted to the exigencies of vocal communication, but rather that language adapted to our pre-existing auditory biases.[8]

Thinking in terms of languages adapting to humans has profound implica-tions for the way we think of language universals: it suggests that it might be more revealing to view them not as a set of constraints defining a possible human language encoded in the genome, but rather as the result of convergent evolution. Deacon (1997) develops this idea at length, concluding that:

> universal rules and implicit axioms of grammar aren't really stored or located anywhere, and in an important sense, they are not *determined* at all. Instead, I want to suggest the radical possibility that they have emerged spontaneously and independently in each evolving language, in response to universal biases in the selection processes affecting language transmission. They are *convergent* features of language evolution in the same way that the dorsal fins of sharks, ichthyosaurs, and dolphins are independent convergent adaptations of aquatic species. Like their bio-logical counterparts, these structural commonalities present in all lan-guages have each arisen in response to constraints imposed by a common adaptive context. Some of the sources of universal selection on the evo-lution of language structures include immature learning biases, the con-straints of human vocal articulation and hearing, and the requirements of symbolic reference ... Because of these incessant influences, languages independently come to resemble one another, not in detail, but in terms of certain general structural properties, and any disruption that under-mines a language's fit with its host will be selected against, leading to reconvergence on universal patterns. (Deacon 1997: 116)

There is considerable evidence for such external forces acting on and shaping grammars. Functional linguists have long argued that many cross-linguistic patterns arise as a result of discourse pressures (Du Bois 1987; Foley and Van Valin 1984) and a general preference for iconic structures (Givón 1989; Haiman 1985). Even more direct are pressures on the processing system, which appear to be responsible for constraints on long-distance dependency constructions (Kluender 1998; Kluender and Kutas 1993) and many word order universals (Hawkins 1994; Kirby 1998). One should also note in this connection that *absolute universals* – properties which are shared by all languages – are hard to find, and they tend to be rather uninteresting: they are statements like 'all languages have vowels and consonants', 'all languages have nouns (words prototypically referring to things) and relational words', 'all languages have recursion'. The more 'meaty' universals are either statistical (most languages have property X) or implicational (if a language has property X, then it also has property Y). This seems more compatible with the view that universals are a result of languages converging on certain solutions than with the view that universals are innate constraints defining a possible human language.

4. Universal Grammar again

4.1 Problems with the poverty-of-the-stimulus argument

When discussing human adaptations to language earlier in this chapter, I refrained from mentioning any innate syntactic knowledge, or even any specifically syntactic specialisations. This is not to suggest that such adaptations did not take place, but simply that we do not know enough about the evolutionary origin or the genetic basis of syntax to constrain linguistic theory in any meaningful way. The argument for an innate Universal Grammar is essentially a linguistic one. However, because it has played such an important role in contemporary linguistic theory, it is fitting to conclude this chapter with some observations about its validity and explanatory power.

The existence of Universal Grammar is inferred from two premises:

1. Human languages have certain (universal) properties (e.g. restrictions on movement such as the Subjacency Condition).
2. These properties cannot be learned because the relevant information is not available in the input.

Therefore, some linguists have argued, knowledge of these properties must be innate. This, in essence, is the 'poverty-of-the-stimulus' argument, the most powerful and direct argument for the existence of innate syntactic knowledge (Chomsky 1986; Crain 1991; Lightfoot 1989). Other sources of evidence which have been marshalled in favour of the innateness hypothesis (e.g. the speed and alleged uniformity of language acquisition, dissociations between language and other cognitive abilities, the fact that some language impairments are inherited) play only a subsidiary role: while they do suggest the existence of biological adaptations to language, they tell us very little about the nature of these adaptations – specifically, they do not necessarily imply the existence of innate linguistic principles (as opposed to, for example, innate learning biases or an enhanced ability to process hierarchically organised structures).

To appreciate the validity of the poverty-of-the-stimulus argument, it is important to note that it relies on certain assumptions about the properties of the adult system, the kind of information that is available to learners, and the abilities that they bring to the learning task. It is to these that we now turn.

4.1.1 Properties of the adult system

The argument from the poverty of the stimulus is predicated upon the claim that all speakers have the abstract linguistic knowledge embodied in the principles of Universal Grammar. However, this supposed universality of abstract linguistic knowledge is an assumption, not an empirically established result. It is true that virtually all neurologically unimpaired adults are proficient language users. This, however, does not entail that they are all equally proficient, or that they all rely on the same abstract rules; and there is accumulating evidence that individuals with little formal schooling have considerable difficulty processing complex syntactic structures (Chipere 2003; Dąbrowska 1997; see also the evidence for shallow processing in Chapter 2).

Another important point to bear in mind is that many of the principles which are supposed to constitute our innate language endowment are theory internal. As Tomasello put it:

> Many of the Generative Grammar structures that are found in English can be found in other languages – if it is generative grammarians who are doing the looking. But these structures may not be found by linguists of other theoretical persuasions because the structures are defined differently, or not recognized at all, in other linguistic theories. (Tomasello 1995: 138)

The fact that restrictions on movement cannot be learned (if indeed this is a fact) does not entail that they must therefore be innate: it could also mean that we need a better linguistic theory – one which does not require movement. Of course, linguistic theory still needs to account for the dependency phenomena that movement rules were postulated to explain; the point here is that the alleged unlearnability of a particular grammatical rule or principle cannot be taken as evidence for the innateness of Universal Grammar unless we have independent evidence for the psychological reality of that rule or principle.

4.1.2 Information available in input

The second premise of the argument from the poverty of the stimulus is that certain crucial kinds of information are not available to the learner. The problem is that this is often asserted rather than actually demonstrated. Consider Chomsky's favourite illustration, the fact that children seem to acquire a relatively complex structure-dependent rule of auxiliary fronting ('move the first auxiliary after the subject to the beginning of the sentence') rather than a simpler structure-independent rule ('move the first auxiliary to the beginning of the sentence'): thus, when forming interrogatives corresponding to example (1), English speakers produce (3) rather than (2), which is what the structure-independent rule would produce.

(1)   *Everything that has been damaged will be paid for.*
(2)   **Has everything that been damaged will be paid for?*
(3)   *Will everything that has been damaged be paid for?*

This, Chomsky asserts, occurs in spite of the fact that utterances that would enable them to distinguish between the two hypotheses are so rare that 'a person might go through much or all of his life without ever having been exposed to the relevant evidence' (Chomsky 1980a: 40). However, the assertion is not supported by any data on how frequent or infrequent the relevant utterances actually are, either here or in the many other subsequent rehashings of the argument. Other linguists have taken the trouble to look at the corpus data, and found that relevant examples constitute about 1 per cent of all interrogative utterances in a wide range of corpora (Pullum and Scholz 2002). Now 1 per cent may not seem like a lot – but since children are exposed to vast amounts of input (cf. Chapters 2 and 3), it is 1 per cent of a very large number: Pullum and Scholz estimate that by age 3, a typical child will have heard between 7,500 and 22,500 relevant instances.[9]

The tendency to assert that some aspect of linguistic knowledge could not possibly be learned from the input, without providing any supporting evidence, is endemic in the nativist literature (see Pullum and Scholz 2002 for further examples). This seriously undermines the poverty-of-the-stimulus argument, since there is accumulating evidence that the information available in the input is richer than previously thought (Redington and Chater 1998). For example, lexical co-occurrence patterns can be used to classify words into grammatical categories, and prosodic phrasing provides clues about constituency. Also, in spite of frequent claims to the contrary, it appears that children receive plenty of negative evidence, that is to say, evidence that an utterance they have just produced is ill-formed by adult standards (see Chouinard and Clark 2003 for an up-to-date discussion). It is true that some kinds of knowledge (e.g. properties of the various kinds of empty categories) cannot be acquired from the input available to children. But again, this does not necessarily mean that the child must have innate knowledge of these: an alternative conclusion would be that we need to look for ways of accounting for the same phenomena which do not postulate such invisible and inaudible constructs.

4.1.3 The child's language learning abilities
However rich innate linguistic knowledge may be, there are many idiosyncratic properties of individual languages which it cannot specify: the actual words in the language and their meanings, the grammatical markers and their

functions, subcategorisation requirements of particular verbs, various 'quirky' constructions which violate the usual grammatical patterns, morphological classes, and so on. All of these must be acquired using some mechanism other than setting the parameters of Universal Grammar.

Many of these language-specific aspects of linguistic knowledge are abstract and quite complex – in fact, they appear to be every bit as complex as the 'core' properties which are deemed to be specified in Universal Grammar (Culicover 1999; Dąbrowska 2000; see also next chapter for a discussion of the complexities of lexical meaning and Chapter 8 on knowledge about the distribution of inflectional endings). It follows, therefore, that the learning mechanisms necessary to acquire language-specific knowledge must be quite powerful – possibly powerful enough to learn at least some aspects of 'core' grammar.

4.2 Some new questions

Arguments for an innate Universal Grammar often take the form of a challenge to anti-nativist researchers to explain some particularly esoteric aspect of grammatical knowledge. For example, Bickerton (1996) proposes that students of human behaviour who believe in the creation or invention of language should be required to take an examination in which they would have to answer questions such as the following:

> Question 1: Explain how, and why, the inventors of language arranged things so that *John wants someone to work for* means 'John wants someone such that he, John, can work for that person' while *John wants someone to work for him* means 'John wants someone such that that person will work for him, John'. State how you yourself learned the reversal of meaning in the subordinate clause and show how its invention was culturally and/or biologically adaptive. (Bickerton 1996: 34)

Bickerton's formulation is a caricature of the 'invention' view. Those who maintain that language was 'invented' do not claim that it was designed at the drawing board, but that it emerged gradually, over a number of generations, as a consequence of being used to solve specific communicative problems. However, Bickerton does make a valid point: namely, that existing empiricist/constructivist theories of language acquisition have not dealt with many issues which are central to the generative enterprise, such as how people use grammatical cues to recover pronoun reference and missing arguments. The problem is that the generativists also fail to provide a satisfactory explanation of how the relevant knowledge is acquired. This is easiest to see if we turn the tables on Bickerton and ask him to take the nativist version of the same exam. The first question would be the following:

Question 1: Explain how evolution arranged things so that *John wants someone to work for* means 'John wants someone such that he, John, can work for that person' while *John wants someone to work for him* means 'John wants someone such that that person will work for him, John'. State how, and where, the reversal of meaning in the subordinate clause is encoded in the human genome and how and by what physical and/or chemical processes it comes to be represented in the human brain.

Posing the question in this way is just as unfair to the nativists as Bickerton's original question was to the opposite camp. No sane nativist believes that the difference in meaning exemplified in Bickerton's sentences is directly encoded in our genes. But this raises the question of what actually *is* encoded: does the human genome contain statements to the effect that a trace must be properly governed? Does it contain instructions for finding traces? What form do these take? The point, of course, is that proclaiming that some aspect of our linguistic knowledge is innate does not answer the question of how we come to have it – it merely raises three new ones:

1. How did our species come to have this innate knowledge?
2. How is the knowledge encoded in our genes, and how does the genetic information translate into linguistic representations in the brain?
3. How do learners access innate knowledge when constructing a grammar of the language they hear?

As we will see shortly, all of these questions have yet to receive a satisfactory answer.

4.2.1 Evolution
For someone who attaches so much importance to innate linguistic knowledge, Chomsky is remarkably reticent about how the capacity for language evolved. In 1980, he side-steps the issue by stating that:

These skills [i.e., the ability to acquire language] may well have arisen as a concomitant of structural properties of the brain that developed for other reasons. Suppose that there was selection for bigger brains, more cortical surface, hemispheric specialisation for analytic processing, or many other structural properties that can be imagined. The brain that evolved might well have all sorts of special properties that are not individually selected; there would be no miracle in this, but only the normal workings of evolution. We have no idea, at present, how physical laws apply when 10^{10} neurons are placed in an object the size of a basketball, under the special conditions that arose during human evolution. (Chomsky 1980b: 321)

More recently, he has expressed a similar opinion:

> Perhaps these [properties of language] are simply emergent physical properties of a brain that reaches a certain level of complexity under the specific conditions of human evolution. (Chomsky 1991: 50)

Other researchers (e.g. Calvin and Bickerton 2000; Jackendoff 2002; Pinker and Bloom 1990) have been considerably more explicit. However, although the scenarios they have proposed are not unreasonable, they are still very sketchy, mutually incompatible, and, worst of all, unverifiable. This is unavoidable: since languages do not fossilise, accounts of language evolution are necessarily little more than scientific just-so stories.

4.2.2 Genetics and neurogenesis

We also know very little about which genes are relevant to the development of language, let alone about how they actually do their job, although in this case we are almost certain to learn a great deal more in the future. The most promising avenue of research is the genetics of developmental language disorders. We already know from twin studies that such disorders do indeed involve a significant genetic component, since concordance rates for linguistic problems are considerably higher for identical twins (who share all their genes) than for fraternal twins (who share only 50 per cent of their genes) – that is to say, given one twin with a language impairment, the likelihood that the other twin will also be impaired is much higher if they are identical than if they are fraternal (Bishop et al. 1995; Stromswold 2001; Tomblin and Buckwalter 1998).

However, there is little research linking specific linguistic deficits to specific genes or groups of genes. The first – and, at the time of writing, only – unambiguous link of this kind was established by Lai et al. (2001), who showed that the severe speech and language difficulties found in many members of the so-called KE family were associated with a mutation in one particular gene, FOXP2.[10] This discovery is sometimes regarded as providing direct support for the claim that Universal Grammar is encoded in the human genome. There are, however, several reasons to be sceptical about such an interpretation. First, the effects of the genetic anomaly in the KE family are relatively non-specific: the affected members have problems with pronunciation, morphology and syntax as well as with sequencing fine non-linguistic movements of the mouth and face muscles; and their non-verbal IQs are, on average, 18 points lower than those of non-affected members, though still within the normal range (Vargha-Khadem et al. 1995). Secondly, FOXP2 is also found in other mammals, and the human version of the gene differs at only three amino-acid positions from the corresponding mouse gene, and at only two positions from the analogous gene in chimpanzees, gorillas and rhesus macaques (Enard et al. 2002). Thirdly, the gene appears to be involved in the development of the lungs, heart and gut as well as several regions of the brain (Marcus and Fisher 2003).

Thus, while something about the normal version of human FOXP2 seems to help an individual to develop language, the gene itself does not contain a blueprint for grammar. FOXP2 is a transcription factor, or a gene which regulates the functioning of other genes. It is possible that these other genes are responsible for encoding the principles of Universal Grammar into the developing brain – but if so, they have not been found yet. Another possibility is that FOXP2 exerts its influence in a much more roundabout way, for example by controlling the amount of brain tissue available for sequencing fine facial movements.

4.2.3 *Accessing innate knowledge*

To be able to use innate knowledge about syntactic categories and relations, children must be able to identify instances of these categories in the language they hear. However, they cannot rely on some invariant features of the input to do this, since the relevant categories are highly abstract and do not share any perceptual features.[11] This raises the question of how children link the speech they hear with innate syntactic knowledge – a fundamental problem for nativist theories of acquisition which has received relatively little attention in the literature, and, as yet, no satisfactory solution.

The most serious attempt to deal with the linking problem is Pinker's semantic bootstrapping hypothesis (Pinker 1984, 1987). Pinker proposed that, in addition to innate syntactic categories such as 'noun', 'subject' and 'sister of X', children are also equipped with innate semantic categories such as 'thing', 'agent' and 'argument of X', as well as innate linking rules connecting the two ('words for things are nouns', 'agents are normally subjects' and so on). Linking rules make it possible for children to identify examples of the relevant syntactic categories and relations. Once they have done this, children can induce their language-specific distributional characteristics, which in turn enables them to identify other category members, such as abstract nouns, passive subjects and so on.

There are several problems with Pinker's proposal. First, it requires further innate knowledge in addition to Universal Grammar. Secondly, because it exploits correlations between semantic and syntactic categories, it requires such correlations to be universal – but, as Pinker himself acknowledges, they are not (for example, agents do not match up with prototypical subjects in ergative languages, so in these languages innate linking rules would not only not help, but actually be a hindrance). Thirdly, as Tomasello (2000) points out, the theory's empirical predictions are incorrect: children's earliest subjects include some agents, but also many other semantic roles.

5. Conclusion

There is a growing consensus that language – an evolutionary late-comer – piggybacks on structures which originally evolved for other purposes (Hauser et al. 2002; Lieberman 1991, 1998; Tomasello 1999; Worden 1998), such as producing and recognising sounds, planning motor sequences, categorisation, storage and retrieval of information, predicting the actions of other individuals, and cultural learning. Many researchers maintain that we also have some language-specific adaptations, although there is considerable disagreement about what these are and how they may have evolved. However, it should be clear that, for reasons discussed earlier, a good theory of language will keep such stipulations to a bare minimum. Furthermore, they should be treated as tentative hypotheses to be confirmed or rejected by biological research rather than as central tenets of the theory.

Notes

1. Humans do have some innate representations. For example, human infants preferentially look at face-like stimuli, suggesting that they have an innate representation of a human face. The latter is, however, highly schematic (something like an oval with three blobs corresponding to the eyes and the mouth), and appears to be encoded in subcortical structures, not the cortical structures that are involved in face processing in adults (Johnson 1998). Its function, it seems, is to ensure that infants pay attention to human faces, which guarantees that the cortical system responsible for face recognition in mature individuals has plenty of opportunity to learn about them.
2. Similar conclusions can be drawn from research on the formation and subsequent development of creole languages (see e.g. Mühlhäusler 1986).
3. The ubiquity of imitation does not, of course, rule out the possibility of innovation. If the linguistic system is to develop, at least some members of the community must occasionally produce novel signs or novel sign combinations. Note, however, that for the innovation to become part of the shared system, it must be imitated by others.
4. The shift is not complete, so oral muscles in humans are actually under dual control. The viscero-motor system continues to control the more 'primitive' vocalisations such as laughter or crying; it is for this reason that laughter and crying are difficult to suppress in certain emotional states and even more difficult to fake convincingly.
5. It is also possible that the two regions are simply located next to each other, and consequently both are often damaged as a result of the same injury. However, there is evidence that the same regions are involved in both functions. Electrical stimulation studies conducted by Ojemann and his team, for example, found that there was 86 per cent overlap in the sites where the sequencing of oral-facial movements and phoneme perception was disrupted (Calvin and Ojemann 1994).
6. They are also not very good at throwing, which supports Calvin's scenario.

7. Humans are very good at monitoring the interlocutor's understanding and adjusting their speech accordingly. For example, adults, and even children as young as 4 or 5, produce simplified, redundant speech when conversing with children under 3 (Snow 1986).

8. Some phonemic distinctions, for example the contrast between voiced and prevoiced sounds found in Thai, are acquired. However, languages across the world 'prefer' those distinctions to which we are innately sensitive, so the voiced/voiceless contrast is used phonemically much more frequently than the voiced/prevoiced contrast.

9. Note, too, that the whole argument rests on the assumption that interrogatives are formed by moving the auxiliary from the position it occupies in declaratives. Learners would also avoid making the error in (2) if they learned a question-formation rule which did not involve movement, for example a simple template like AUX + Subject NP + nonfinite VP. As shown in Chapter 9, there is considerable evidence that children do in fact acquire such templates.

10. Recent genome-wide scans found four more regions on four different chromosomes that appear to be involved in another kind of language disorder (Fisher et al. 2003). However, the specific genes responsible for the disorder have not yet been identified.

11. Note that the evolution of Universal Grammar raises an analogous problem. All known examples of innate and domain-specific knowledge have some physical invariant (a motor program or a perceptual representation) which gives evolution something concrete to work on. However, because the form–meaning mapping in human languages is arbitrary, it differs from language to language, and it is not clear what could be selected for in the course of evolution.

Part II

The Building Blocks of Language

7 Words

The standard argument for the innateness of syntax goes something like this: children acquire the grammar of their native language remarkably quickly, on minimal exposure, and with no overt teaching. Moreover, they go through the same developmental stages and make relatively few errors. Most importantly, some aspects of language (e.g. knowledge about empty categories, constraints on movement) are acquired without any experience. Since no known learning theory could begin to explain how this happens, linguistic knowledge must be innate.

With this argument in mind, consider the following facts about lexical development:

1. In early and middle childhood, children learn about ten new words a day – approximately one in every waking hour (Carey 1978; Miller 1986; Miller and Gildea 1987).
2. Words are often learned after a few presentations in ambiguous conditions, and sometimes after only one presentation (Carey 1978; Dickinson 1984; Heibeck and Markman 1987; Markson and Bloom 1997).
3. Most words are learned without overt teaching, and attempts to teach vocabulary at school sometimes lead to very strange results.[1]
4. Lexical development exhibits some striking regularities. For example, colour terms are acquired at a specific maturational stage; and dimensional adjectives and other spatial terms are acquired in a fairly uniform order.
5. Most words are acquired without effort and almost without errors, in spite of the fact that lexical meanings are often very difficult to pin down. (Many dictionary definitions are grossly inadequate, and even philosophers find it difficult to explicate our tacit knowledge of everyday concepts.)
6. Children can acquire words from domains of which they have no experience. For example, blind children have been shown to acquire visual terms without much difficulty (Landau and Gleitman 1985).

Applying the same logic to these facts, the conclusion seems inescapable: lexical knowledge, or at least a significant part of it, must be innate. In fact, this is precisely the conclusion drawn by Chomsky:

Barring miracles, this means that the concepts must be essentially available prior to experience, in something like their full intricacy. Children
must be basically acquiring labels for concepts they already have.
(Chomsky 1991: 29)

Piattelli-Palmarini (1989) has expressed similar views:

The process of 'learning' just picks them [i.e. innate lexical meanings] out
en bloc, once the phonetic *label* is assigned to the concept. Association
now becomes a very minor component of the mechanism: What is being
associated is just the sound *for that* concept and the innately available
concept itself . . . Association is marginal to the process: it boils down
to a heavily constrained pairing of certain labels to certain innate concepts. (Piattelli-Palmarini 1989: 31)

The problem with this conclusion, impeccable as the logic may be, is that it is
patently absurd, since it commits us to the belief that humans are born with
innate concepts such as *innings, poppadom, widget, aerobics, Internet, baptise*
and *overdraft*. While such a position is logically consistent, I suspect that
anyone who has ever tried to explain what an innings is to a person with no
experience of baseball or cricket, or what an overdraft is to someone from a
culture that does not use banks, will be rather sceptical.

Furthermore, as Gleitman (1990) convincingly demonstrates, matching the
concept and the phonological label is not as trivial a task as Piattelli-Palmarini
makes it out to be. Determining which aspect of the world a particular part of
a parental utterance refers to is difficult enough even when it refers to something in the child's immediate environment; but most parental speech is not a
running commentary on situations observed by the child. Utterances such as
Eat your peas, Let's go to the park or *It rained last night* do not co-occur with
episodes of pea-eating, going to the park, and rainy weather; and episodes of
thinking, knowing, understanding, hoping, wondering, guessing and suppos-
ing all look quite similar. More damaging still, asserting that lexical concepts
are innate hasn't quite eliminated the miraculous: it has merely shifted it to
another domain. We still need to explain how the species acquired these innate
abilities (cf. Chapter 6, section 4.2). A moment's reflection will reveal that they
could not have come into being through any known evolutionary process –
unless thousands of years ago evolution 'knew' that someday we were going
to invent baseball, banks and fitness clubs. Hilary Putnam makes a similar
point:

To have given us an innate stock of notions which includes *carburettor,
bureaucrat, quantum potential*, etc., as required by Fodor's version of
the Innateness Hypothesis, evolution would have had to be able to anticipate all contingencies of future physical and cultural environments.

Obviously it didn't and couldn't do this. (Putnam 1988, quoted in Chomsky 1991: 32)

Chomsky finds this argument unconvincing: evolution didn't need to anticipate all contingencies, only those required for concept formation in the real world; and we shouldn't worry if the idea seems absurd since many claims which originally seemed highly implausible have been shown to be true. Besides, it is misleading to compare ordinary language acquisition with the acquisition of scientific concepts. The mind has other capacities for the formation of concepts – used, for example, during the construction of scientific theories – so 'concepts that do not fall within the range of [the language faculty] might be constructible by the mechanisms of [general cognition]' (Chomsky 1991: 33).

So at least some concepts (for example, scientific concepts such as *quantum potential*) are not innate and the mind has non-linguistic mechanisms capable of constructing them. The obvious question to ask at this juncture is which category *peek-a-boo, weekend* and *table* belong to? If Chomsky wishes to claim that they are innate, then he needs to explain how they could possibly have been written into the human genome – and divine creation seems to be the only possible explanation. If they are not, then why should other lexical concepts be unlearnable? There is no evidence whatsoever that such culturally specific notions are any more difficult to acquire than universal or near-universal concepts as *person, three* or *hot.*

Chomsky's views on the innateness of lexical concepts are admittedly extreme; most psycholinguists would maintain that lexical concepts themselves are not innate, but their acquisition is tightly constrained by various cognitive mechanisms which are. I have no quarrel with the claim that lexical development is constrained by innate factors. What remains unclear, however, is how tightly constrained it is: that is to say, how much detective work the child needs to do to establish the meanings of the words she hears around her.

1. The semantics of locative terms

To address this question, we will examine the meanings of words belonging to a particular domain – namely, locative terms – and then briefly review what we know about their acquisition. Locative terms, or words like *in* and *behind*, which specify the location of one object (the **trajector**) with respect to another object (the **landmark**), provide a particularly interesting test case for research concerning the role of innate factors in lexical development. If any lexical concepts are innate, or strongly constrained by innate factors, locative concepts should be among them. They relate to universal aspects of human experience, and they have obvious survival value for the species, so it is not difficult to envisage why evolution might have favoured encoding them in the genome.

Moreover, they would also have been useful to our prehuman ancestors, so evolution would have had plenty of time to operate.

Locative expressions are also comparatively easy to study because they have fairly concrete meanings, so there is a large body of research on their meanings and their acquisition which can be interpreted in the context of research on infant spatial cognition and infant perceptual processing mechanisms and their neurophysiological bases.

Moreover, it is possible that children's knowledge of spatial terms helps them to learn other aspects of their language. It is well known that spatial terms are often the starting points of grammaticalisation processes which eventually produce tense, aspect and case markers, complementisers, comparatives, morphemes expressing causal relations, and other grammatical functors (see Casad 1996a; Comrie 1976; Dąbrowska 1996; Heine 1997; Rudzka-Ostyn 1985; Traugott 1978). This suggests a conceptual affinity between spatial terms and various grammatical notions, and in fact some linguists have argued that grammatical notions should be interpreted in localistic terms even when there is no historical evidence that they derive from spatial concepts (Anderson 1971, 1994; Hjelmslev 1935; Jackendoff 1983; Miller 1972, 1974). If such conceptual affinities do exist, children could use their knowledge of spatial concepts to get a handle on the more abstract notions encoded by various grammatical functors.

The conventional wisdom on the acquisition of locative terms is that it involves 'learning how to apply them to . . . prior knowledge about space' (Clark 1973: 62; see also Johnston and Slobin 1979; Levine and Carey 1982; Slobin 1973) – that is to say, to prelinguistic concepts of containment, support, occlusion etc. (In this context, 'prelinguistic' doesn't necessarily mean 'innate': the concepts could emerge out of prelinguistic sensorimotor experience.) There is good supporting evidence for this view:

1. Locative expressions are acquired very early. The first terms usually appear at 16–17 months, and they have been reported as early as 12–14 months (Choi and Bowerman 1991: 100); by the time the child goes to school, the system is firmly in place.
2. Children acquiring different languages acquire equivalent words in roughly the same order. The order of acquisition is determined by non-linguistic knowledge, though acquisition may be delayed if the linguistic form is difficult (Johnston and Slobin 1979).
3. Errors in the use of basic spatial terms are extremely rare in spontaneous speech (Choi and Bowerman 1991; Sinha et al. 1994; Tomasello 1987).
4. Children generalise newly acquired concepts to new contexts very quickly, often within days of the first use (Choi and Bowerman 1991; Tomasello 1987).

In spite of this, I will argue that learning locative terms does *not* consist simply in matching linguistic labels to pre-existing concepts. The main reason for this is that although we may well have pre-linguistic concepts of containment, support etc., these do not correspond in any direct way to linguistic expressions such as the English *in*, *on* etc. The relevant evidence will be discussed under three headings: conventional construal, polysemy, and cross-linguistic variation.

1.1 Conventional construal

Objects in the real world come in all shapes and sizes and can participate in an indefinite number of spatial relationships. On the other hand, the linguistic resources available to code these relationships are generally quite limited: in English, about two dozen basic spatial expressions. This means that the same locative term must be used to refer to a variety of relationships between very different objects, and the fit of words to the world is often rather less than straightforward.

Take the English preposition *in*. One can define *in* as 'within an inside region'; but what counts as an 'inside region' is anything but obvious. For example, if the landmark, or reference object, does not define an enclosed space, the conceptualiser must project virtual boundaries. With a landmark such as a bowl, the inside is partly defined by the wall and the bottom, but to get an enclosed space you need to add a 'virtual lid', which would normally be the plane containing the top edge of the bowl. This might seem to be a trivial point, but consider the configurations depicted in Figure 7.1.

In (a), the banana is said to be *in* the bowl even though it is not actually located in the region defined by the walls of the container and the projected 'lid'; in (b) it is located within this region, but you can only say it is *under*, not *in*, the bowl. Moreover, in some cases there is more than one way to define the

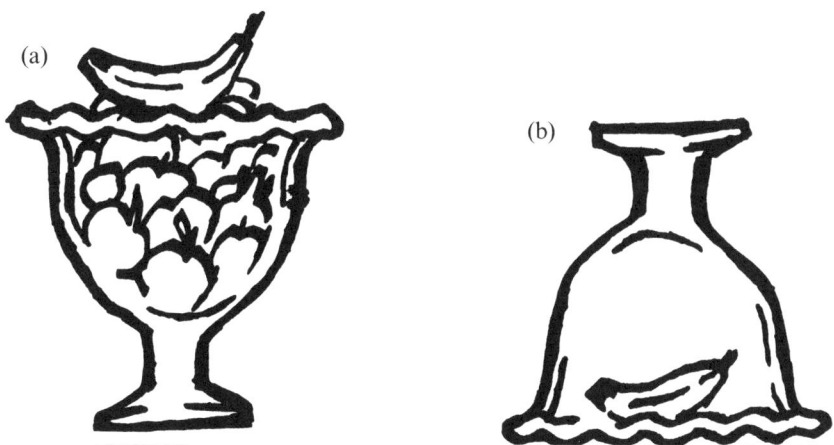

Figure 7.1 Is the banana 'in the bowl'? (adapted from Herskovits 1985: 19)

inside region: compare *There is a banana in the bowl* and *There is a crack in the bowl*. Or consider the expression *The bird is in the tree*: in this case, all the boundaries of the 'container' are virtual. (All three examples are taken from Herskovits 1985, 1986.)

Making words fit the world also involves a fair amount of idealisation, as objects need to be assimilated to the abstract geometric descriptions embodied in the semantics of locative expressions. Thus a frying pan might be idealised as a container (cf. the expression *in the frying pan*); a river as a line (*along the river*) and a table as a horizontal surface (*on/under the table*) (Dąbrowska 1993; Herskovits 1985; Talmy 1983).

The crucial point here is that all of these are conventional, and hence *linguistic*, phenomena. This can be easily demonstrated by showing that different languages require different construals. In English, a bird is *in* the tree, but many other languages require different terms (usually the equivalent of *on*; notice that even in English, an apple would be *on*, not *in*, the tree, in spite of the fact that the relationship between the apple and the outer boundary of the tree is exactly the same as that between the bird and the outer boundary of the tree). In English, the 'inside' of a bowl can be either the region defined by the wall, the bottom and the 'virtual lid' (of whatever shape) or the bowl itself, but many languages allow only the former conceptualisation. Hence, if you want to say *There is a crack in the bowl*, you either have to use another preposition (e.g. the equivalent of *on*) or a non-spatial paraphrase (something like *The bowl is cracked* or *The bowl has a crack*). Furthermore, different languages require different idealisations of the same objects. English idealises a frying pan as a container, so your fried eggs are *in the pan*; in Polish, they would be *on* the frying pan (*na patelni*). If a ball rolls between the legs of a table and emerges on the other side, an English speaker will say that it rolled *under the table*: English requires that the table be construed as a horizontal surface. In contrast, in Atsugewi, the ball would roll *through* the table because the table is thought of as a three-dimensional object (Talmy 1983). Sometimes even different dialects of the same language require different conventional construals. In Britain, you leave your car *in the street*. In America you leave it *on the street*, but your neighbours' children playing near it would be *in the street*; and if you decided that the driveway would be a safer place to park, your car would *in the driveway*, not *on* it.

As a final illustration, let us consider an extended example from Cora, an Uto-Aztecan language spoken in a mountainous region of Mexico. Cora has an extremely rich system for encoding spatial relationships which includes spatial adverbs, particles, and verbal prefixes which are used in various combinations to convey elaborate descriptions of spatial configurations. Cora locatives have been extensively studied by Eugene Casad (1977, 1982, 1988), and the reader is referred to these works for a comprehensive description. Because the system is so rich, it cannot be described in any detail here; but its very richness and utter foreignness are an excellent illustration of the central theme of this chapter, namely, that humans possess complex abstract systems which are extremely unlikely to come prewired.

The following discussion is based on data from Casad and Langacker (1985), which describes the semantics of just two morphemes, *u* (which can be glossed as 'inside') and *a* ('outside'). Because of space limitations, I cannot justify the analysis proposed by the authors. However, it should be stressed that Casad and Langacker do not ask the reader to take the analysis on faith; as demonstrated throughout the paper, various quirks and idiosyncrasies of Cora locationals make perfect sense given the construal described here.

Although *a* means 'outside', it can also be used to refer to location *inside* a shallow container such as a basin or pan (as opposed to, say, a jar, which requires *u*). In other words, as far as the *u/a* distinction is concerned, shallow containers do not count as containers: any object located near the outside surface of the landmark is considered 'outside' the landmark.

As in the case of the English *in* and *out*, the container with respect to which things are located can be virtual. Consider the complex expressions *mah* 'away up there to the side in the face of the slope' and *muh* 'away up there near the centre line of the face of the slope'. Both of these locationals consists of three morphemes. The first morpheme, *m*, is a deictic prefix which can be glossed as 'at a medial distance from the speaker' (in contrast to other prefixes meaning 'near the speaker' and 'far from the speaker'). The final *h* means 'on the face of the slope' and contrasts with suffixes meaning 'at the foot of the slope' and 'at the top of the slope'. Between the two come *u* and *a*, which mean 'inside' and 'outside' – but 'inside' and 'outside' what? Casad and Langacker argue that the landmark region is defined relative to the line of sight:

> A conceived situation of some complexity is required [to define the boundary]. This situation . . . is sketched in [Figure 7.2]. It involves a vantage point (VP) somewhere in the area at the foot of the slope; when no semantic conflict results, this vantage point is generally equated with the position of the speaker. From this vantage point, a viewer (normally the speaker) is presumed to be looking directly up the face of the slope. The broken arrow in [Figure 7.2] represents the viewer's line of sight in relation to the slope – observe that this line of sight runs from the foot of the slope, along the face, up to the horizon line between the face and top, but does not curve to include the region on top. The landmark enclosure for *u/a* is defined relative to this line of sight: it includes a narrow region along either side of the line as well as a restricted area at the foot of the slope surrounding the vantage point. (Casad and Langacker 1985: 262)

The following sentences provide an even more striking example of the importance of conventional construal:

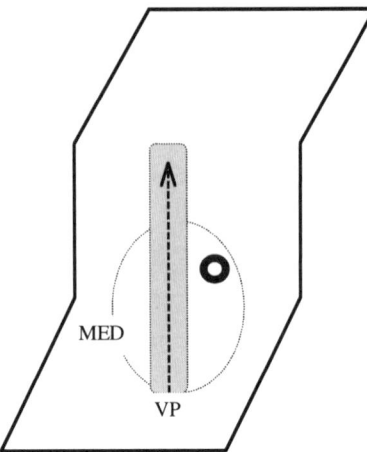

Figure 7.2 *mah* 'away up there to the side in the face of the slope' (adapted from Casad and Langacker 1985: 262)

(1)   a. *u-   h-   kí-   tʸa-   pu'u*
            inside slope   short middle   BE:planted upright
            'Its [the dog's] tail is chopped short.'

        b. *a-   h-   kí-   tʸa-   pu'u*
            outside slope   short middle   BE:planted upright
            'Its [the dog's] tail is chopped short.'

Both sentences can be used to describe the same objective situation: namely, to state that the dog's tail has been lopped off. But what does a short tail have to do with slopes and containment, and why does the sentence with *a* mean the same thing as the sentence with *u*?

In fact, they don't mean quite the same thing, as they would be appropriate in different contexts. (1a) would be used to describe a situation in which the dog is viewed from behind, as in Figure 7.3a, while (1b) describes a dog viewed from the side, as in Figure 7.3b. The motivation for using *a* and *u* should now be apparent. In (1a), the 'slope' facing the observer is the dog's rump, and the tail is 'inside' the region defined with respect to the observer's line of sight. In (1b), the 'slope' is the dog's side, and the tail sticks out outside the region defined by the line of sight.[2] Notice that this usage requires a (metaphorical) projection of a term normally used to refer to parts of a mountain onto a body part, motivated by the topographical similarity of a slope and an animal's rump and conventionalised in the grammar.[3] While the Cora *u* may be said to expresses 'containment', containment is very much in the eye of the beholder.

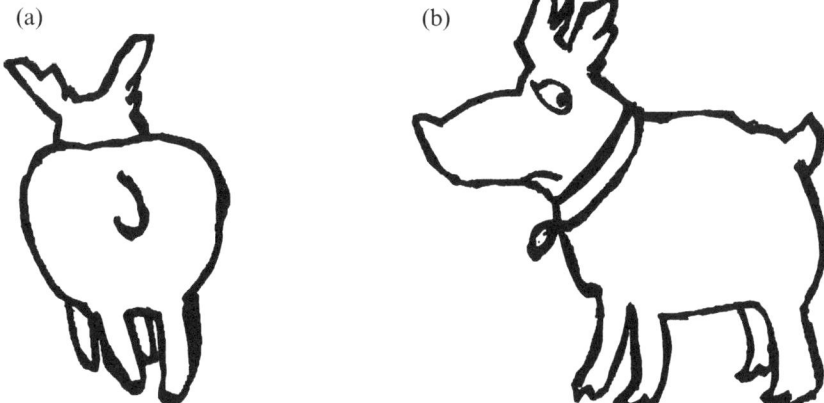

(a)　　　　　　　　　　(b)

Figure 7.3 Another virtual container

1.2 Polysemy

Most locative expressions are massively polysemous. For example, according to Brugman (1988; see also Lakoff 1987) the English preposition *over* has nearly 100 distinct senses, of which 24 designate various spatial relationships. A few of these are exemplified in (2) below.

(2)　　a. *There is a lamp over the table.* [= 'above']
　　　　b. *He spread a cloth over the table.* [= 'on']
　　　　c. *He jumped over the stream.* [= 'across']
　　　　d. *He has travelled all over Europe.* [= 'all around']
　　　　e. *He lives over the hill.*　[= 'on the other side of']

Polysemy is a sensible way of dealing with the conflicting demands imposed by the great diversity of spatial relationships to be described and by the fact that the lexicon must be finite (cf. Geeraerts 1988; Lakoff 1987; Rosch 1975, 1977). What is relevant for the present discussion is that different languages choose different solutions to this problem: that is to say, they carve up the semantic space in diverse and often incompatible ways. This becomes obvious when we compare the uses of *over* exemplified in (2) with the corresponding locative expressions in another language. Each of these senses of *over* corresponds to a different preposition in Polish (*nad*, *na*, *przez*, *po* and *za*, respectively). Moreover, each of the Polish prepositions is also polysemous, and the distinctions they express cross-cut those encoded in the English system.

For a more dramatic illustration of such cross-linguistic differences, consider the relationships depicted in Figure 7.4.[4] English classifies them into three categories – CONTAINMENT, SUPPORT and UPNESS WITHOUT CONTACT – and

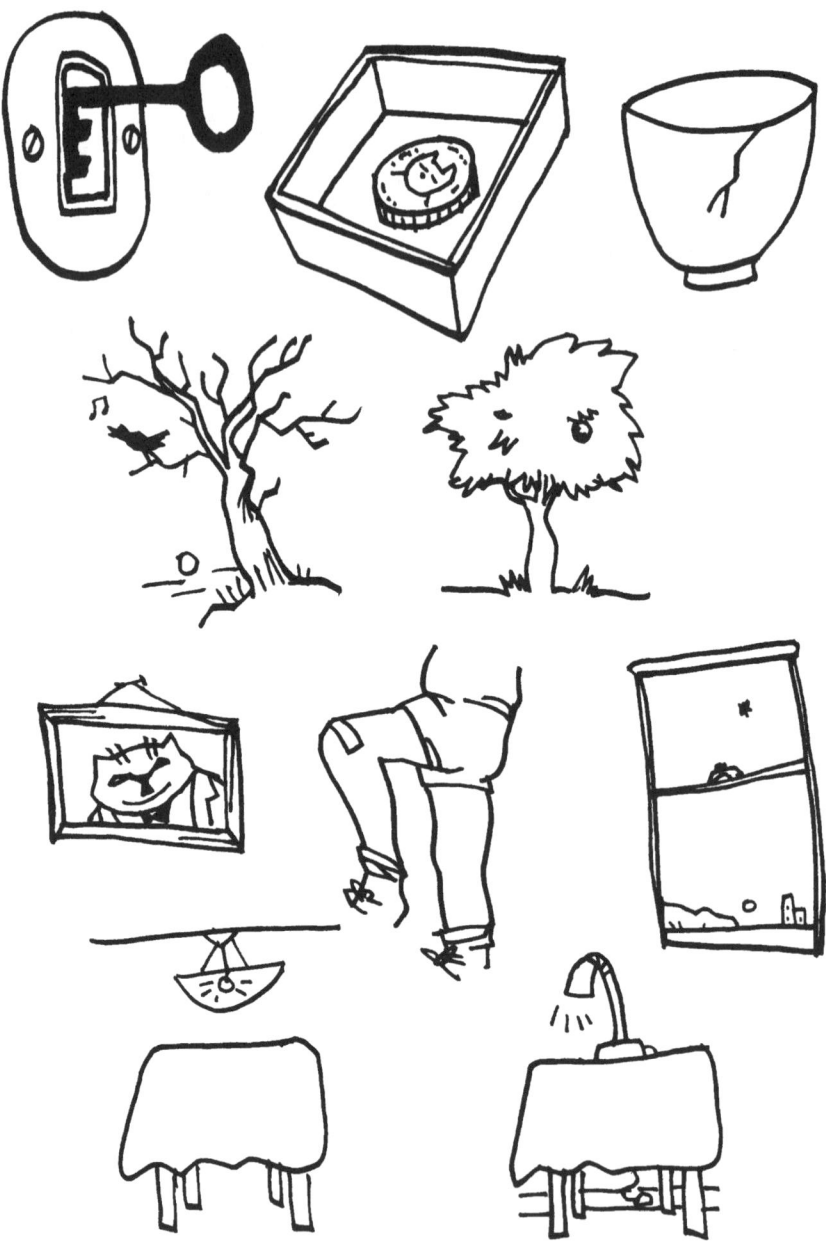

Figure 7.4 Some 'in', 'on' and 'above' relationships: key in a door, coin in a box, crack in a bowl, bird in a tree, apple on a tree, picture on a wall, plaster (Band-Aid) on a leg, fly on a window, lamp above a table, lamp on a table

codes them by means of three prepositions, *in*, *on* and *above*. Some other languages (e.g. Greek and Spanish) conflate CONTAINMENT and SUPPORT and code ABOVENESS separately. Kikuyu also has only a two-way distinction, but it conflates the prototypical *on* (as in *The lamp is on the table*) and *above*, and expresses everything else with a generalised locative morpheme. Italian, Portuguese, Swedish, Indonesian, Mandarin and Finnish all make a three-way distinction, but each carves up the semantic space in a slightly different way. Dutch and German divide the set of relationships into four categories, and Japanese into eight.

It is clear, then, that having innate categories corresponding to specific locative lexemes would be of little use to learners, since the detective work involved in determining which categories out of the thousands of possible ones were actually employed in their language would not be much easier than creating them on the basis of the evidence.

On the other hand, innate concepts need not coincide with specific lexemes. One could claim, for example, that what is innate is category prototypes (archetypal configurations around which future categories will grow) or some more basic dimensions along which lexemes differ ('semantic features'). I will discuss the latter possibility later on. The former may initially seem quite attractive, since there is considerably less variation between languages in the configurations that they choose for category centres. For example, although the English preposition *on*, the Polish *na* and the French *sur* all designate different categories, the prototypical sense (a trajector object located on top of, and supported by, a horizontal landmark) is the same in all three languages. However, a moment's reflection will reveal that this theory suffers from exactly the same problems as the more radical view espoused by Chomsky, Fodor and Piattelli-Palmarini. As the discussion below will make clear, the number of distinct concepts that would have to be encoded in the genome would still be intractably large; and the learner would still need to determine category boundaries.

1.3 Cross-linguistic variation

The differences in the ways languages carve up space are enormous. Depending on the language, locative meanings can be expressed by adpositions, nouns, adverbs, particles, verbs, adjectives, verb affixes or noun inflections, or they may be distributed across lexemes belonging to different classes (Sinha and Kuteva 1995). Moreover, spatial meanings are often integrated with other semantic systems (Brown 1994; Sinha et al. 1994; see also the Tzeltal data below). Consider, for example, Japanese. Japanese has three means of conveying locative meanings:

1. Verbs which code path of motion, e.g. *hairu* 'go in', *deru* 'go out', *ireru* 'put in', *dasu* 'take out', *agaru* 'go up', *oriru* 'go down'. Functionally, this is the

most important part of the system, as most locative information is conveyed by this means.

2. Relational object-part terms, e.g. *naka* 'inside', *soto* 'outside', *ue* 'top', *shita* 'bottom'. For example, *tsukue no ue ni* means 'on the desk' (lit. 'at the top of the desk').

3. Locative particles such as *ni*, *de* 'at, in', *o* 'through, from', *e* 'to', *kara* 'from', *made* 'to'. Functionally, this is the least important part of the system, as the particles are highly polysemous and generally add little or no new information to that already conveyed by other elements of the sentence.

This system makes it possible to code aspects of the situation in several parts of the sentence (often redundantly):

(3)   *Hon-wa   hako-ni haitte   imasu.*
        book-TOP box-AT entering is
        'The book is in the box.'

(4)   *Hon-wa   hako-no   naka-ni   haitte   imasu.*
        book-TOP box-GEN inside-AT entering is
        'The book is inside the box.'

The first sentence literally means something like 'The book, having entered the box, is (there)': the verb *hairu* conflates the idea of motion and the path of motion (from outside inwards). The semantic contribution of the particle *ni* is entirely redundant: it does not add any information to that expressed by *haitte imasu*. The same information can be expressed using (4), which is even more redundant, since the locative information is distributed across three morphemes: the particle *ni* 'at', the relational noun *naka* 'inside', and the verb *hairu* 'enter'.

Other languages have locative systems which differ even more from those found in the familiar European languages. To appreciate the cross-linguistic diversity, in this section we will look at a few rather exotic systems: the Mixtec system of body-part terms, Tzeltal dispositional adjectives, and absolute systems in several languages.

1.3.1 Metaphorical projection of body-part terms
In Mixtec, an Otomanguean language spoken in Oaxaca in Mexico, locative relationships are described by using body-part terms (Brugman 1983; Brugman and Macaulay 1986; Lakoff 1987). For example, someone who has just climbed a mountain would be located at 'mountain's head' (5). *On* relationships are described by using several different expressions, depending on the shape of the landmark object: *on the mat* would be translated 'mat's face' (6); *on the table* would be 'at the table's (animal) back' (7); and *on a branch* becomes 'at tree's arm' (8). (All the Mixtec data cited in this section come from Brugman 1983 and Brugman and Macaulay 1986.)

(5) *hížaa-re*   *šini* *žuku*
    be+located-3SgM head mountain
    'He's at the top of the mountain.'

(6) *se?e-rí*   *hítú nǔǔ yúu*
    son-1Sg lie   face mat
    'My son is lying on the mat.'

(7) *hísndee sɨkɨ*   *mesá wãã*
    be+on animal+back table that
    'It's on that table.'

(8) *ndukoo-rí nda?a yúnu*
    sit-1Sg   arm   tree
    'I am sitting on the branch of the tree.'

Body-part terms are used to refer not only to the relevant part of the land-mark object, but also to the neighbouring region in space: 'at mountain's head' could mean 'over the mountain' as well as 'on top of the mountain'. Some of the terms in the system designate human body parts, some animal body parts, and some can refer to either, which results in rather strange (to us) patterns of polysemy. For example, the term *čìì* 'belly' can be used to refer to the middle of the front surface of a vertically oriented object (the region where the belly would be in an upright human) or the underside of a horizontally oriented object (where the belly would be in a four-legged animal), or the vicinity of either of these. Thus, with a horizontal landmark such as a table, *čìì* can be translated as 'under' (9).

(9) *yuù wǎ híyaà*   *čìì* *mesá*
    stone DET be+located belly table
    'The stone is under the table.'

It should be obvious from this brief description that English and Mixtec carve up spatial scenes in very different ways, and, consequently, the informa-tion conveyed by a Mixtec sentence and its English translation is not strictly equivalent. English is quite explicit about the position of the trajector with respect to the landmark (contact/no contact) but does not specify the shape of the landmark, while the opposite is true in Mixtec.

On second thoughts, the use of body-part terms to express locative mean-ings is not as exotic as it might at first seem. The American English expression *in back of* is also a metaphorical extension of a body-part term, and the same metaphor is (just about) accessible, though much less transparent, in the prep-osition *behind*. The word *front* in the complex preposition *in front of* comes from Latin *frons* 'forehead', though in this case the link is purely etymological and unknown to most speakers. In fact, body-part terms are common sources of locative expressions (see Svorou 1994 and the extensive literature cited there). What is special about Mixtec is that the use of body-part terms is much more systematic and more transparent synchronically.

However, the extension of body-part terminology to the locative domain is conventional: that is to say, although there are broad similarities between languages in the way they effect the mapping, the details are language-specific and must be learned. For example, the words for eye, face, forehead, head, breast and chest are all common sources for the spatial meaning of 'in front of' (Svorou 1994); but different languages make different choices from this list. In this connection, it is also instructive to compare Mixtec and Cora: while Mixtec projects body-part terms onto inanimate objects such as mountains,[5] Cora sometimes projects 'hilly' terms onto parts of the body.

1.3.2 Dispositional adjectives

Like Mixtec body-part terms, dispositional adjectives in Tzeltal code more than the position of one object with respect to another (Brown 1994). Tzeltal does not have words corresponding to the English *on* or *in*, and information about CONTAINMENT and SUPPORT is always co-lexicalised with much more specific information about shape, size, orientation, mode of support or attachment, subject category, and other semantic dimensions in dispositional adjectives which can be translated by such complex English expressions as 'mounted on top of', 'positioned at right angles to', 'hanging down from', 'glued to the surface of', 'spirally wound around' etc. There are several hundred roots which encode very specific shape information about location. Some examples of these are presented in Figures 7.5 and 7.6.

Tzeltal dispositional terms actually designate the overall configuration of the trajector and the landmark rather than the relationship between the two; information about the locative relationship itself is usually conveyed by implication rather than directly. This leads to interesting ambiguities, which Brown calls 'figure/ground ambiguities', deriving from whether the adjective is taken as describing the figure (i.e. trajector) or the ground (the landmark; see Figure 7.7). For example, *waxal ta X Y* 'standing at X Y' can mean either '(vertically aligned) Y is on X' or 'Y is in a (vertically aligned) X'. The dispositional adjective merely indicates that something is in a vertical position; it is the following NPs which specify which of the two objects is the figure (trajector) and which is the ground (landmark). From this we can infer whether the figure is 'on' or 'in' the ground.

1.3.3 Absolute systems

The final example in this brief survey of locative systems in the world's languages concerns relationships between objects located in the horizontal plane. English uses four contrasting terms to designate such relationships (*in front of*, *behind, to the left of, to the right of*), as well as more general terms like *near* and *beside*. Systems such as this are called **relative** because, when the landmark

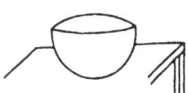

PACHAL TA table, bowl 'be-located', of wide-mouthed container canonically 'sitting'

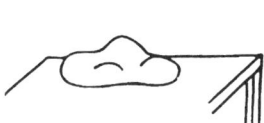

PAKAL TA table, dough 'be-located', of blob with distinguishably flat surface lying 'face'-down

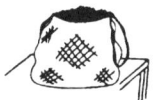

CHEPEL TA table, netbag 'be-located', of a full (bulging) bag supported underneath

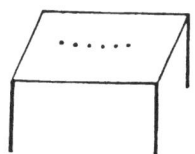

CHOLOL TA table, beans 'be-located', of multiple objects arranged in a row

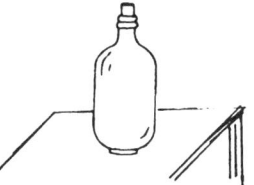

WAXAL TA table, bottle 'be-located', of tall oblong-shaped container or solid object canonically 'standing'

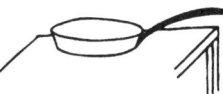

LECHEL TA table, frying pan 'be located', of wide flat object lying flat

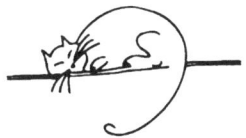

MOCHOL TA table, cat 'be-located', of animate object lying curved on its side

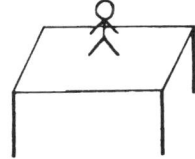

TEK'EL TA table, toy man 'be-located', of a vertically standing (on hind legs) animate creature or a long/thin object

Figure 7.5 Some ways of encoding 'on' relationships in Tzeltal. Source: Brown (1994: 760)

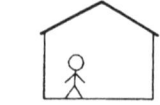

...TA *Y-UTIL* house, man
'AT its-inside'

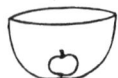

PACHAL TA bowl, apple
'be-located', of bowl-shaped container
canonically 'sitting'

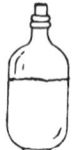

WAXAL TA bottle, water
'be-located', of taller-than-wide
rectangular or cylindrical object
vertically 'standing'

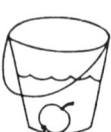

T'UMUL TA water, apple
'be-located' immersed in liquid in a
container

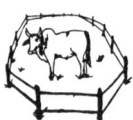

TIK'IL TA corral, bull
'be-located' by having been inserted
into a container with a narrow opening

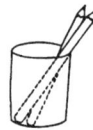

XIJIL TA cup, pencils
'be-located', of long/thin object, by
having been inserted carefully into
bounded ground

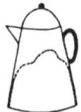

XOJOL TA pot, coffeebag
'be-located' by having been inserted
singly into closely fitting container

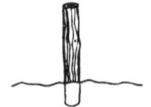

TZ'APAL TA ground, stick
'be-located' by having been inserted at
end into supporting medium

Figure 7.6 Some ways of encoding 'in' relationships in Tzeltal. Source: Brown (1994: 767)

object does not have an inherent front, the position of the trajector is described relative to the location of an observer, usually the speaker. Thus, depending on where the observer is, the same situation can be truthfully described by saying *The mouse is in front of/behind/to the left of/to the right of the fish* (cf. Figure 7.8).

English also uses an **absolute** system of geographical terms (*north*, *south*, *east* and *west*) to describe macrolocations, or locations of large figures such as towns and villages with respect to large reference objects. When I say *Doncaster is east of Sheffield*, I am using the absolute system.

Some languages use an absolute system to describe microlocations as well. In such languages, the configuration represented in Figure 7.8 will be

Shape/orientation/position characteristics may apply to *EITHER* the figure *OR* the ground object

to FIGURE: to GROUND:

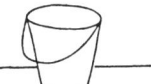

waxal ta mexa te baltie
standing AT table bucket
'The bucket is on the table.'

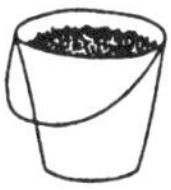

waxal ta balti ixim
standing AT pail corn
'The corn is in the bucket.'

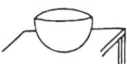

pachal ta mexa bojch
sitting AT table gourd bowl
'The gourd is on the table.'

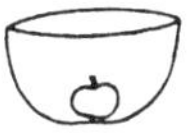

pachal ta bojch te mantzanae
sitting AT gourd the apple
'The apple is in the gourd bowl.'

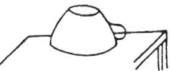

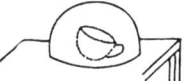

nujul ta mexa te basoe
inverted AT table the cup
'The cup is inverted on the table.'

nujul ta bojch te basoe
inverted AT gourd bowl the cup
'The cup is inside/underneath (the) gourd bowl.'

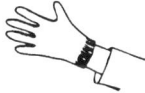

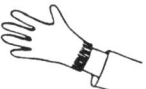

xojol ta sk'ab te spotzil sk'abe
inserted AT his-hand the covering his-hand (i.e. the glove)
'The glove is inserted onto his hand.'

xojol s-k'ab ta y-util ala tzajal tzotz
inserted his-hand AT its-inside red yarn (= glove)
'His hand is inside the glove.'

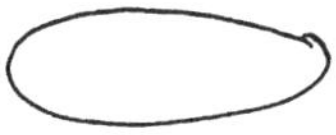

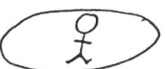

joyol ta lum te ch'ajan tak'in
circle-shaped on the ground the wire
'The wire is in a circle on the ground.'

joyol ta ch'ajan tak'in te ach'ixe
encircled by wire the girl
'The girl is encircled by (the) wire.'

Figure 7.7 Figure/ground 'ambiguities'. Source: Brown (1994: 776)

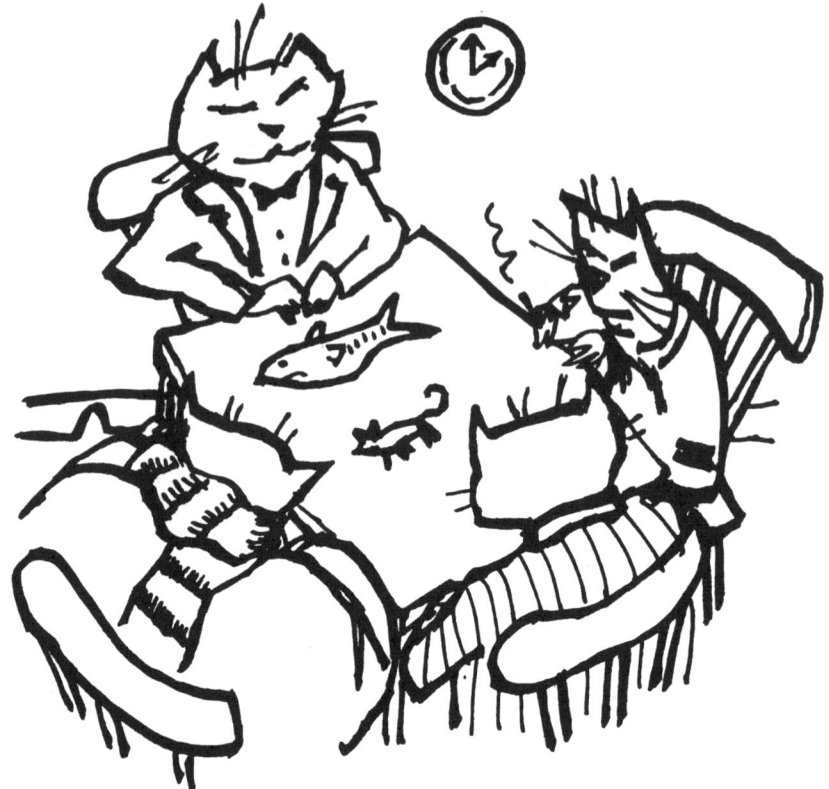

Figure 7.8 A spatial scene and four observers

described by saying something like *The mouse is east of the fish.* Note that
because the coordinates of the system are fixed rather then being projected
from the speaker, the mouse is always 'to the east' of the fish, regardless of the
position of the speaker/observer.

Absolute systems sometimes use the four compass points, and sometimes
other cardinal directions defined by the direction of the prevailing winds
(Guugu Yimidhirr) or some feature of local topology such as a large river
(Yupno) or the sea (many Oceanic languages). In Tzeltal, the relevant topo-
logical feature is the general inclination of the land, which slopes down
towards the north, so anything south of the reference object is said to be
'uphill' and anything towards the north is 'downhill'. (This is just the overall
direction of the inclination: there are many local irregularities, but the general
direction of the slope fixes the system of coordinates. See Brown and Levinson
1993 for further details.) These two opposing directions define the strong axis
of the system. The system also has a 'weak' axis perpendicular to the strong
axis which lacks opposing poles. Together, the two axes define a three-way dis-

tinction: up v. down v. across the slope. In Figure 7.9, the saucer is 'uphill', the
spoon is 'downhill' and the two coasters are both 'across the slope' from the
glass.

It should be clear from the above discussion that absolute systems are not
only quite different from relative systems; they are also different from each
other in that they use different reference points and different numbers of cardinal directions.[6] While 'east' and 'west' always refer to the same direction,
'inland' and 'seawards' do not: if you live on an island, 'inland' means 'east'
on the western coast and 'west' on the eastern coast.

1.3.4 Interim conclusion

In spite of the fact that spatial conceptualisation is strongly constrained by the
nature of the world and by our psychobiology, there is tremendous variation
in the way that different languages structure space. This makes the hypothesis
that locative concepts are innate extremely implausible.

A less extreme version of nativism in lexical semantics is the claim that all
humans are born with a set of semantic primitives ('features', 'atoms' etc.)
which can be combined in various ways to construct the meanings of all lexical
concepts in all the world's languages. This approach suffers from most of the
problems that plague the holistic approach, plus some of its own, and is thus
even less attractive. Some of these problems will be discussed later, in section
3.1 of this chapter; for the present, we may just note that for our purposes,
most versions of the atomistic approach are indistinguishable from holism
because the primitives postulated by the atomists correspond to lexical categories in familiar European languages: *in* corresponds to the semantic primitive IN, or the notion of CONTAINMENT, *on* expresses ON or SUPPORT, and so on.

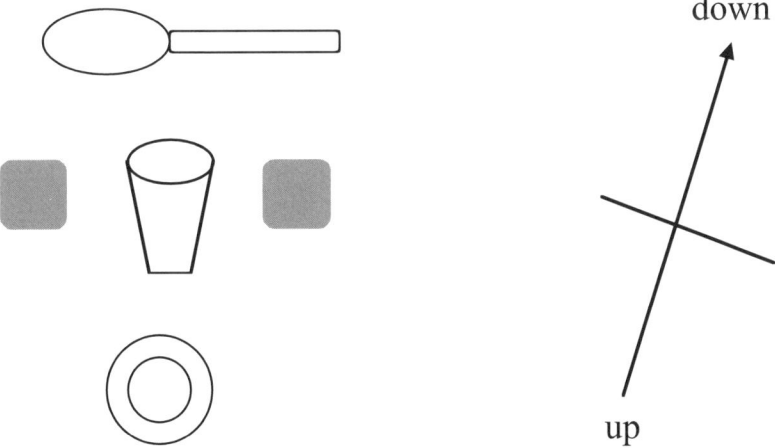

Figure 7.9 The Tzeltal geocentric system of projective relationships

For example, Jackendoff (1983) notes that the English preposition *under* can designate a place (*The mouse is under the table*), a path (*The mouse ran under the table* 'The mouse traversed the region under the table') or the endpoint of a path (*The mouse ran under the table* 'The mouse ran to the region under the table'), and proposes the following conceptual structures to capture the distinctions:

(10)   a. $[_{Place}$ UNDER $([_{Thing}$ TABLE$])]$
       b. $[_{Path}$ TO $([_{Place}$ UNDER $([_{Thing}$ TABLE$])])]$
       c. $[_{Path}$ VIA $([_{Place}$ UNDER $([_{Thing}$ TABLE$])])]$

The expression *up the hill* (as in *The house is up the hill*) receives the following analysis:

(11) $[_{Place}$ ON $([_{Path}$ UP $([_{Thing}$ HILL$])])]$

Thus, according to Jackendoff, ON, UP and UNDER are semantic primitives whose meanings correspond to the basic meanings of the English prepositions *on*, *up* and *under*. Now there is nothing incoherent about the claim that the meaning of a particular expression is paraphrasable by means of a single semantic primitive. However, as Bowerman points out, there are reasons to worry about such glib formulations:

> I find it sobering that the 'non-linguistic spatial concepts' often hypothe-sised to underlie spatial prepositions – e.g. 'containment' and 'support' – lend themselves much more readily to shaping into spatial categories of English than, say, Tzeltal. In other words, our ideas about plausible 'primitives' in the language of thought may themselves be conditioned by the language we have learned. (Bowerman 1996: 160)

2. The acquisition of locative terms

As explained earlier, the conventional wisdom on the acquisition of locative terms is that it involves matching linguistic labels to pre-existing concepts. Now that we have seen the diversity in locative systems across languages, this position is rather less appealing: it is extremely unlikely that children are equipped with innate concepts corresponding to locative terms in all the world's languages, and even if they were, such a vast inventory of possible meanings would be of little help in fixing the meanings of the words which actually occur in the child's language.

However, it is possible, in principle, that children come equipped with basic locative concepts which happen to correspond rather closely to the meanings of English prepositions. If this were the case, then locative terms which do not correspond to the innate concepts should be considerably more difficult to acquire. In this section, therefore, we briefly examine some research devoted to the acquisition of locative systems which structure space in radically different ways from English and other familiar Indo-European languages.

2.1 Warlpiri

We will begin by looking at the acquisition of locative terms by Warlpiri children. Warlpiri is interesting from our point of view because it does not have terms corresponding to *in, on* and *under*. It does, of course, have terms which can be used to talk about scenes which in English would be described using these prepositions, but these are extended senses of expressions whose primary meanings are rather different. The terms are *kanunju-mparra* 'down-along' or, in certain contexts, 'under'; *kaninja-rni* 'down-hither' or, with the right kind of landmark, 'in'; and *kankarla-rra* 'up-thither' or 'on'. All three expressions are bimorphemic and consist of a locative stem and a directional affix. It is not very clear what the exact semantic contribution of each morpheme is – the traditional glosses are not very helpful in this regard – but it is evident that Warlpiri spatial categories are different from those found in English and other familiar languages.

Bavin (1990) conducted a simple experiment testing the comprehension of locative terms by Warlpiri children aged from 3;11 to 8. The experimental task involved placing an object as instructed by the experimenter – in, on or under a landmark object. The landmarks used were a toy *yunta* (a shelter consisting of a flat top with four poles for support), a toy *yujuku* (a shelter with sides, open at the two ends), and a toy pick-up truck.

The results were quite intriguing. *Kankarla-rra* 'up-thither' was fairly consistently interpreted as 'on' by all the children, but responses to instructions with the other two terms were varied, and depended on properties of the reference object. *Kanunju-mparra* 'down-along' was interpreted as 'under' when the reference object was a *yunta*; but when the landmark was a truck, 39 per cent interpreted it to mean 'in' the open back of the truck. *Kaninja-rni* 'down-hither' was interpreted as 'in' when the landmark was a *yujuku*, but when the landmark was a truck, the children gave inconsistent responses: some placed the object in the cabin, some on the tray in the back and some under the truck. In other words, there is no evidence in Bavin's data that Warlpiri children are sieving through the language input looking for labels for their prelinguistic concepts IN, ON and UNDER. In fact there is no evidence that they make these distinctions at all.[7]

2.2 Tzotzil

Tzotzil is a Mayan language, closely related to Tzeltal. Like Tzeltal, it uses geocentric coordinates defined by the general incline of the land, but in the region where Tzotzil is spoken the land slopes westwards, so 'uphill' means 'east', not 'south'.

De León (1994) found that Tzotzil caregivers use geocentric terms ('uphill/east' and 'downhill/west') with children as young as 2, and children are expected to understand the terms. (One mother in the study rebuked her 3-year-old son for not knowing where east was!) Children know the basic principles of the system by around 4;6 (i.e. before European children reliably distinguish left and right), though they generally use local landmarks rather than geocentric terms: that is, instead of saying 'The basket is uphill/east', they might say something like 'The basket is towards the market town'. They start producing the terms for 'sunset' and 'sunrise' around 9, which 'suggests that around this age the child shifts the local centre of the orientation grid to the absolute co-ordinate provided by the sun' (de León 1994: 876).

Like Mixtec, Tzotzil also uses body-part terms to describe more immediate locations. Preliminary work carried out by de León (1991, cited in Levinson 1994) suggests that this system is acquired even earlier: Tzotzil children begin to use body-part locatives well before the age of 3.

2.3 Japanese

In Japanese, we saw earlier, locative meanings are distributed across three form classes: motion verbs, relational nouns and particles, with the first of these doing most of the work. Sinha et al. (1994) report on a longitudinal study of one Japanese child, Adam, observed by the team from age 1;3 to 2;11.

Adam's first locative terms were motion verbs such as *dasu* 'take out', *toru* 'take off', *hameru* 'fit in' etc. The first recorded usage of a locative verb occurred at 1;3.28; and they are recorded in every session from 1;6 onwards. Locative nouns (*soto* 'outside', *naka* 'inside', *ue* 'top' etc.) emerged shortly afterwards, around the time of his second birthday. The last to appear were the particles *ni*, *de* 'at, in', *kara* 'from', and *e* 'to'. All four particles first emerged in collocation with *koko* 'this place', and their use remained highly formulaic throughout the period of study. This pattern of acquisition makes sense, since it is motion verbs and relational nouns that convey specific information – but it is rather difficult to explain if you believe that children are simply looking for labels for pre-existing locative concepts corresponding to 'in', 'on' etc. If Adam were simply looking for labels for 'in' and 'on', he should have learned the locative particles much earlier, since they occurred fairly frequently in the input (in fact, the frequency of locative particles in the speech of Adam's mother was four times that of locative relational nouns, which he acquired earlier).

This acquisition pattern, incidentally, also argues against the idea that children construct meanings out of a universal set of primitives. If this were the case, more specific concepts should be more difficult to acquire than concepts which directly correspond to the putative primitives. The data collected by

Sinha and his colleagues suggests the opposite: the verb *hameru* 'fit in', which co-lexicalises the action of inserting and the destination of the trajector, is acquired earlier than the general locative particle *ni* 'at, in'; *toru* 'take off', which co-lexicalises causative movement and direction, comes long before *kara* 'from', and so on.

2.4 Korean

Another series of studies conducted by Melissa Bowerman and Soonja Choi (Bowerman 1996; Choi and Bowerman 1991; Choi et al. 1999) compared the acquisition of morphemes specifying the path of a moving object by English- and Korean-speaking children. The relevant parts of the locative systems of the two languages are quite different. English path morphemes are prepositions, while in Korean the shape of the path is co-lexicalised with other notions in the verb. Furthermore, English path morphemes are indifferent as to whether the movement is spontaneous or caused (the same preposition is used with both transitive and intransitive verbs: *go in*, *put in*), while in Korean the corresponding meanings are expressed by different verbs. Finally, Korean path-incorporating verbs make distinctions which cross-cut those made by English prepositions: e.g. *kkita* 'fit a three-dimensional object into or onto another object' can be translated as *put in* (for example, when describing the action of putting glasses inside a case), *put on* (when a cap is put on a pen), or *put together* (when two Lego pieces are fitted together). Conversely, the meanings expressed by *put in* and *put on* are coded by a number of different verbs in Korean: *kkita* when two three-dimensional objects fit closely, *nehta* when the fit is loose, *pwu-thita* when two flat surfaces are joined, *kkotta* when an elongated object is put into/onto a base, and so on. In addition, there is another set of verbs for designating the action of putting clothing on various parts of the body.

Choi and Bowerman report that the first locative expressions usually appear between 14 and 16 months, and that children use them productively by 16–20 months. The children's use of locative expressions is generally correct, and it follows language-specific patterns from the very beginning. English-speaking children acquire their first path morphemes (*up*, *down*, *in*, *out*, *on*, *off*) very early (usually between 16 and 17 months, and sometimes as early as 12–14 months) and almost immediately generalise them to spontaneous and caused motion and to changes of body posture. For example, they might say *in* when putting something into a box or when they themselves are climbing into a box; *up* when they want to be picked up, when going up stairs, and when standing up. Korean children, in contrast, always use different verbs to refer to caused motion and to spontaneous motion. Thus, they will say *kkita* when fitting an object into a hole, but they never overextend this term to describe a situation when they themselves creep into a narrow space; and they never overgeneralise *ancta* 'sit down' and *anta* 'pick up and carry' to situations involving upward or downward motion.

Furthermore, English-speaking children distinguish CONTAINMENT (*in*) and SUPPORT (*on*) relations, and do not worry about details of trajector and landmark geometry, or whether the fit is tight or loose. Korean children do not make this distinction: they use *kkita* 'fit' for putting things into tight containers and for tight attachment to a ground object, *nehta* for loose containment, *kkota* for putting an elongated object into/onto a base, and so on.

In short, Bowerman and Choi found no evidence that children begin by mapping prelinguistic spatial concepts onto the words they hear. In spite of this, the children in their study made few errors. When errors did occur, they tended to be language-specific, showing that the children had difficulty with working out the details of a system they had already acquired. Korean children, for example, had problems with words that encode pure path notions, which is an English lexicalisation pattern. This shows that even at this very young age (under 2), they had already formed some generalisations about what was likely to be lexicalised in their language and what was not.

2.5 General discussion

The developmental studies summarised here clearly show that children acquire the rudiments of the locative system of their language very early – well before the age of 3, though some distinctions may take somewhat longer to learn. Moreover, they appear to be sensitive to language-specific categories from the very beginning, and the pattern of acquisition observed in naturalistic studies is virtually error-free (Choi and Bowerman 1991; Sinha et al. 1994; Tomasello 1987). The developmental research, then, shows that children are extremely good learners.

I observed at the beginning of this chapter that several studies (Carey 1978; Dickinson 1984; Heibeck and Markman 1987) have shown that children can form partial semantic representations of new words after only a few exposures, or even just one exposure, to the new word. These 'fast-mapping' studies have been used as evidence that lexical knowledge must be innate (though the authors themselves did not necessarily advocate such conclusions). However, the existence of fast mapping does not necessarily imply that children are endowed with innate lexical knowledge. It could also be interpreted as further evidence that they are good learners. This conclusion appears to be confirmed by a study by Markson and Bloom (1997), which showed that fast mapping is not confined to word learning.

Markson and Bloom asked their subjects (3- and 4-year-old children and adults) to use unfamiliar objects to measure the length of another object. In one version of the task, the objects were referred to as *kobas* ('Let's use the kobas to measure which is longer. Line up the kobas so we can count them. We can put the kobas away now.'). In another version, participants were simply told that the objects were given to the experimenter by her uncle ('We can use the things my uncle gave me to measure which is longer. My uncle gave these to me. We can put the things my uncle gave me away now.'). This was followed by a testing phase, which occurred immediately, after a week's delay, or a month later. In the testing phase, participants were shown an array of objects and were asked to pick out the koba or the object given to the experimenter by her uncle.

Markson and Bloom found that adults performed significantly better than children on the word-learning task when they were tested immediately after training, but the differences between age groups disappeared after a week. About 70 per cent of the participants could still point to the correct object when tested a month after training. This replicates the results obtained in earlier fast-mapping studies. The new finding was that participants were equally good at remembering which object was given to the experimenter by her uncle; in fact, when tested immediately after the training phase, children performed significantly better on this task than on the word-learning task.[8] Fast mapping, then, is not restricted to word learning.

On the other hand, Markson and Bloom also found that people are not equally good at remembering any arbitrary fact about an object. In another experiment, participants watched as the investigator placed a sticker on one of the unfamiliar objects and heard a similar commentary ('Watch where this goes. This goes here [placing sticker on one of the objects]. That's where this goes.'). In this version of the experiment, recall was significantly poorer. It is not clear whether this was due to the fact that the information was presented visually or whether the location of a sticker was deemed less relevant by the participants than the identity of an object. Whatever the reason, their findings suggest that fast mapping, though not unique to language, does not apply to all memorisation tasks. Children are good learners, but not equally good at learning anything. Something about the human cognitive apparatus makes certain associations easier to acquire than others.

3. Innate structure, yes – but of what kind?

The general conclusion, then, is that children are good learners, but they are not unbiased learners. In fact, many would argue that they are good learners *because* they are biased towards certain solutions. It is important to realise that rejecting the notion that lexical concepts are built in does not entail rejecting the existence of innate structure of any kind. Clearly, children must have *some* innate predispositions which make language learning possible. Learning is impossible without experience, but an organism needs a great deal of innate structure before it can have any experience, and even more to be able to extract patterns from it. There is considerable empirical evidence for various constraints on lexical development in general (Dockrell and Campbell 1986; Markman 1987, 1990; Smith et al. 1992; Tager-Flusberg 1986) and for prelinguistic biases on the perception of space which shape the acquisition of locative terms (E. V. Clark 1973a, 1976, 1980; H. Clark 1973; Huttenlocher et al. 1983). The question, then, is not whether children are endowed with innate structure, but rather what form their innate predispositions take, and it is to this question that we now turn.

3.1 Semantic primitives

A less extreme version of nativism in semantics is the claim that what is innate is not lexical concepts themselves, but semantic primitives or 'atoms' of meaning like ADULT, MALE or CAUSE. These can be combined to form complex concepts such as BACHELOR [ADULT & MALE & NEVER MARRIED] and KILL [CAUSE-BECOME-NOT-ALIVE] (see Bierwisch 1970; Bierwisch and Schreuder 1992; Jackendoff 1983, 1990; Katz 1972, 1987; Katz and Fodor 1963; Miller and Johnson-Laird 1976). On this view, lexical acquisition involves discovering which combinations of primitives are lexicalised in a given language (Clark 1973b, 1975; Clark and Clark 1977).

Although the approach may initially seem quite attractive, it is plagued with problems, many of them of a rather fundamental nature. Perhaps the most serious of these is that most lexical concepts cannot be analysed into primitives. Semantic decomposition works reasonably well for a few lexical fields such as kinship terms and farmyard animals, but attempts to extend it beyond these have been unsuccessful. As noted by Fodor et al. (1980), the number of convincing exhaustive decompositions in the literature is vanishingly small. Most decompositions are partial: some aspects of meaning are captured by means of semantic primitives, but when these are factored out, we are left with an unanalysed residue. Take the word *red*, for example. *Red* is a colour term, so we could say that its semantic representation contains the feature [COLOUR]. Let us factor this out of the meaning of *red*. What do we do with the residue? Is it coherent to talk of redness minus colour (cf. Fodor et al. 1980; Jackendoff 1983)?

There are problems even with traditional mainstays of semantic decomposition. As several researchers have pointed out, *kill* is not synonymous with 'cause to become not alive' or even 'cause to die': you can cause someone to die on Tuesday by shooting him on Monday, but you cannot kill someone on Tuesday by shooting him on Monday (Fodor 1970; Lakoff 1987). In a similar vein, there are various connotational differences between the terms *bachelor* and *spinster* which are not captured by the traditional feature definitions (*bachelor:* [ADULT & MALE & NEVER MARRIED]; *spinster* [ADULT & NOT MALE & NEVER MARRIED]): spinsters are supposed to be old, sexually unattractive and desperate to get married, while bachelors are either young and eligible or happily single and not interested in marriage.[9] Worse still, some unmarried adult males – for example, priests, homosexuals, and male partners in cohabiting heterosexual couples – cannot be felicitously described as bachelors, except in a strictly legal context (Lakoff 1987: 70ff).

Another difficulty concerns the meaning of the features themselves. As many critics have pointed out, proponents of semantic decomposition have failed to provide a satisfactory account of how speakers translate perceptual information into semantic primitives (see Johnson 1987; Lakoff 1987); and attempting to define words by using meaningless features is a rather pointless exercise.

Semantic feature theory also has little to recommend itself in the way of psychological reality. Intuitively, concepts such as FATHER and MOTHER are, if anything, more basic than the supposed primitives MALE and PARENT.[10] Such intuitions are corroborated by psycholinguistic evidence. A number of experimental studies attempted to determine whether lexical decomposition is a prerequisite to comprehension by comparing reaction times to sentences containing words expressing 'simple' concepts (e.g. MOVE) with those containing more complex concepts such as RUN or FLY (both of which refer to a particular kind of motion). If comprehension involves lexical decomposition, the latter should take longer to process. Most studies, however, have failed to find any differences, and some have found the reverse of the expected result: reaction times to complex concepts were shorter than to concepts defined using fewer features (Bierwisch and Schreuder 1992; Fodor et al. 1975).

Developmental studies also fail to provide support for the notion of semantic primitives. As pointed out by Taylor (1989), the semantic feature hypothesis predicts initial overextension followed by contraction, in discrete steps, of category boundaries (as the learner adds new features); the categories the child uses during the overextension phase should be similar to adult superordinate categories. Neither of these predictions is confirmed by developmental data. Early usage is often characterised by *underextension*, which is followed by a period of gradual extension and contraction during which usage at category boundaries oscillates while the category centre remains stable. This developmental pattern is consistent with the predictions of prototype theory but not of semantic feature theory. Furthermore, children's first words rarely express primitive notions. On reflection, this is hardly surprising, since 'complex' notions – those expressing meanings defined by a combination of features – tend to be more concrete and hence evoke richer imagery (cf. MOVE and FLY, TOOL and HAMMER, CONTAINER and BOTTLE).

3.2 Perceptual primitives

The semantic primitives approach, then, though it may initially seem quite promising, turns out to be unworkable. This brings us back to the question of how we come to have concepts in general, and spatial concepts in particular. If they are not innate, they must be learned from experience – but how? The traditional empiricist answer is that complex concepts are constructed out of simpler concepts which ultimately derive from sensorimotor experience. Is this solution at all feasible?

Most cognitive scientists would argue that it is not. The following quotation from Fodor et al. (1980) sums up the prevailing views on the matter quite well:

> It's thus important to emphasize that the Empiricist version of TSP [The Standard Picture, i.e. semantic decomposition theory] is *not* plausible. If there are few convincing examples of definitions, there are literally *no* convincing examples of definitions which take *prima facie* non-sensory/motor terms into a sensory/motor vocabulary. There is, indeed, no reason to believe even that the definitions we have examples of generally exhibit an epistemically interesting direction of analysis. On the contrary, the 'right hand' (definiens) side of standard examples of definitions does not tend, by and large, to be more sensory/motor than the 'left hand' (definiendum) side. So, for example, the conventional wisdom has it that 'grandmother' means 'mother of father or mother'; 'ketch' means 'two-masted sailing vessel such that the aft (or "mizzen") mast is stepped forward of the helm'; 'bachelor' means 'unmarried man'; 'kill' means 'cause to die', etc. It's hard to discern a tendency toward the sensory/motor in these examples, and these examples are quite typical. Surely, no one could seriously argue that words like 'mother, father, mast, vessel, cause, die, married and man', all of which occur in the definiens, are somehow closer to transducer language, than, say, 'grandmother', 'ketch', 'kill' or 'bachelor' are. (Fodor et al. 1980: 268)

Fodor et al. are right, of course, when they argue that, for the overwhelming majority of lexical concepts, verbal definitions are no nearer to sensorimotor experience than the terms defined. However, there is no reason to think that the semantic representations of lexical concepts are verbal definitions. Let us take one of their own examples: the meaning of *ketch*. While it is true that terms such as *mast* or *vessel* are no more 'perceptual' than the term defined, it does not follow that our mental representation of the concept KETCH does not include a perceptual component. In fact, I would argue that a visual image is a central part of the meaning of the term. One acquires the concept that goes with the phonological label *ketch* by seeing exemplars and extracting their shared properties. A verbal definition is helpful to the extent that it draws attention to the relevant characteristics, but it is neither necessary (since it is possible to acquire the concept without ever hearing the definition) nor sufficient (a person who had been presented with a definition but never seen the real thing would have an underspecified representation of the concept).

One might argue that knowing the meaning of *ketch* involves much more than knowing what it looks like: equally relevant are the knowledge that it is a type of ship (and hence that it is used for travelling over water), an understanding of how it moves, and so on. While these observations are undeniably true, they would only constitute a valid objection if this kind of knowledge could not be represented using symbols derived from perceptual experience.

Up until the mid-1980s, most cognitive scientists regarded it as axiomatic that indeed it couldn't: perceptual representations were considered as no more than attenuated copies of sensory states produced by external stimulation, and hence in principle incapable of representing abstract concepts of any kind.

However, recent work in cognitive linguistics (Johnson 1987; Lakoff 1987; Lakoff and Johnson 1980; Langacker 1987, 1991a, 1991b; Rudzka-Ostyn 1988; Talmy 1983, 1985), cognitive psychology (Barsalou 1993, 1999; Barsalou et al. 1993; Gibbs and Colston 1995; Jones and Smith 1993; Mandler 1992; Paivio 1986), and artificial intelligence (Regier 1996) shows that symbol systems grounded in perceptual experience are much more powerful than previously believed. Their new power derives from shedding two traditional assumptions about sensory experience: the ideas that perceptual images are mental pictures, and that they are unstructured holistic representations.

The impetus for the new work came from a number of studies of perception which showed that certain neurons in the brain respond selectively to different aspects of the stimuli perceived. For example, some neurons in the visual cortex respond to the presence of a line irrespective of its length, orientation or position; other neurons fire only in response to stimuli with a specific orientation; and so on. If different aspects of a visual image (shape, orientation, colour, movement etc.) are processed separately during perception, there is no reason to assume that they must be accessed together during conception. This implies that perceptual images can be partly indeterminate, and that they are componential.

Barsalou (1999) provides an excellent synthesis of much of the new work on perceptual symbol systems and argues that knowledge derived from perception can support a fully blown conceptual system with the capacity to represent abstract concepts, combine concepts productively, and produce inferences. In his framework, a perceptual symbol is a record of the neural activity that occurs during perception. Patterns of activation in the sensorimotor areas of the brain are captured in the association areas during perception. In conception, the association areas partially reactivate sensorimotor areas to simulate the sensorimotor experience. Thus, concepts are mental simulators which can give rise to slightly different simulations on different occasions.

As suggested earlier, these new perceptual symbols are componential (different aspects of concepts are represented separately) and schematic (indeterminate with respect to some properties). Another important characteristic is that they are multimodal: they combine information from the various sensory modalities, proprioception and introspection. Introspective information (i.e. information about the conceptualiser's own mental states) is particularly important, as it provides the foundation for the development of abstract concepts. Consider, for example, Barsalou's account of how the concept TRUTH could be implemented in a perceptual symbol system. To represent the fact that a particular statement is true, the conceptualiser produces a simulation of the event that it describes and compares it with his own perception of the event; if the two structures map onto each other, the sentence can be described as true. While performing the comparison, the conceptualiser develops perceptual symbols for the simulation of the event, the process of comparing the simulation to the perceived scene, and the outcome of the comparison (a successful mapping). If the process is repeated on a number of occasions, a simulator will develop for the concept TRUTH: that is to say, the conceptualiser will have learned to simulate the experience of successfully mapping a simulation onto a perceived situation (Barsalou 1999).

This proposal, though admittedly sketchy and speculative, shows that it is possible to represent abstract concepts using experientially grounded symbols, at least in principle, and hence the pessimism expressed by Fodor and others is unfounded. A different, but not necessarily incompatible approach to abstract concepts is to be found in the work of many cognitive linguists, who have argued that these concepts are understood at least partly in metaphorical terms, that it to say, by importing structure from more basic domains. For example, it has been suggested that ANGER is understood partially through the metaphor ANGER IS THE HEAT OF A FLUID IN A CONTAINER: hence, when people get angry, we say that they *get hot under the collar*, that *their blood boils*, that they *get all steamed up*, and eventually, they may *explode* (Kövecses 1986; Lakoff 1987; Lakoff and Johnson 1980; Matsuki 1995). Other linguists have proposed that mental processes such as understanding and reasoning are understood in terms of more accessible concepts such as SEEING and PHYSICAL MANIPULATION (see Jäkel 1995; Lakoff and Johnson 1980).

It seems, then, that the idea that meanings are built up from perceptual primitives does offer a feasible solution to the problem of how we come to have concepts. Clearly, many problems remain to be solved and many important details still need to be elaborated. However, the considerable progress that has already been made suggests that this is a very promising avenue of research. It should also be emphasised that, other things being equal, there are several reasons for preferring theories which use perceptual primitives over those which appeal to amodal systems. First, using perceptual primitives solves the symbol-grounding problem. Theories which postulate amodal symbols must provide an account of how these are mapped onto perceptual states and entities in the world.[11] This problem never arises in a system which uses perceptual symbols, since these are built bottom-up from perceptual states. Secondly, using perceptual primitives dispenses with the need to postulate biologically implausible innate structures with no obvious evolutionary antecedents. Perceptual systems have been around for a long time and the neurological structures that they use provide an obvious source of building blocks for higher-order concepts. Last but not least, perceptual primitives, while constraining learning in highly specific ways, offer enough flexibility to support the wide variety of lexical concepts that we encounter in the world's languages.

All this said, the proof of the pudding is in the eating, and a fitting way to conclude this chapter is to ask whether a system equipped only with perceptual structures and a general learning mechanism could acquire the locative terms of the various languages that have been discussed earlier. The ultimate test of the proposal would be to design a computer model which had the basic perceptual structures built in and see how well it would perform on spatial categorisation tasks. As it happens, such a model has been built, thus offering us an opportunity to evaluate the proposal.

4. Lexical learning in a constrained connectionist network

The model alluded to was developed by Regier (1996). Regier used an approach he calls 'constrained connectionism', which differs from ordinary 'unconstrained' (i.e. parallel distributed processing) approaches in that it contains structures dedicated to specific tasks. The structures bias the learning process, making some things easy and others very difficult or impossible to learn. However, the constraints are perceptual, not linguistic; and unlike the innate structures postulated by generative linguists, they are independently motivated.

Regier's model contains three built-in structures: an orientation-combination structure, which extracts various orientational features; a map-comparison structure, which detects quasi-topological features such as contact and inclusion; and a motion-trajectory structure, which parses events into source, path and goal and calculates the overall path of the trajector. The first two structures are loosely motivated by their functional similarity to known neural structures (orientation-sensitive cells, topographic maps of the visual field, cells with centre-surround receptive fields); the motivation for the motion trajectory structure is less direct (see Regier 1996). All three structures are embedded in a traditional connectionist network.

Regier presented the network with 'movies' consisting of sequences of trajector–landmark configurations. Some of these depicted stationary configurations; in others, the trajector moved relative to the landmark. Each 'movie' was paired with a linguistic label (*in*, *on*, *through* etc.). The network was trained using English, German, Russian, Japanese and Mixtec terms (on different runs) and then tested on a novel set of movies.

The results were very encouraging. The network was able to learn to respond with the appropriate terms in all five languages and showed excellent generalisation to novel configurations. As we have seen earlier, the languages used in the experiment carve up the semantic space in different ways, and hence the network had to learn to 'attend' to different features of the input, depending on the language. For example, consider the terms for 'above' and 'on' relationships. In English, the relevant feature is contact: if the trajector touches the landmark, it is *on* it; otherwise, it is *above* the landmark. In Mixtec, the contrast hinges on the orientation of the landmark: *šini* 'head' is used when the landmark is vertical and *sɨkɨ* 'animal back' when it is horizontal, regardless of whether there is contact or not. German requires its speakers to pay attention to both features: *auf* is used when the trajector is in contact with a horizontal surface, *an* when it is in contact with a vertical surface, and *über* when there is no contact. Finally, Japanese has only one term, *ue ni*, which is insensitive to either distinction. The network, like a human child, learned whichever system it was exposed to. The built-in perceptual structures offered enough constraints to make learning possible and enough flexibility to allow learning systems based on different principles.

It should be emphasised that Regier's network is not a realistic model of human spatial cognition. The structures built into the model are only loosely motivated by known neural structures, the relationship being one of analogy rather than exact correspondence. The network did not have to solve all the complexities discussed earlier in this chapter: its input was highly idealised (the objects in the movies were simple, two-dimensional figures labelled 'trajector' and 'landmark') and it did not have to deal with the additional complications posed by polysemy or virtual boundaries. Furthermore, the network lacked the prelinguistic knowledge that we know children bring to the acquisition task, and it had no social experience (it did not interact with other agents). However, the fact that it was able to extract the relevant features of spatial configurations and succeeded in generalising them to novel instances shows that it is possible to build semantic representations from perceptual primitives, and thus offers indirect support for the conjecture that this is what children do as well.

5. Conclusion

A common argument for the innateness of syntax is that children could not learn certain aspects of the grammar of their language through any known learning process, and therefore at least some syntactic knowledge must be innate. This is an example of what Dawkins (1986) calls an argument from incredulity: I don't see how children could possibly learn syntax, and therefore they cannot learn it – it must be innate.

Explaining language acquisition by appealing to innate knowledge does not answer the question of how we came to have language; it just shifts it from an ontogenetic to a phylogenetic level. Saying that the species acquired language through some unknown evolutionary process is not an advance on saying that children acquire language through some unknown learning process. The unlearnability argument was generally accepted partly because the generative tradition in psycholinguistics has tended to overestimate children's grammatical accomplishments (that is to say, impute to them knowledge that they do not have: cf. Dąbrowska 1997) and underestimate their lexical accomplishments (what is actually involved in learning a word) – thus sending several generations of generative linguists on a dubious quest for Universal Grammar.

I hope to have demonstrated that locative terms, and by implication, lexical concepts in general, must be learned, and learning them is no easy matter. It requires some rather sophisticated detective work, including the ability to project virtual boundaries which are not given in the input. In spite of this, children begin to use the spatial terms of their language very early, and their usage is overwhelmingly correct. This suggests that the early and largely error-free development of grammatical knowledge need not be taken as evidence that it is innate: if children are intelligent enough to learn lexical concepts, they might be intelligent enough to learn grammar as well. In fact, considering the complexity and sheer magnitude of the task (at least partial entries for 60,000 words!), the reader might well conclude that learning syntax is the easy part.

Of course learning grammar is different from learning vocabulary: grammar isn't just about the relationship between form and meaning, but also about how smaller units are put together to form more complex expressions. In the following chapters, I will address some of these differences, but I will also argue that the differences have been overemphasised. We will see that learning grammar resembles lexical development in many important respects, and conversely, that learning words entails a fair amount of syntactic learning.

Notes

1. For example, Miller and Gildea (1987) found that children participating in vocabulary-building programmes at school produced sentences such as *I was meticulous about falling off the cliff* and *Our family erodes a lot*. They were puzzled by these until they consulted the dictionary that the children were using and learned that *meticulous* means 'very careful' and *erode*, 'to eat out'.

2. Presumably, one can use both forms when describing a currently invisible dog: in this case, the speaker would assume the vantage point of a virtual observer. Virtual observers also figure in the semantics of English expressions. Imagine you are describing a family photograph depicting Grandpa Watkin standing beside Granny Watkin. You can say either *Grandpa Watkin is to the left of Granny Watkin* or *Grandpa is on Granny's right*, depending on whether you are assuming the point of view of the person looking at the photograph or of the people in it.

3. This is not an isolated example of such projection: other 'hilly' topographic adverbs also have extended senses relating to body parts (Casad, personal communication).

4. The following discussion is an adaptation and extension of a similar discussion in Bowerman (1993, 1996). I would like to acknowledge my debt to her.

5. Historically, Mixtec locatives seem to have arisen through metaphorical projection of body-part terms onto inanimate objects. It is unclear, however, to what extent the metaphor is still alive in speakers' minds today. Brugman maintains that speakers do indeed project body-part structure onto inanimate objects; others (e.g. Levinson 1994; Regier 1996) have argued that the relationship between the body-part and locative senses is purely diachronic, and that speakers choose the appropriate locative term by performing a complex analysis of the shape of the ground object. However, Levinson studied a different language – Tzeltal – whose body-part locatives are subtly different from those of Mixtec. Unlike Mixtec, the Tzeltal system is object internal, not relational: that it to say, the body-part construction specifies that the figure is located at a particular part of the ground, regardless of the ground's orientation (for example, 'at the ear of the table', i.e. its corner), not that it is located in a particular position relative to the ground located in a larger reference frame (e.g. on top of/underneath the table). Thus, 'at the butt of the bottle' always means 'at the end opposite the neck', even when the bottle is upside down or horizontal. Furthermore, when Tzetzal body-part terms are applied to inanimate objects, they refer to object parts, and cannot be projected to regions around them: 'at the nose of' means 'contiguous to a pointed part of', not 'in front of'. (To talk about regions, speakers must use other systems: relational nouns or a geocentric system – see below.) Regier's argument is based on the fact that his connectionist network learned Mixtec locatives in spite of the fact that it knew nothing about body parts. This shows that it is possible to use body-part locatives appropriately without performing the metaphorical mapping; but of course it does not prove that this is what humans do. Note, too, that the point that the data was used to illustrate remains valid whatever the synchronic status of the metaphor: the Mixtec locative system is fundamentally different from the systems employed by familiar European languages.

6. Relative systems, incidentally, also differ in how they project orientations from objects which do not have an inherent front or back. If an English speaker stands facing a tree with a ball between her and the tree, she would say that the ball is *in front of the tree*: the tree's front is the side that is facing the observer. In some other languages – for example, in Hausa – the tree's front is the side facing in the same direction as the observer, so the ball would be *behind the tree*.

7. Bavin does not tell us what the correct adult response would have been in each case, so we do not know whether the children had acquired the target system. It is clear, however, that they were not operating with concepts corresponding to the English prepositions *in*, *on* and *under*.

8. The word-learning task requires participants to learn a new phonological form, so it could be argued that it is in fact more difficult than the 'uncle' task. To see if this affected performance, Markson and Bloom introduced

a new non-lexical condition which required participants to store a lexical form: participants were told that one of the unfamiliar objects 'came from a place called Koba'. Performance was still good, and after a month's delay, there were no significant differences between recall in this condition and the 'koba' and 'uncle' conditions.

9. The social stereotypes enshrined in the word *spinster* are no longer applicable, which is why the term is becoming obsolete. On the other hand, we have a new term which, according to the traditional feature analysis, should be contradictory: *bachelor girl*.

10. See Lakoff (1987) for an in-depth discussion of how our understanding of the concepts FATHER and MOTHER is bound up with knowledge of complex domains such as biological parenthood, nurturance, legal responsibilities etc.

11. This is another aspect of the linking problem discussed in Chapter 6.

8 On rules and regularity

1. Words and rules

As we saw in the last chapter, learning the basic lexical units of a language is a daunting task. But to know a language, one must also be able to produce and understand larger expressions: morphologically complex words, phrases and sentences. Such complex structures can be assembled by combining smaller units according to the rules of grammar.

Intuitively, grammatical rules and words seem to be very different kinds of things. Words are form–meaning pairings, learned by associating stretches of sound with meanings. Rules, on the other hand, are procedures for manipulating words – or rather, classes of words. A simple, and rather hackneyed, example is the rule for forming the past tense of regular English verbs, which adds the *-ed* suffix to the verb stem. Linguists usually represent this procedure with a formula such as this:

(1)   V [Past] → V + *-ed*

Simple though it is, the past-tense rule is abstract, in that it can apply to any (regular) verb; consequently, unless its application is pre-empted by the existence of a stored irregular form, speakers can use it to produce the past tense of any verb in their vocabulary, and of any new verb that they might encounter.

It is rules which allow us to go beyond the expressions we have actually heard and produce novel forms. Thus, to become competent speakers of their language, children must acquire some mental analogue of rules. And in fact, there is plenty of evidence that they do. Sticking to the English past-tense rule, a classic study conducted by Jean Berko in 1958, and numerous replications by other researchers since then, have demonstrated that children are able to inflect novel verbs in experimental conditions: for example, when presented with a nonsense verb like *zib* they are able to form the past tense form *zibbed.* Outside the laboratory, nearly all children occasionally produce regularisation errors such as *breaked* and *catched*, sometimes after a period of correct production. Until the mid-1980s, nearly everyone agreed that these well-known facts provided direct evidence that children learn symbolic rules of the kind postulated by linguists.

2. The connectionist bombshell

This seemingly unshakeable view was challenged in 1986 by Rumelhart and McClelland, who reported that they had trained an artificial neural network to produce the past-tense forms of English verbs. Their network took phonological representations of verb stems as input and produced phonological representations of past-tense forms as output. It had been trained on a large set of stem–past pairs, and was subsequently tested on a new set of verbs which it had not encountered before.

The network consisted of a set of input units and an identical set of output units, with each input unit connected to each output unit. The entire assembly could be thought of as an extremely simple model of the brain in which the units correspond to neurons and the connections to axons and dendrites. Its most interesting property was that it could learn: the connections varied in strength and could be modified during training.

Rumelhart and McClelland trained the network by presenting it with a pattern of activation representing an English verb stem and allowing it to produce an output – that is to say, a pattern of activation on the output units representing the past-tense form of that stem. The training algorithm then compared the actual pattern of activation of the output units to the target pattern and modified the connection weights so as to minimise the difference. This procedure was repeated many times with all the verbs in the training set until the network was able to supply the correct past-tense forms of most of them.

In the next phase, Rumelhart and McClelland tested the model using the verbs in the original training set as well as a new set of verbs which it had not encountered before. They found that it was able to provide the past-tense form of many (though not all) of the novel verbs – in other words, that it was able to generalise beyond the verbs it had been trained on. Furthermore, the network sometimes regularised the irregular verbs it had learned earlier, producing forms like *catched* and *digged*, even though it had supplied the correct irregular forms before. Thus, in two important respects, the network's behaviour resembled that of human language learners.

As noted earlier, the occasional occurrence of regularisation errors in children's spontaneous speech and the fact that they are able to inflect novel words in an experimental setting have long been considered as direct evidence that children learn symbolic rules of the kind that have been proposed by linguists (e.g. 'add -*ed* to any V'). Such rules make use of abstract symbols, such as noun and verb, and formal operations, such as suffixation, which are specific to language. The apparent ease with which children learn them has been taken as evidence that they are equipped with a powerful learning mechanism dedicated specifically to acquiring language. Rumelhart and McClelland's network used a relatively simple, general-purpose learning mechanism to extract patterns from the input, and produced the same kind of behaviour simply by forming low-level associations between representations, without any explicit rules. This raised the possibility – attractive for some, unpalatable for others – that the rule-like behaviour seen in humans might also be a product of such a general-purpose, 'low-tech' mechanism.

3. The linguists strike back

As critics were quick to point out, there were many problems with this early model (Lachter and Bever 1988; Pinker 1991; Pinker and Prince 1988). The network could learn rules that are not attested in any human language (e.g. 'form the past tense by mirror-reversing the order of segments'), but it could not learn some fairly common patterns (such as reduplication of the stem). It sometimes produced blends which sound extremely strange to human ears (e.g. *membled* for *mailed*, *conflafted* for *conflicted*). Because it only represented phonological properties, it could not handle homophones with different past tense forms such as *lie* 'to recline' (past tense *lay*) and *lie* 'tell lies' (past tense *lied*). It was strongly dependent on phonological similarity, and hence unable to inflect novel regulars which did not resemble regulars in the training set. Most damning of all, critics argued, Rumelhart and McClelland got their model to generalise the regular pattern by manipulating the input. The network was initially trained on just ten verbs, eight of which were irregular. When these had been learned, Rumelhart and McClelland increased the training set to 420 verbs, of which the overwhelming majority were regular. It was this vocabulary discontinuity – or, to be more precise, the fact that it was suddenly swamped by regular mappings – that caused the network to generalise.

Some of these problems were addressed in later models (e.g. Daugherty and Seidenberg 1992; Hare and Elman 1995; Hare et al. 1995; MacWhinney and Leinbach 1991; Marchman 1993; Plunkett and Marchman 1991, 1993). The later models incorporated one or more layers of hidden units between the input and the output units, allowing the network to form internal representations, and hence making it less dependent on surface similarity. They also adopted more realistic training regimes, and some represented aspects of semantic structure, which enabled the network to distinguish homophones.

However, the critics also struck at an idea that lies at the very heart of the connectionist approach to modelling morphological rule learning – namely, the claim that regular and irregular inflections are handled by a single mechanism – by drawing attention to significant psychological and neuropsychological differences between regular and irregular forms (see Pinker 1998, 1999; Pinker and Prince 1992; Prasada and Pinker 1993). As pointed out earlier, children learning English sometimes apply the regular inflection to irregular stems, producing errors like *comed* and *bringed*. On the other hand, errors of the opposite kind – i.e. 'irregularisations' such as *bat* for *bit* (on analogy with *sat*) or *truck* for *tricked* (on analogy with *stuck*) – are exceedingly rare. Likewise, when overgeneralisations are induced during psycholinguistic experiments with adult participants (for example, by forcing them to supply the past-tense form under severe time pressure), regularisation errors are vastly more frequent than irregularisations.

Secondly, irregular verbs are more sensitive to frequency than regulars. In psycholinguistic experiments, reaction times to low-frequency irregulars are slower than reactions to irregular forms of high frequency. Also, when forced to produce past-tense forms very quickly, people tend to make more errors with low-frequency irregulars (Bybee and Slobin 1982). Results for regular past-tense forms are mixed. In some studies (Pinker and Prince 1992; Ullmann 1999) participants reacted equally fast and equally accurately to high-frequency and low-frequency regulars. Other studies, however, do report frequency effects for regulars, although, in English, these were observed only for relatively high-frequency forms (Alegre and Gordon 1999; see also the discussion in Chapter 2, section 3.1.4).

Thirdly, regular and irregular inflections may be differentially affected in various special populations (Marslen-Wilson and Tyler 1997, 1998; Ullman, Corkin et al. 1997). Anomic aphasics and Alzheimer's patients seem to have particular problems with irregularly inflected words, while regular processes are largely unaffected. In contrast, in agrammatic aphasics, Parkinson's patients, and children with SLI the regular system is disrupted, while performance on irregulars remains relatively good.

Finally, some imaging studies (Jaeger et al. 1996; Ullman, Bergida and O'Craven 1997) suggest that different areas of the brain are active when processing regular and irregular inflections. These results, however, are problematic, as it is not always the *same* areas that are associated with the processing of regular verbs on the one hand and irregular verbs on the other in different studies; moreover, not all researchers have found such differences (see Seidenberg and Hoeffner 1998).

4. The dual-mechanism model

We have seen that there is good evidence that regular inflections are different from irregulars in several important ways – although it is worth noting at this juncture that most of the evidence relates to just one morphological subsystem, namely, the English past tense. On the other hand, even die-hard critics of connectionism like Pinker and Marcus acknowledge that artificial neural networks can model some aspects of human linguistic knowledge and are able to generalise previously learned patterns to novel input. These critics argue, however, that the productivity exhibited by network models is fairly limited because it is constrained by phonological similarity: the models generalise a pattern to a novel word when it resembles something they have encountered before. This kind of productivity, Marcus and Pinker suggest, is characteristic of *irregular* processes in human language. They are adamant that connectionist networks cannot adequately model regular inflections, which do not depend on memory for previously encountered forms and can apply to any stem, regardless of its phonological properties. Regular inflections, they propose, rely on a different psychological mechanism: symbolic rules. To explain human behaviour, then, we need two mechanisms: an algorithmic device capable of implementing symbolic rules, which is responsible for regular inflections; and associative memory, which supplies irregular forms and, occasionally, novel forms which resemble irregulars (Marcus et al. 1995; Pinker 1998, 1999).

Thus, the basic premise of the dual-mechanism model is that regular inflections are different because they can apply as a default to any stem. Children are able to learn the regular inflection because they are endowed with a mental mechanism specifically dedicated to manipulating abstract symbols; connectionist models, which lack such a mechanism, cannot acquire a true default.

But is it true that they cannot? This might have been true of the Rumelhart and McClelland model, but not of more recent models which incorporate hidden units. Hidden units, as pointed out earlier, allow networks to form their own representations of the input, which makes them less dependent on surface similarity. Furthermore, connectionist nets are very sensitive to frequency information, and tend to develop stronger representations for patterns which are frequently represented in the input. Because regular inflections apply to more words than irregular patterns, the nodes representing them become very excitable, and hence more likely to become active when a novel stem is presented. Thus, networks can exploit statistical properties of the language to learn the regular inflection.

But this is not good enough for proponents of the dual-mechanism theory, who insist that regularity in the psychological sense has little to do with frequency. It is true that regular inflections tend to apply to more stems than irregular patterns – but this is a consequence, not the cause, of their being regular. Regular inflections become common because they are applied to new words that enter the language, and occasionally to low-frequency irregulars. In other words, they are not regular because they are frequent; they are frequent because they are regular.

What then is regularity in the psychological sense, and how do speakers know that an inflection is regular? Since regular inflections do not depend on access to memory, the theory predicts that *the regular inflection will apply in all circumstances in which memory cannot be or is not accessed*. Marcus et al. (1995) and Pinker (1998) list a number of such circumstances; they are summarised in Table 8.1.

Table 8.1 Circumstances in which memory is not accessed and the default inflection is applied (adapted from Marcus et al. 1995)

Circumstance	Examples
Novel words	*wugs, zibbed*
Low-frequency words	*stinted, eked*
Borrowings	*latkes, cappuccinos*
Unusual-sounding words	*ploamphed, krilged*
Words with irregular homophones	*lied* (cf. *lay*), *hanged* (cf. *hung*)
Words which rhyme with irregular words	*blinked* (cf. *sank*), *glowed* (cf. *grew*)
Names	*the Childs, the Manns*
Truncations	*synched, specs*
Acronyms	*PACs, OXes*
Onomatopoeic words	*dinged, beeps*
Words which are mentioned rather than used	*I checked the article for sexist writing and found three* man*s in the first paragraph.*
Derivation from different category:	
(a) denominal verbs	*spitted* 'put on a spit'
(b) deadjectival verbs	*righted* 'returned to an upright position'
(c) nominalisations	*ifs, ands, buts*
Derivation via different category:	
(a) via noun (V → N → V)	*costed* 'calculated the costs'
(b) via verb (N→ V → N)	*wolfs* 'instances of wolfing'
Derivation via name:	
(a) eponyms	*Mickey Mouses, Batmans*
(b) products	*Renault Elfs*
(c) teams	*Toronto Maple Leafs*
Bahuvrihi compounds	*sabre-tooths, low-lifes*

The clearest example of such a situation is when speakers inflect nonce words like *wug* or *zib* in a psycholinguistic experiment. Since such words are made up by the experimenter for the purpose of the experiment, speakers obviously cannot rely on stored representations of their inflected forms; yet they happily provide regular past-tense forms like *zibbed* and regular plurals such as *wugs*. A similar situation arises in real life when speakers have to inflect low-frequency words or words which have only recently been borrowed from another language; and these, too, usually receive regular endings.

The next three items in the table illustrate the fact that the use of the regular inflection does not depend on similarity to stored exemplars. Speakers apply the regular infection to unusual-sounding nonce words like *ploamph* or *krilg*, for which there are no similar-sounding entries which they could analogise from, and also to verbs that are similar or even identical in sound to well-established irregular forms. Thus, the past tense of *blink* is *blinked*, not *blank*, in spite of the existence of irregular forms like *stank*, *sank* and *drank*; and the past tense of *lie* 'to tell untruths' is *lied*, not *lay*, in spite of the fact that its homophone *lie* 'to recline' is irregular. Hence, *Yesterday I lay on the sofa and lied to my boss.*

The regular inflection is also used with various non-canonical roots, including names, truncations, acronyms and phonological sequences which represent noises or which stand for the word itself rather than its referent – that is to say, when the word is mentioned rather than used. (The sentence *I checked the article for sexist writing and found three* man*s in the first paragraph* means that the speaker found three occurrences of the word *man*, not three adult male human beings pressed between pages 1 and 2: the form *man* refers to the word, not its referent.)

Finally, the regular inflection is used with several categories of derived words. Typically, derived words inherit the grammatical properties of their head, so if the latter is irregular, the derived word, too, is irregular. Thus, the past tense of *overdo* is *overdid* because the past tense of its 'parent', the verb *do*, is *did*; and the plural of *stepchild* is *stepchildren* because the plural form of *child* is *children*. Some derived words, however, cannot inherit their grammatical properties from their parent because they have the wrong kind of parent. For example, a verb derived from a noun or an adjective cannot inherit its past-tense form from the original word because nouns and adjectives do not have past-tense forms. When this happens, the derived word is inflected regularly: the past-tense form of the verb *to spit*, meaning 'to put on a spit', is *spitted* (not *spat*); and the past tense of *to right* 'return to an upright position' is *righted* (not *rote* or *wrote*). This principle also applies to nouns derived from other categories: we speak of *ins and outs* and *ifs and buts*.

Some words have more convoluted – and more interesting – genealogies. Sometimes a verb is derived from a noun which itself was derived from a verb (in other words, the verb has a noun as parent and a verb as grandparent), or a noun might be derived from a verb which was derived from a noun. What is interesting about such cases is that the intervening category (the 'middle generation') makes it impossible for the new word to inherit the inflectional properties of its grandparent. For example, the verb *cost* 'calculate the costs', as in *She costed the proposal*, is derived from the noun *cost* 'the amount of money needed for a particular purpose', which in turn comes from the irregular verb *cost* meaning 'be worth a particular amount of money'. However, *cost* 'calculate the costs' cannot inherit the irregular past-tense form from *cost* 'be worth a particular amount' because it was derived via the noun, and nouns are not marked for tense; consequently, the information about the irregularity of the original verb is not accessible to the processing mechanism, and the default inflection must apply. The same phenomenon can be observed in words derived via a name. The common noun *Mickey Mouse* (meaning 'simpleton') is derived from the name of the Disney character, and since names don't have plural forms, it cannot inherit the irregular plural of its 'grandparent', the common noun *mouse*. Hence, the plural of *Mickey Mouse* is *Mickey Mouses*, not *Mickey Mice*.

The last item on the list – bahuvrihi compounds – is another category of words with a mixed-up family background. Bahuvrihi compounds are compounds which refer to a different class of things from either of the compounded words: for example, a *pickpocket* is a kind of thief, not a kind of pocket or of picking; a *bluebell* is a kind of flower, not a bell, and so on. The plural forms of bahuvrihi compounds in English are always regular, even when the rightmost element is irregular: *sabre-tooths* (not a tooth but a tiger), *low-lifes* (not a life but a person).

As the reader has no doubt noticed, the circumstances listed in Table 8.1 are an odd collection, and some of them are rather exotic. It is also clear that the use of the default inflection in these circumstances does not depend on phonological similarity to stored forms. Therefore, Pinker and Marcus argue, connectionist models, which map phonological representations of stems onto phonological representations of target forms, will not be able to learn to supply the regular inflection when required – unless, of course, they are specifically designed to deal with each of these circumstances individually.

Learners equipped with symbolic rules in addition to associative memory never face this problem. Once they have identified the regular inflection, they apply it as a default in all circumstances except when they have specifically learned to use an irregular pattern. In other words, they don't need any special knowledge about the circumstances in Table 8.1, whether innate or acquired: the whole list falls out naturally from the division of labour between the symbol-manipulation device and associative memory.

Or does it? It is possible that English speakers almost always use -*s* and -*ed* to signal plurality and past tense in the circumstances described earlier because they are equipped with a special mental device which takes over in such circumstances. On the other hand, it is also possible that they apply the regular inflection simply because, in practice, it is the only one available. The irregular past-tense and plural inflections in English are restricted to specific words or very narrow classes of words having certain phonological properties, and hence are not readily extendable to new contexts. Thus, the fact that the 'default' endings are generally used in the special circumstances enumerated in Table 8.1 could be due simply to the lack of any other truly productive pattern in the language.

One of the consequences of the fact that the irregular past tense and plural in English are extremely restricted in their applicability is that the regular inflections apply to the vast majority of types. This introduces another confound: speakers may be more willing to extend the regular inflection to new words simply because it is more frequent, and hence more deeply entrenched in their minds, than any of the irregular patterns.[1] As indicated earlier, according to the dual-mechanism theory regularity in the psychological sense has little to do with frequency; but the fact is that the vast majority of English nouns and verbs *are* regular.

There is yet another confounding factor in addition to the differences in frequency and applicability. In both the plural and the past tense in English, the regular and the irregular inflections rely on different morphological processes. Regular past-tense and plural forms are formed by suffixation, which results in inflected forms which are easily segmentable into a morpheme that signals a type of activity and a morpheme that signals tense (e.g. *play* + *ed*) or a morpheme that designates a type of thing and a morpheme that indicates plurality (*cat* + *s*). Most irregular inflections, in contrast, involve stem changes: *ring–rang, catch–caught, man–men, mouse–mice*. The stem-change mechanism is less transparent, and hence probably more difficult to generalise. Furthermore, because there are several different patterns of stem changes competing with each other, learners are forced to attend to the individual properties of each word, rather than to similarities between words, and this is clearly not conducive to unconstrained generalisation.

To summarise: it is undeniable that regular inflections in English are very different from the irregulars. Unlike the irregular patterns, they are not restricted to a narrowly defined group of stems, but apply 'elsewhere', when no other pattern can be used; and there are sharp contrasts in the way that regular and irregular inflections are acquired, processed and affected in language impairment. What is not clear is whether these differences are a result of the fact that regular and irregular inflections rely on different mental mechanisms, or whether they are attributable to the idiosyncratic properties of the English system of marking past tense and plurality – specifically, to the effect of differences in frequency, applicability, morphological process, or some combination of these factors. Because of these confounds, the English past-tense and plural inflections are simply not very good testing grounds for theories dealing with the mental status of rules.

But the dual-mechanism theory, of course, is not just about English inflections: it is about language in general. The circumstances in which the default inflection applies are supposed to fall out automatically from the organisation of the human capacity for language; hence, the same set of circumstances should be associated with the regular inflection in all languages. What we must do, then, is to test this prediction against data from other languages. Ideally, we would want to find an inflectional system in which there are at least two truly productive endings and in which the regular inflection (i.e. the inflection that speakers use in the circumstances enumerated in Table 8.1) applies to a minority of types. The existence of such 'minority default' systems would show conclusively that regularity does not depend on high type frequency, and hence provide strong evidence in favour of the dual-mechanism theory.

Do we know of any such systems? Marcus et al. (1995) argue at length that in the German plural and past-participle inflections the regular patterns apply to a minority of forms, and offer the Arabic plural as a third example. Unfortunately, the last two of these putative cases are problematic for two reasons. First, it is not clear that the regular patterns in these subsystems do in fact apply to a minority of types (see Boudelaa and Gaskell 2002; Bybee

1995), and in any case, they certainly apply to more types than any one irregular pattern, of which there are a number in both languages. Secondly, like the English past tense and plural inflections, these systems use different morphological mechanisms for regulars and irregulars. The past participle of regular (or weak) verbs in German is formed by adding a suffix (-*t*) and in most cases also a prefix (*ge-*), while most irregular (or strong) past participles, like irregular past-tense and past-participle forms in English, require stem changes (and a different suffix, -*en*, as well). In the case of the Arabic plural, the regular mechanism (the so-called sound plural) simply adds an affix to a stem, while the irregular mechanism (the broken plural) involves modifying the stem in various ways, sometimes quite dramatically. The German plural, on the other hand, appears to be a perfect test case for the dual-mechanism theory, and it is to this inflection that we now turn.

5. The German plural: a minority default?

German has five plural suffixes (-*e*, -*en*, -*er*, -*s* and zero), three of which (-*e*, -*er* and zero) are sometimes accompanied by umlauting of the stem. Clahsen (1999), Clahsen et al. (1992), Marcus et al. (1995), Pinker (1999) and others have pointed out that one of the suffixes, -*s*, has a special status. Like the regular plural affix in English, it is used in the special circumstances enumerated in Table 8.1: with novel words, names, borrowings, onomatopoeic words, acronyms, etc. This, they argue, shows that -*s* is the regular or default ending for the German plural.

What makes the -*s* ending particularly interesting is the fact that it applies to a small number of nouns – only about 4 per cent (Marcus et al. 1995: 227) – which makes it a minority default *par excellence*. Furthermore, most other plurals are also formed by suffixation, thus eliminating the morphological process confound; and at least two other endings are productive – that is to say, they apply to fairly large and open-ended classes of nouns.

Proponents of the dual-mechanism theory have proposed that German-speaking adults and children learning German know that -*s* is the default ending and therefore apply it whenever a plural form cannot be retrieved from memory. They support this claim with three types of evidence. First, children learning German often overgeneralise -*s*; and although they also overgeneralise the other endings, regularisation errors (i.e. overgeneralisations of the regular ending) are 'an order of magnitude' more frequent than irregularisations (Clahsen et al. 1992: 247). Secondly, adult speakers tend to use -*s* with novel words, particularly unusual-sounding novel words (Marcus et al. 1995). Finally, some researchers have argued that -*s* plurals are processed in a qualitatively different way (see Clahsen 1999 and the work cited there).

Hence, the German plural has come to be regarded as the definitive evidence for the dual-mechanism theory, 'the exception that proves the rule' – and also the final blow for connectionist models of inflection. Connectionist networks are strongly dependent on frequency and consequently, say the 'dualists', they are unable to learn to freely generalise an infrequent pattern. Furthermore, since they have no default mechanism to fall back on when memory cannot be accessed, they would be unable to apply the regular ending in the special circumstances listed in Table 8.1, unless they were specifically trained or actually hard-wired to deal with every single circumstance individually (Marcus et al. 1995).

It should be pointed out at this juncture that the claim that connectionist networks are unable to learn a minority default is actually incorrect, as shown by network simulations described by Hare et al. (1995), Plunkett and Nakisa (1997) and Pulvermüller (1998). However, it is true that systems of this kind are more difficult for networks to learn; and clearly, networks trained on phonological representations of stem–past or singular–plural pairs cannot 'know' that conversions, words which are mentioned rather than used etc., all require the default ending, even when homophonous with words that take irregular inflections. We will return to these and other problems with network models later in this chapter; in this section, I focus on the problems that the German plural poses for the dual-mechanism theory.

First, the evidence that German speakers treat *-s* as the default is far from conclusive. Let us begin with the language acquisition data. Clahsen et al. (1992) report that in their sample, the overgeneralisation rate for *-s* (25 per cent) was somewhat higher than the corresponding figure for *-en* (22.5 per cent) and 'an order of magnitude' higher than overgeneralisation rates for *-e* and *-er* (2.73 per cent and 0.95 per cent, respectively). This finding is at odds with other studies of the acquisition of plural marking in German, which report that *-en* and *-e* overgeneralisations are much more frequent than *-s* overgeneralisations, particularly in younger children (see Behrens 2001, submitted; Ewers 1999; Gawlitzek-Maiwald 1994; Köpcke 1998; Mills 1985; Park 1978).[2] Moreover, on closer scrutiny, it emerges that the high figure for *-s* overgeneralisations was arrived at by using a non-standard method of calculating overgeneralisation rates. These are usually computed by dividing the number of overgeneralised forms by the number of opportunities for overgeneralisation, that is to say, the number of plural forms that require some other affix. Clahsen et al. calculated what we might call relative overgeneralisation rates: for each affix, they divided the number of overgeneralised forms with that affix by the total number of forms (overgeneralisations and correctly inflected stems) with that affix. Thus, the figure they cite does not mean that *-s* was used with 25 per cent of the words that required some other affix, but that 25 per cent of all *-s*-suffixed plurals in their data were overgeneralisations. This shows that *-s* overgeneralisations are quite frequent relative to the frequency of this affix. However, if we use the more common method of calculating overgeneralisation rates, the figure for *-s* drops to 1.9 per cent, which is rather similar to the overgeneralisation rate for *-e* (1.2 per cent) and much lower than that for

-en (11.7 per cent). In other words, *-s* overgeneralisations are more frequent than we would predict on the basis of the frequency of the affix alone, showing that frequency is not the *only* factor determining overgeneralisation rates; they are not, however, more frequent in any absolute sense.

In fact, overgeneralisation rates for *-en*, the most frequent affix, are very high whichever method we use to calculate them: in Clahsen's own corpus, the relative overgeneralisation rate for *-en* is 22.5 per cent – almost the same as that for *-s*. Clahsen et al. do not regard this as a problem; in fact, they manage to turn it into an argument in favour of the dual-mechanism theory, arguing that children overgeneralise *-en* because they *think* it is the default ending. As evidence for this, apart from the high overgeneralisation rates, they point out that regular plurals do not occur inside compounds,[3] and the children in their sample who had high overgeneralisation rates for *-en* tended to leave it out in compounds, even when the adult form contained a plural marker. For example, instead of saying *Dose-n-öffner* 'can-s-opener', *Bauer-n-hof* 'farmer-s-yard', *Küche-n-fenster* 'kitchen-s-window', their subjects said *Dose-öffner*, *Bauer-hof* and *Küche-fenster.* However, there are some serious problems with this argument. First, the children did not invariably leave *-en* out in compounds: in fact, they supplied it most of the time. Secondly, the *-en* in compounds does not necessarily have a plural meaning: note, for example, that *Bauernhof* is prototypically a yard belonging to a single farmer, not several farmers; likewise, *Küchenfenster* is a window in a kitchen, not kitchens. This suggests that the *-en* in compounds is not a plural marker, but either a historical residue or a linking morph inserted for phonological reasons (cf. Wegener 1999). Last but not least, the finding that children are particularly prone to overgeneralise the plural marker which they leave out in compounds has not been confirmed by other researchers (see Gawlitzek-Maiwald 1994).

The claim that German adults treat *-s* as the default is equally problematic. It is true that speakers tend to use *-s* more often with nonce words than with real words. However, they do not apply it indiscriminately to all, or even most, novel forms. In Köpcke's (1988) experiment, for example, *-s* plurals accounted for only 17 per cent of the responses. Furthermore, speakers used different affixes with different nonce words, depending on the words' gender and phonological make-up: for example, they preferred *-en* with feminine nouns ending in *-ung* and *-schaft* and masculine nouns ending in schwa, *-e* with masculine nouns ending in *-ling*, *-s* with nouns ending in a full vowel, and so on. By and large, the likelihood of a particular plural marker appearing after a particular nonce word depended on how frequently that marker occurred with real words similar to the nonce word (i.e. real words with the same endings, the same number of syllables, and so on). Other researchers (e.g. Gawlitzek-Maiwald 1994) have obtained similar results. Thus, nonce-word experiments show that German speakers are aware that each of the five plural affixes has a different domain of application, and that they apply the affixes accordingly.

Another source of evidence for the special status of -*s* comes from two psycholinguistic experiments tapping speakers' performance online, i.e. while they are actually processing plural forms. The first of these, by Clahsen et al. (1997), found that people processed high-frequency irregular nouns faster than low-frequency irregulars while no such differences were found with regular nouns. The second, by Sonnenstuhl et al. (1999), used the cross-modal priming technique to investigate the effect of singular versus plural primes on lexical decision tasks involving singular nouns. In experiments using this technique, people are asked to decide as quickly as possible whether a visually presented target (in this case, a singular noun) is a word. It is well known that reaction times are shorter when participants hear a related word (called a prime) immediately before seeing the target, and the experimenter can vary the kind of prime and measure the effect on reaction times to the target word. Sonnenstuhl et al. used two kinds of prime: the noun stem itself and the plural form of the noun. Their results showed that a plural form with -*s* was as good a prime for the singular as the singular form itself (reaction times to a singular form like *Karton* 'box' were the same when it was preceded by *Karton* or by *Kartons*); but for -*er* plurals, the singular was a better prime than the plural (participants reacted faster when *Kind* 'child' was preceded by *Kind* than when it was preceded by its plural *Kinder*). The authors' interpretation of this result is that regulars, but not irregulars, are morphologically decomposed during processing: in other words, when processing regular nouns, speakers obligatorily access the stem form and hence react as if they had actually heard the stem.

Several researchers have pointed out various problems with these experiments, some methodological and some pertaining to the interpretation of the results (Drews 1999; Sereno et al. 1999). Perhaps the most serious problem is that both studies compared -*s* with -*er*, the one plural affix which everyone agrees is not productive. Of all the German plural affixes, -*er* is the most restricted in applicability (it is used only with strong masculine and neuter nouns) and the least predictable in distribution, so each -*er* plural must be stored in the lexicon. It is the only affix which was almost never used by subjects in Köpcke's (1988) nonce-word production task, and in an acceptability judgement study conducted by Marcus et al. (1995), most nonce words with -*er* were judged to be the least acceptable of all affixed plurals. Finally, -*er* is very rarely overgeneralised by children (Behrens submitted; Ewers 1999; Gawlitzek-Maiwald 1994; Köpcke 1998). Thus, the differences between -*s* and -*er* could be due to the special characteristics of -*er* rather than the properties of the default plural. To test the predictions of the dual-mechanism theory, it would have been much more appropriate to compare -*s* with the more productive affixes (-*en* and -*e*).

Yet another problem with treating the German -*s* as a default analogous to the English -*s* plural is that, unlike its English counterpart, the German ending does not invariably apply in all the circumstances in Table 8.1. One systematic exception, acknowledged by Marcus et al. (1995), is bahuvrihi compounds, which take whichever plural ending is required by the rightmost element: for example, the plural form of *Großmaul* 'big mouth, braggart' is not **Großmauls* but *Großmäuler* because the plural of *Maul* 'mouth' is *Mäuler*. Another obvious exception is rare words: since *-s* applies to only 4 per cent of German nouns, the vast majority of all nouns, rare or frequent, take other plural affixes.

In the remaining circumstances, *-s* is the usual ending, but it is not the only option, a fact which raises serious doubts about the viability of the dual-mechanism explanation. Consider plural marking on borrowings, for example. Marcus et al. (1995), citing Köpcke's (1988) data on recent borrowings, point out that about 50 per cent of them take the *-s* plural. They regard this as satisfactory evidence that *-s* is used with borrowings. However, as a matter of arithmetical necessity, if 50 per cent of borrowings take *-s*, the other 50 per cent do not. With such a high proportion of exceptions, plural marking on borrowings should be something for Marcus and his co-authors to worry about, not cite as support for their theory. Note, too, that a large proportion of recent borrowings in German are either English words or words that entered German via English. Since many German speakers, particularly of the younger generation, have a good working knowledge of English, it is not unreasonable to assume that at least some of the new words were borrowed with their English plural. Languages do sometimes borrow foreign plurals along with the singular (cf. English *criteria, alumni, seraphim*), and this is more likely when the suffix also exists in the borrowing language.

Other exceptions include nominalised verbs, which inflect like ordinary nouns (*Essen-Ø* 'meals', from *essen* 'to eat'; *Schau-en* 'shows', from *schauen* 'to look'; *Käuf-e* 'purchases', from *kaufen* 'to buy'), and some nominalised VPs (e.g. *Tunichtgut-e* 'ne'er-do-wells', *Habenichts-e* 'have-nots'). It is not true, therefore, that nouns derived from other categories always take the regular plural. Nor is *-s* invariably used with names and abbreviations. The latter can take *-en* when the final vowel is stressed: for example, the plural of *LPG*, from *Landwirtschaftliche Produktionsgenossenschaft* 'farming cooperative', is either *LPGs* or *LPGen* (Wegener 1994: 269). And although *-s* is strongly favoured with names, the preference is much stronger with surnames than with place names (which often take *-Ø* rather than *-s*), product names (which can take *-Ø*, and sometimes also *-en* or *-e*: see Wegener 1999), or first names (so we have *Emil-e* and *Beate-n* alongside *Emil-s* and *Beate-s*). Finally, *-en* and *-e* plurals are applied in default circumstances when the noun stem ends in *-s* (Indefrey 1999).

To conclude: it is undeniable that *-s* has a somewhat special status among the plural affixes in German. The acquisition and nonce-word data shows that it is generalised more readily than one would expect, considering its low frequency, and it is the usual plural ending in most of the circumstances listed in Table 8.1. Both of these findings call for an explanation.[4] However, the fact that other endings are also found in default contexts raises serious doubts about the explanation put forward by proponents of the dual-mechanism theory; and there is little evidence that German speakers, either child or adult, treat it as a default.

The German plural, then, is certainly not the definitive proof of the dual-mechanism theory that it is sometimes claimed to be. To evaluate the claims made by the theory, we need to examine still more data. In the following sections, we will consider two further inflectional subsystems – the Polish genitive and dative – whose properties, as we shall see, make them particularly interesting test cases.

6. The Polish genitive: an inflectional system without a default

6.1 The system

The Polish genitive marking system is complex and fairly irregular. The genitive singular is normally signalled by one of three endings, *-i* (or its variant *-y*),[5] *-a* or *-u*. Some nouns, however, take adjectival endings (*-ego* for masculines and neuters, *-ej* for feminines), and some do not decline at all (see below). Which ending is actually used depends on several factors. The single most important of these is gender, which can be fairly reliably predicted from the nominative singular form.[6] Feminine nouns almost always take *-i* or *-y* (depending on the phonological properties of the final consonant of the stem), neuter nouns usually take *-a*, and masculine nouns usually take either *-a* or *-u*.

All three endings are readily applied to new words, but each is restricted to a particular subset of nouns. Thus, there is no single suffix which could be considered the regular or 'default' genitive ending for all nouns. However, the feminine and neuter inflections are regular in the sense that they apply to the vast majority of feminine and neuter nouns respectively, and this generalisation can be easily captured by means of two symbolic rules, one which adds *-i/-y* to any stem with the features [N, GENITIVE, FEMININE] and another which adds *-a* to any stem with the features [N, GENITIVE, NEUTER].

On the other hand, the distribution of the two masculine endings, *-a* and *-u*, is fairly arbitrary, although there are some broad regularities. Almost all animate nouns, as well as most nouns which designate tools, body parts, the names of the months, units of measurement and most brand names require *-a*, while nouns designating substances, large objects, locations and abstract concepts generally take *-u*. Some derivational affixes and stem-final consonants and consonant clusters are also associated with one or the other of the two endings (see Kottum 1981; Westfal 1956).[7]

Most of these criteria, however, are not very reliable: there are many exceptions, and they are often in conflict. The noun *tytoń* 'tobacco' designates a substance, and hence should take *-u*; but it ends in an '*a*-friendly' consonant. In this case, the semantic factor gets the upper hand: the genitive form is *tytoniu*, not *tytonia*. In contrast, *mózg* 'brain' designates a part of the body and hence should take *-a*, but the final consonant cluster is strongly associated with *-u*, and in this case, phonology wins. The noun *rozpuszczalnik* 'solvent' provides an example of a case where morphological and semantic criteria are in conflict: the suffix *-nik* favours *-a*, and the noun designates a substance, so according to the semantic criterion, it should take *-u*. In this case, the morphological factor is decisive: the genitive form is *rozpuszczalnika*.

There are some complications in addition to the problems with inanimate masculines. Some nouns require endings which are normally used with adjectives. These include deadjectival nouns such as *uczony* 'scholar' (lit. 'learned'), many native surnames, and foreign names ending in *-e* (e.g. *Goethe, Rilke*). Furthermore, some masculine nouns designating humans decline like feminine nouns, and some nouns, mostly borrowings and foreign proper names, especially those that that do not resemble Polish words, are not inflected at all.

In summary, there is no single default inflection which, unless blocked, applies freely to all nouns, although one could say that feminine and neuter nouns do have default endings, namely, *-i/-y* and *-a* respectively. However, it is not clear which, if any, of the masculine endings is regular. Traditionally, this status is assigned to *-a*, because it is more frequent than any of the other endings, but according to the dual-mechanism theory, regularity in the psychological sense (i.e. default status) does not depend on frequency, and hence we need to consider other criteria.

As explained earlier, one of the central tenets of the dual-mechanism theory is that regular inflections must apply in the default circumstances discussed earlier, so we can use this set of circumstances as diagnostic contexts for identifying the default. If only one masculine ending occurs in these circumstances, we can conclude that it is the regular ending in the technical sense of the theory; otherwise, both endings must be regarded as irregular.

6.2 Genitive masculine forms in default contexts

We must begin by noting that some of the criteria listed in Table 8.1 are either not applicable to the Polish data or do not allow us to distinguish regular and irregular forms. The former include onomatopoeic words (*tik-tak* 'tick-tock', *dzyń-dzyń* 'ding-dong', *kukuryku* 'cock-a-doodle-doo' etc.), which are neuter and hence cannot take a masculine ending,[8] and names and words derived from them, which inflect for case just like ordinary nouns. The latter category includes homophones and rhymes. It is relatively easy to find pairs of lexemes which share the same phonological form but take different endings (2) and pairs of rhyming words which take different endings (3):

(2) a. *tenor* 'tenor (voice)', gen. *tenoru*   *tenor* 'tenor (singer)', gen. *tenora*
    b. *tłok* 'crowd', gen. *tłoku*   *tłok* 'piston', gen. *tłoka*

(3) a. *motor* 'motorcycle', gen. *motoru*   *traktor* 'tractor', gen. *traktora*
    b. *smak* 'taste', gen. *smaku*   *ssak* 'mammal', gen. *ssaka*

The problem is that the mere existence of such pairs does not help us to determine which ending is regular, since both homophony and rhyme are symmetrical relations: for every -*a* noun which has a homophone that takes -*u*, there is an -*u* noun which has a homophone that takes -*a*; likewise, for every -*a* noun that rhymes with an -*u* noun there is an -*u* noun that rhymes with an -*a* noun. The remaining nine criteria, however, can be applied to the Polish genitive, and it is to these that we now turn. (Novel words and overgeneralisations in child language will be dealt with in the following subsections.)

Low-frequency words are equally likely to take either ending. Of the 100 least frequent masculine nouns from a frequency list compiled by Kurcz et al. (1990), 48 take -*a* and 46 take -*u*.

Borrowings usually take -*a* if animate and mostly -*u* if inanimate. Some, however, are not inflected at all, usually because they are in some way non-canonical and hence cannot be assimilated to any of the established templates. For example, *guru* and *urdu* do not sound like Polish nouns, which never end in -*u* in the nominative. *Kamikadze, attaché,* and *dingo* are phonologically similar to Polish neuters, but they are assigned the masculine gender because of their meaning (*kamikadze* and *attaché* prototypically refer to males, and *dingo* inherits its gender from its superordinate *pies* 'dog'). Because of this, the neuter pattern is not applicable and such nouns remain uninflected. The word *boa* is even more interesting. It inherits its gender from its superordinate *wąż* 'snake', which is masculine. Although words ending in -*a* in the nominative are usually feminine, there is a sizeable group of masculine nouns with this ending (e.g. *poeta* 'poet', *artysta* 'artist', *logopeda* 'speech therapist'); these, in spite of their gender, are inflected like feminines. However, such nouns invariably refer to human beings, and because of this semantic discrepancy, the pattern cannot be applied to *boa*, an animal.

The fact that some words, particularly non-canonical-sounding words, are left uninflected is difficult to accommodate in the dual-mechanism theory, according to which the default inflection must apply if there are no similar examples stored in memory which the speaker could analogise from. One could argue, of course, that the default ending in this case is zero. The problem with this is that such non-canonical words are found in all three genders, and they are left uninflected in all cases, not just in the genitive. Following the same logic, we would have to conclude that zero is the default ending for all cases and genders. This would amount to saying that in a richly inflected language like Polish, all the real work is done by associative memory, while the rule system is on hand to add zero – that is to say, do nothing – when memory fails. This is clearly not a very attractive proposal.

Unusual-sounding words: as explained earlier, words which cannot be accommodated in any established template are simply left uninflected.

Words which are mentioned rather than used can occur in the citation form (4), in the form in which they appeared in the text quoted (5), or in the form required by the syntactic context of the sentence in which they are mentioned (6). In the latter case, the usual ending is used: *-a* nouns such as *autor* 'author' take *-a* and *-u* nouns like *rasizm* 'racism' take *-u*.

(4)   *Jak się pisze 'autor'?*
       'How do you spell "autor" (author:NOM)'?

(5)   *Skreśl wszystko od 'autorowi' do 'rasizm'.*
       'Cross out everything from "autorowi" (author:DAT) to
       "rasizm" (racism:NOM).'

(6)   *Nie mogę znaleźć tego drugiego 'autora'/'rasizmu'.*
       'I can't find the other (occurrence of the word) "autor"
       (author:GEN)/"rasizm"(racism:GEN).'

Truncations usually take the same endings as the words from which they are derived – either *-a* or *-u*, depending on the base noun. Thus, *dyr* (from *dyrektor* 'director') and *merc* (from *mercedes*) both take *-a*, like their full forms; while *hasz*, like its base *haszysz* 'hashish', takes *-u*. When the truncated stem is not a noun, the choice of ending is determined by semantic factors. For example, *sam* 'supermarket' is derived from (*sklep*) *samoobsługowy* 'self-service (shop)'. *Samoobsługowy* is an adjective and hence takes the adjectival ending *-ego* in the genitive, which *sam* cannot inherit because it is not an adjective and does not sound like one, so in this case, the usual semantic criteria apply: *sam*, like most nouns designating large objects most naturally conceptualised as locations, takes *-u*.

Acronyms are often left uninflected; but when they do take an ending, it is nearly always *-u*. By this criterion, then, the default ending is *-u*. However, the overwhelming majority of acronyms designate organisations and institutions, i.e. abstract entities, so the choice of ending can be explained by appealing to semantic criteria.

Words derived from a different category: when the noun is derived from a different category (e.g. a verb or an adjective), the choice of ending depends primarily on the morphological process used in the derivation. Most masculine nouns derived from verbs designate either the agent of the action (e.g. *pisarz* 'writer') or the instrument used to perform the action (*zszywacz* 'stapler'), while those derived from adjectives tend to designate individuals possessing a particular characteristic (e.g. *dziwak* 'an eccentric' from *dziwny* 'strange, eccentric'). These nouns invariably take *-a*. As mentioned earlier (see note 7), in such cases semantic and morphological factors work together: derivational suffixes come to be associated with a particular inflectional ending because of the meaning of the words formed with the suffix; and the same inflectional ending is used even when the derived word doesn't have the right semantic properties. On the other hand, nouns derived using the three *u*-friendly affixes, *-unek*, *-ot* and *-izm*, take *-u*. This is also compatible with their semantics, as nearly all nouns with these affixes are abstract.

Nouns can also be derived from words belonging to other categories by removing the verbal or adjectival suffix from the base. Most words derived in this way take -*u*: *bieg* 'a run' from *biegać* 'to run', *wykład* 'lecture' from *wykładać* 'to lecture', *brąz* 'the colour brown' from *brązowy* 'brown (adj.)' etc. Again, this is largely attributable to semantics, since such words tend to designate abstract concepts. However, the use of -*u* with back-formations is not universal: -*a* is used when the resulting noun refers to an animate being (e.g. *psuj* 'a clumsy person who is always breaking things' from *psuć* 'to break', *brutal* 'a brutal person' from the adjective *brutalny* 'brutal') and very occasionally with inanimates as well, especially when the derived noun refers to a concrete object (*gryz* 'a bite' from *gryźć* 'to bite', *skręt* 'roll-up' from *skręcać* 'to twist').

The last possibility for deriving new nouns from other categories involves conversion. This option is available only with adjectives such as *uczony* 'learned' or *służący* 'serving' which can also be used as nouns meaning 'scholar' and 'servant'. Such nouns invariably keep their adjectival inflection.

Words derived via a different category can take both endings, and the choice depends on the morphological processes used in the derivation. If the derived noun is formed with an *a*-friendly affix like -*acz*, -*nik*, or -*arz*, it takes the ending preferred by the affix. For example, the noun *utleniacz* 'oxidant' is derived from the verb *utleniać* 'to oxidise', which in turn was derived from the noun *tlen* 'oxygen', and it takes -*a* in spite of the fact that *tlen* takes -*u*. On the other hand, nouns derived from denominal verbs by back-formation require -*u*. Thus, *dodruku* is the genitive form of the noun *dodruk* 'an additional print run', derived from the verb *dodrukować* 'to print additional copies', which in turn comes from *drukować* 'to print', which is derived from the noun *druk* 'print'.

Bahuvrihi compounds referring to inanimate objects typically take -*u*, although there are many exceptions; animates, on the other hand, always take -*a*. Here are some examples:

(7)   -*u* inanimates:
        piorunochron 'lightning rod' (lit. 'lightning-protect'), gen.
        piorunochronu
        równoległobok 'parallelogram' (lit. 'parallel-side'), gen. *równoległoboku*

(8)   -*a* inanimates:
        kątomierz 'protractor' (lit. 'angle-measure'), gen. *kątomierza*
        trójkąt 'triangle' (lit. 'three-angle'), gen. *trójkąta*

(9)   -*a* animates:
        garkotłuk 'a clumsy cook' (lit. 'pot-break'), gen. *garkotłuka*
        stawonóg 'arthropod' (lit. 'joint-leg'), gen. *stawonoga*

Particularly relevant for our purposes are compounds which have a masculine noun as the rightmost element but require a different ending from the noun. As the following examples illustrate, neither ending has a special status: a compound containing an -*a* noun may require -*u* and vice versa.

(10)   *-a* noun in *-u* compound:
         ząb 'tooth', gen. *zęba*
         trójząb 'trident' (lit. 'three-tooth'), gen. *trójzębu*

(11)   *-u* noun in *-a* compound:
         strajk 'strike', gen. *strajku*
         łamistrajk 'scab' (lit. 'break-strike'), gen. *łamistrajka*

The distribution of genitive masculine endings in the various circumstances which, according to the dual-mechanism theory, call for the default inflection is summarised in Table 8.2. As the summary demonstrates, no single ending is associated with all of these circumstances. In fact, most default contexts allow more than one ending, and which one is actually chosen depends on the properties of the noun. Since, by definition, the use of the default cannot depend on lexical properties of the noun, we must conclude that all masculine endings are irregular.

6.3 Adult productivity with genitive endings

It will be clear from the preceding discussion that the confounds which make the English data difficult to interpret are absent in the Polish genitive marking system: the irregular inflections apply to large and phonologically unrestricted noun classes and, like the regulars, involve suffixation. Thus, the Polish genitive case offers us an excellent opportunity to test a central tenet of the dual-mechanism theory: that symbolic rules are the main mechanism underlying our capacity for producing and understanding novel forms, while associative memory is only marginally productive. If this claim is correct, speakers should be more productive with the feminine and neuter inflections than with the irregular masculines.

This prediction was tested in a nonce-word experiment in which Polish-speaking adults were asked to supply the genitive form of nouns of all three genders (see Dąbrowska 2004: study 1).[9] As explained earlier, there is a strong tendency for masculine nouns designating small, easily manipulable objects to take *-a* and for nouns designating substances to take *-u*. In order to determine whether Polish speakers are sensitive to this distinction, one-third of the nonce words were presented in a sentential context suggesting they referred to concrete objects, e.g.:

(12)   *Ale malutki **figoń**! Nigdy nie widziałem takiego malutkiego _____.*
         'What a tiny **figoń**! I have never seen such a tiny _____.'

and one-third in a context inviting participants to conclude that they designated substances, e.g.:

(13)   *Na przeziębienie najlepszy jest **progonys**. Wypij dwie łyżki _____.*
         'If you've got a cold, **progonys** is best. Take two tablespoons of
         _____.'

Table 8.2 Genitive inflections on masculine nouns in 'default' circumstances

Circumstance	Required ending	Examples
Low-frequency words	*-a* or *-u*	*szańc-a* 'bulwark' *częstokoł-u* 'palisade'
Borrowings	*-u*, *-a* or Ø	*fonem-u, pub-u drink-a, jeep-a guru-Ø, boa-Ø, swahili-Ø*
Unusual-sounding words	Ø	*guru-Ø, boa-Ø, swahili-Ø*
Words which are mentioned rather than used	Form in which the word was originally used, citation form, or whatever ending the noun normally takes	*Nie mogę znaleźć tego drugiego 'autor-a'/ 'rasizm-u'.* 'I can't find the second (occurrence of) "author"/"racism".'
Truncations	*-a*, sometimes *-u*	*merc-a* 'Mercedes' *spec-a* 'specialist' *hasz-u* 'hashish'
Acronyms and abbreviations	Ø or *-u*	*PCK-Ø* (*Polski Czerwony Krzyż* 'Polish Red Cross') *PAN-u* (*Polska Akademia Nauk* 'Polish Academy of Sciences')
Derivation from different category:		
(a) affixation	*-a*, sometimes *-u*	*zszywacz-a* 'stapler' *rasizm-u* 'racism'
(b) back-formation	*-u*, sometimes *-a*	*skręt-u* 'twist', *skręt-a* 'roll-up' (both from *skręcać* 'to twist')
(c) nominalised adjectives	*-ego*	*uczon-ego* 'learned, scholar'
Derivation via different category	*-a* or *-u*	*utleniacz-a* 'oxidant' *dodruk-u* 'additional print run'
Bahuvrihi compounds	*-a* for animates; mostly *-u* for inanimates	*łamistrajk-a* 'scab' ('break-strike') *trójzęb-u* 'trident' ('three-tooth')

The remaining words were introduced as place names, which show no preference for either ending, thus providing a base-line condition.

Of the 24 masculine items, four ended in consonants or consonant clusters which, in the real lexicon, are strongly associated with *-a*, and four in consonants or consonant clusters strongly associated with *-u*. The remaining words had a variety of offsets typical for masculine nouns.

Table 8.3 Response types in the nonce-word production study (%)

Gender	Expected responses	(*SD*)	Gender errors	NOM errors	Other responses
Masculine	93.5	(8.4)	2.6	3.9	0.0
Feminine	92.4	(10.7)	1.5	5.0	1.1
Neuter	65.0	(21.8)	16.1	18.3	0.6

Performance on words of each gender (i.e. the number of expected responses, standard deviations, and the major error types) is summarised in Table 8.3. As we can see, the number of expected responses for masculine nouns is no lower – in fact, slightly higher – than the corresponding figure for feminines. Performance on neuter nouns, on the other hand, was considerably worse than on nouns belonging to the other genders. The unexpectedly high error rates for neuter words were due partly to overgeneralisation of masculine and feminine endings, and partly to use of the citation form (i.e. the nominative). A possible explanation for the poor performance on neuters will be given in section 7 below.

Out of the 60 participants, 57 used both masculine endings productively, and all nouns were sometimes inflected with -*a* and sometimes with -*u*, confirming that both endings are phonologically unrestricted. However, participants preferred -*a* with words which ended in 'a-friendly' consonants, and -*u* with words ending in consonants or consonant clusters which are strongly associated with this ending in the real lexicon: the proportion of -*a* responses was 64 per cent with the former and only 25 per cent with the latter. The respondents showed an even stronger sensitivity to the meaning of the noun as a determinant of the choice of ending. As shown in Table 8.4, they tended to use -*a* when the noun was presented as an object and -*u* when it was presented as a substance. This pattern was found in 57 respondents; the remaining three gave equal numbers of -*a* responses in both conditions. Nouns presented as place names took both endings with equal likelihood, and thus pattern between the two extremes.

It is clear, then, that regularity in the technical sense of the dual-mechanism theory is not a good predictor of productivity. Polish speakers freely generalise the irregular masculine inflections to novel nouns but do not consistently

Table 8.4 Genitive endings on masculine nouns in the Object, Place and Substance conditions (%)

Ending	Object	Place	Substance	Mean
-*a*	77.3	43.8	19.8	46.9
-*u*	21.9	41.9	76.0	46.6
Other	0.8	14.4	4.2	6.5

supply the neuter ending, in spite of the fact that it is regular. Furthermore, speakers are sensitive to both the semantic and the phonological factors affecting the distribution of masculine endings, confirming that the latter are irregular in the technical sense of the dual-mechanism theory.

6.4 Acquisition of the genitive inflection

Thus, a fundamental tenet of the dual-mechanism theory, the claim that regular inflections are always more productive than irregular ones, turns out to be incorrect. This, however, does not necessarily entail that speakers rely on the same mental mechanism to supply both types of inflections: it is possible that two different but equally productive mechanisms are involved. If this were the case, we would expect to find significant differences in the way the two systems are acquired. It is unlikely that two completely independent systems mature at the same time, so we should be able to observe developmental asynchronies between regular and irregular inflections – in other words, children should acquire one system earlier than the other. Furthermore, the rule system and the memory system should show different patterns of development: specifically, we should see a sudden rise in marking rates coinciding with the onset of overgeneralisation errors for regular inflections, and a slow but steady improvement in performance on irregulars. Finally, we would expect to find differences in overgeneralisation rates similar to those observed in English-speaking children: children should overgeneralise regular inflections considerably more often than irregular ones. In this section, we will examine the developmental evidence in order to determine whether any of these predictions are borne out.

Dąbrowska and Szczerbiński (submitted) used the nonce-word task with Polish-speaking children aged from 2;3 to 4;9 and found that all genitive endings are acquired early: even in the youngest group (mean age 2;6), virtually all children were able to use masculine and feminine endings productively (that is to say, apply them to at least one nonce word), and about 72 per cent were productive with the genitive neuter. Moreover, children in all age groups supplied the correct response more frequently with nonce masculines: in fact, as in adults, performance on masculine nouns was slightly better than on feminines (although the difference was not statistically significant) and considerably better than on neuters (where the difference was highly significant); performance on feminines was also significantly better than on neuters (see Figure 8.1).

Thus, the experimental results show no evidence of a developmental advantage for regular inflections. This is confirmed by an analysis of longitudinal spontaneous speech data. Figure 8.2 shows the overall course of acquisition of the genitive inflection in four of the 'Kraków children', Basia, Inka, Jaś and Kasia.[10] The children began to use genitive endings at about 18 months of age. During the immediately following months, they sometimes used the citation

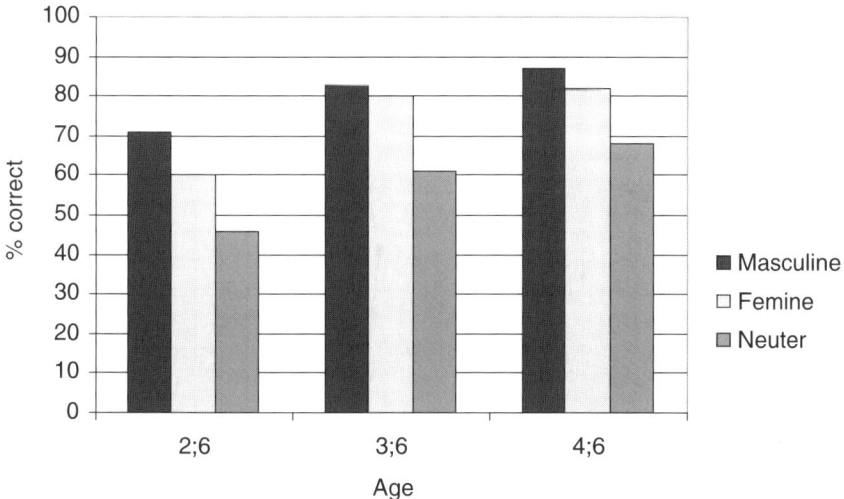

Figure 8.1 Children's performance on the nonce-word production task

form (i.e. the nominative) in contexts requiring the genitive, but such errors gradually disappeared. As can be seen from Figure 8.2, overgeneralisation errors were also relatively infrequent, so from about age 2, the children's use of the genitive is overwhelmingly correct.

Crucially, the pattern of development of the regular and irregular inflections is very similar. Since the masculine and feminine inflections apply to classes of about the same size (44 per cent and 41 per cent respectively of the children's noun vocabulary), the simplest method of measuring growth is to compare the number of noun types used with a particular inflection. Figure 8.3 shows the cumulative number of masculine and feminine nouns used with a genitive ending during the period from emergence (first use) until acquisition (the point at which the child reliably supplies the correct ending) in the four children. It is clear from the figure that both inflections develop at the same rate and show similar patterns of growth: progress tends to be slower at the beginning, then speeds up, but neither inflection shows a sudden 'take-off'. Marking rates on masculine and feminine nouns also show similar patterns of growth (see Dąbrowska 2004: study 2).

We now turn to the children's overgeneralisation errors. According to the dual-mechanism theory, the vast majority of all errors should be regularisations: that is to say, children should overgeneralise the feminine -i/-y and possibly -a (which is the regular ending for neuter nouns as well as an irregular one for masculines). As shown in Table 8.5, -a was indeed overgeneralised more often than -u, but this seems to be better explained as a frequency effect: -a was also 3–4 times more frequent in the children's correct productions, and the relative overgeneralisation rate, which, as explained earlier, factors out the

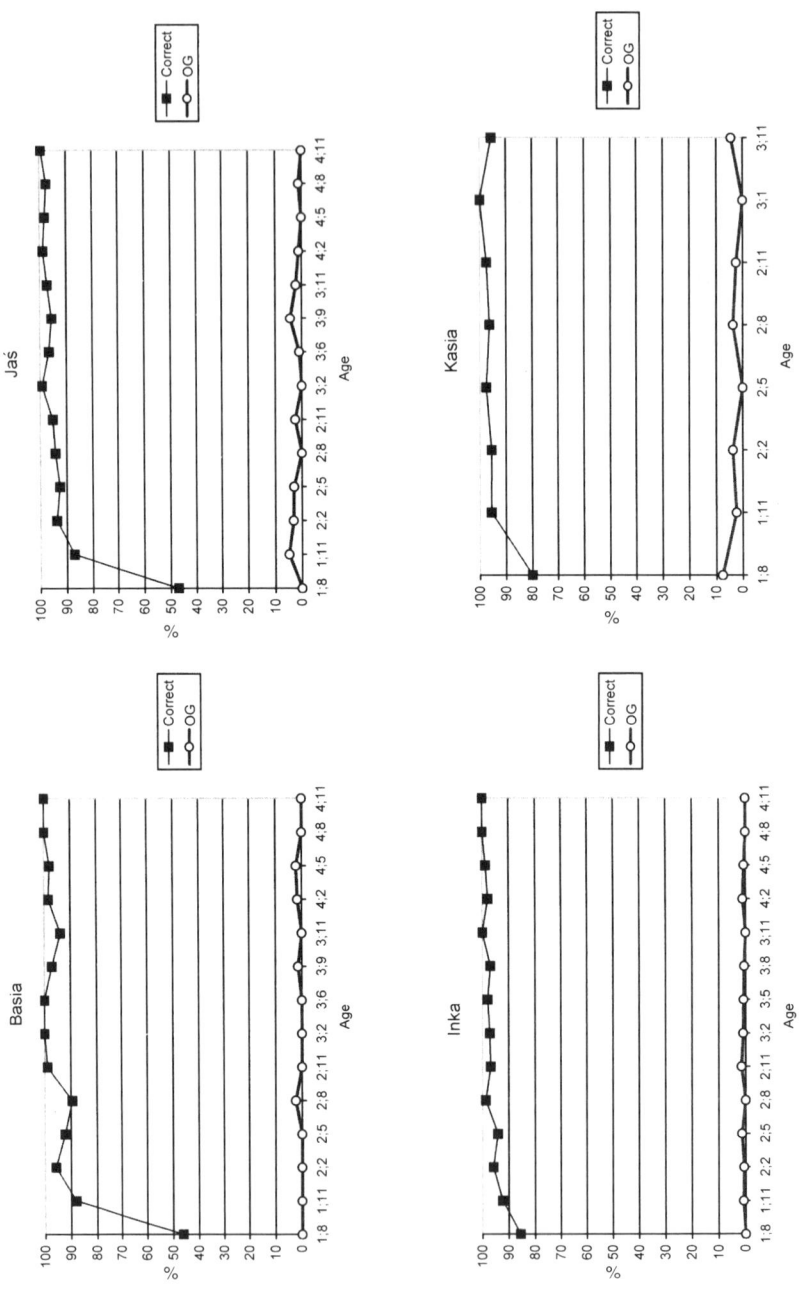

Figure 8.2 Correct uses and overgeneralisations (OG) of genitive endings in the four children.

Note: The ages on the y-axis represent the endpoint of the relevant period. There is no data for Kasia between the ages of 3;1 and 3;11, so the horizontal distances on the y-axis are not proportionate to the time between the data points.

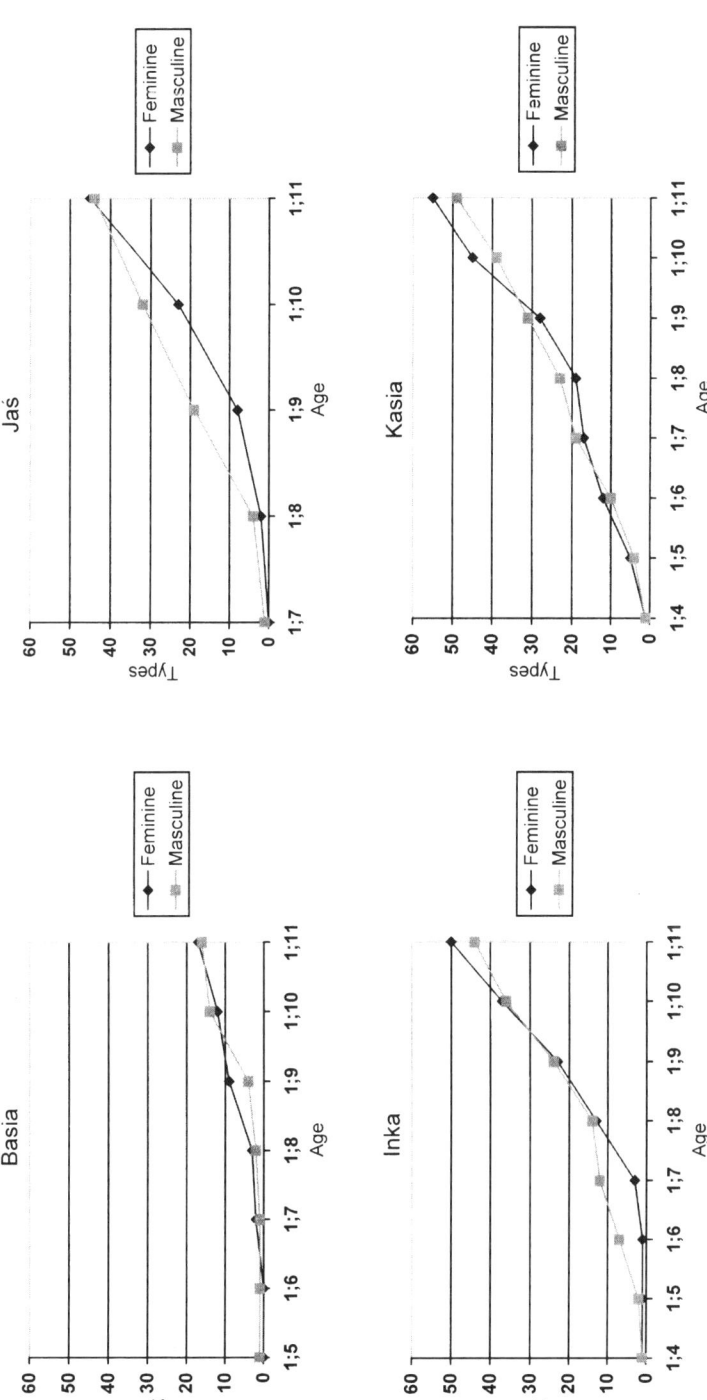

Figure 8.3 Cumulative number of masculine and feminine noun types used in the genitive case

Table 8.5 Overgeneralisation errors in the developmental corpora

Child	Tokens correct			Number of OG errors			AOG rate[a]			ROG rate[b]		
	-a	*-u*	*-il-y*	*-a*	*-u*	*-il-y*	*-a*	*-u*	*-il-y*	*-a*	*-u*	*-il-y*
Basia	387	118	422	2	1	0	0.4	0.1	0.0	0.5	0.8	0.0
Inka	1,050	424	1,187	9	2	3	0.6	0.1	0.2	0.9	0.5	0.4
Jaś	1,137	429	1,264	39	10	1	2.3	0.4	0.1	3.3	2.3	0.1
Kasia	465	119	638	17	15	2	2.2	1.3	0.3	3.5	11.2	0.3
Whole corpus	3,039	1,090	3,511	67	28	6	1.4	0.4	0.1	2.2	2.5	0.2

Notes:

[a] AOG rate (absolute overgeneralisation rate) = overgeneralisation errors as a percentage of the number of noun tokens requiring other affixes

[b] ROG rate (relative overgeneralisation rate) = overgeneralisation errors as a percentage of the total number of tokens with a given affix

effects of frequency, is very similar for both endings. Crucially, the one ending which is uncontroversially regular, namely the feminine *-il-y*, was overgeneralised least often.

The children rarely used any endings in gender-inappropriate contexts: that is to say, they tended to use masculine endings with masculine nouns (though not necessarily the right masculine ending), the feminine ending with feminine nouns, and the neuter ending with neuter nouns. As noted earlier, the gender of most Polish nouns can be reliably predicted from the phonological form of the nominative, so the infrequent occurrence of gender errors suggests that children are sensitive to such cues from a very early age. The picture that emerges, then, is that where there are consistent patterns, children learn them with ease, and overgeneralisation levels are very low; but where the distribution of endings is less predictable, error rates are higher. It should be stressed, however, that these are relative differences: the overall overgeneralisation rates are very low, ranging from 0.5 per cent in Basia to 3.3 per cent in Kasia. Moreover, they remain consistently low throughout the entire period from emergence until age 5;0 (cf. Figure 8.2).

Such low error rates in a system as complex and irregular as the Polish genitive suggest that children's performance relies to a considerable extent on the use of stored forms. A closer analysis of the children's early usage confirms this suspicion. As pointed out earlier, there was a period of about five months after emergence during which children did not always supply the genitive when required: some nouns which should carry the genitive inflection were left in the citation form (the nominative). What is interesting is that during this period of 'inconsistent' usage, genitive and nominative forms were used with different populations of lexemes – that is to say, at any one point in time, each child consistently provided the correct genitive form of some nouns and left others in the citation form. Of course, over time the number of noun types which were consistently inflected in genitive contexts increased, while the number of noun types which were left uninflected got smaller and smaller, so if we consider the entire period, we will find that some nouns were used in both forms in genitive contexts. However, in such cases, all the uses of the citation form generally preceded all the genitive uses. We can see this from Table 8.6, which summarises case marking on all the nouns in each child's transcripts which occurred at least twice in genitive contexts (and hence could have been used in different forms) during the period of 'inconsistent' use. In Basia's transcripts, for example, there are 22 noun lexemes which occurred in genitive contexts during this period at least twice. For eight of the 22 lexemes, there are no attested uses of the nominative form in genitive contexts: that is to say, as far as we know, these nouns were used correctly from the very beginning. Another seven lexemes were never inflected during this period: all the attested forms are nominative. Finally, seven lexemes occurred in both forms. For five of the seven, all the recorded nominative forms precede all the recorded instances of the genitive. For example, there are 21 recorded occurrences of the lexeme *tata* 'dad' in contexts which require the genitive. Fifteen of these are in the nominative case, and they all occurred before the genitive form appeared. The remaining two lexemes were used inconsistently: that is to say, a nominative form occurred at least once in genitive contexts *after* Basia had produced a genitive form of the same noun. There were only six examples of such developmental U-turns in the entire corpus, and four of these were one-off slips (i.e. the child used the nominative after a genitive only once). Thus, during the period when the genitive was not consistently supplied, the children's performance on specific nouns was remarkably consistent, supporting the conjecture that they were acquiring the genitive inflection on an item-by-item basis.

On the other hand, there is also evidence that the children acquired some rule or schema which allowed them to produce inflected forms which they had not heard before. We have already seen that, from about age 2, they marked the genitive virtually 100 per cent of the time, which suggests that they were able to add the inflection to all the nouns in their vocabulary. Furthermore, although overgeneralisation errors were rare, their very existence provides

Table 8.6 Case marking on noun lexemes used in genitive contexts

Child	GEN only	NOM only	All NOM before 1st GEN	At least 1 NOM after 1st GEN	All types with 2+ tokens
Basia	8	7	5	2	22
Inka	32	2	2	1	37
Jaś	19	2	4	1	26
Kasia	25	0	8	2	35

strong evidence of productive use. The distribution of the children's errors also suggests that they were using endings productively: errors occurred most frequently in the most irregular parts of the system, i.e. on masculine nouns.

However, such generalisations are probably quite specific. For example, children might learn to use -*a* with nouns designating animate entities and things that move, or with nouns having certain phonological properties. More general rules (e.g. 'add -*a* to any masculine noun' or 'add -*u* to any inanimate masculine noun') would lead to error, and the fact that errors are rare suggests that children either do not extract such general rules, or if they do, they normally rely on more specific rules in production.

7. The final test case: the Polish dative

The research on the Polish genitive inflection reported in the preceding section brought one unexpected finding: that Polish speakers, adults as well as children, are not fully productive with the neuter ending. This is puzzling, since the genitive neuter inflection is one of the simplest and most regular parts of the case-marking system. Why then do speakers find this relatively straightforward inflection so troublesome? The answer, it seems, is to be found in the peculiar structure of the neuter class.

The majority of neuter nouns are morphologically complex, and most contain one of a few highly productive derivational morphemes. Over a half of all neuter nouns are action nominalisations formed by adding the suffix -*nie* to a verb stem; and another 30 per cent are formed with one of three other highly productive suffixes, -*cie*, -*stwo* and -*ko*. As a result, most neuter nouns are clustered in several small but very crowded regions of phonological space defined by these affixes, and there are relatively few nouns outside these clusters. The masculine and feminine classes, of course, also contain large numbers of morphologically complex nouns; however, none of the clusters is so large, relatively speaking; and there are many nouns distributed fairly evenly throughout the space between the clusters.

If, as suggested above, learners initially extract fairly specific generalisations over clusters of nouns rather than fully abstract rules, then it is possible that in the case of neuter nouns, they might never progress beyond these local generalisations, perhaps because there are not enough nouns outside the clusters to force them to generalise further. This would result in a situation where mature speakers would lack a general rule which applies to all neuter nouns, but would know how to produce the dative forms of words ending in -*nie*, -*stwo*, -*ko* etc. (or, if they pay attention to meaning as well as form, action nominalisations formed with the -*nie* suffix, abstract nouns formed with -*stwo*, -*ko* diminutives, and so on). On the other hand, speakers would extract more general rules in addition to such local regularities for masculine and feminine nouns, which are more evenly distributed in phonological space.

To investigate this possibility, we will look at another adult nonce-word experiment – but one which tested productivity with dative rather than genitive inflections (see Dąbrowska 2004: study 3). There are two reasons for choosing the dative rather than the genitive, or some other inflection, to investigate this issue. First, the dative is the only case in which the neuter ending is different from the case endings characteristic for masculine and feminine nouns as well as the nominative ending, and it is therefore possible to distinguish correct responses, overgeneralisations of masculine and feminine endings, and failures to apply any inflection at all. (As noted in the previous section, the genitive neuter ending, -*a*, is the same as one of the masculine endings, so some of the responses which were coded as correct in the genitive study might in fact have been uses of the masculine ending.) Secondly, using the dative inflection makes it possible to control for a possible confound, namely, type frequency. The neuter class is considerably smaller than the masculine and feminine classes: only about 25 per cent of Polish nouns are neuter, while masculine and feminine nouns make up 41 per cent and 34 per cent of the noun vocabulary respectively. Thus, neuter endings apply to fewer nouns than masculine and feminine endings. There is strong evidence suggesting that type frequency is a major determinant of productivity, so comparing neuter inflections with masculine and feminine inflections would produce ambiguous results: we would have no way of knowing whether any observed differences in productivity were due to class structure or simply class size. However, in the dative case, the feminine class is split between two endings: -*i* (or its variant -*y*), which is used with stems ending in palatalised consonants, affricates and post-alveolar fricatives, and -*e*, which is used with all other feminines; and the number of nouns which take -*e* (18 per cent) is roughly equal to the number of nouns which take the neuter ending.[11]

All four dative endings (the masculine -*owi*, the feminine -*e* and -*il*-*y*, and the neuter -*u*) are regular in the technical sense of the dual mechanism theory: that is to say, all four occur in most default circumstances (see Dąbrowska 2004). Note, however, that, contrary to the theory, both feminine endings are phonologically restricted.

In the experiment, adult native speakers of Polish were given a written questionnaire testing their ability to supply dative endings with nonce nouns. Twenty-four of the nouns (eight masculines, eight feminines and eight neuters) were morphologically simple. There were also 16 complex neuter nouns: eight containing the highly productive nominalising suffix -*nie* and eight containing the diminutive suffix -*ko*, which applies to a much smaller number of nouns. Each item on the questionnaire consisted of a context sentence which introduced the nonce word in the nominative and gave a simple definition of the referent, followed by a test sentence with a blank in a grammatical context which requires the dative. The items containing morphologically complex words also contained an additional clause which gave fairly transparent clues about morphological structure.

The results for the simplex words were similar to those in the genitive study: participants performed close to ceiling on masculine and feminine nouns, but gave the expected response to neuter nonce nouns less than 50 per cent of the time (see Table 8.7). Most errors on simplex neuter nouns involved use of the masculine or feminine endings (which were overgeneralised with approximately the same frequency); but in just under 10 per cent of the trials, participants failed to inflect the nonce word at all, and simply used the nominative form in a grammatical context requiring the dative. This distribution of errors was due to all participants responding inconsistently, rather than some participants consistently using the same incorrect response with all or most of the neuter nouns: in other words, the same respondents used the correct neuter ending with some nouns, the masculine and feminine endings with others, and left some nouns uninflected.

Table 8.7 Response types in the dative study (%)

Condition	Expected	Gender errors			NOM errors	Other errors
		Masculine	**Feminine**	**Neuter**		
Simplex MASC	89.1	–	9.0	0.5	1.1	0.3
Simplex FEM	97.6	1.9	–	0.0	0.0	0.5
Simplex NEUT	46.7	17.9	23.1	–	9.8	2.4
NEUT-*ko*	55.7	28.3	14.7	–	0.3	1.1
NEUT-*nie*	98.4	0.3	0.0	–	0.5	0.8

The figures in Table 8.7 also show that participants supplied the expected ending with morphologically complex neuter nonce words considerably more often than with simplex neuters; in fact, performance on neuters with the nominalising suffix -*nie* was even better than on masculines and feminines. This indicates that speakers do indeed rely on low-level patterns. On the other hand, participants were able to supply the expected ending with morphologically simple neuter nonce words in almost half of the trials, which suggests that they also have a more general rule. This higher-level generalisation, however, is less well entrenched than the more specific patterns, and too weak to be reliably used in production.

It is worth noting that performance on -*nie* nominalisations was much better than on diminutives. This is almost certainly a type frequency effect: as explained earlier, there are about five times as many -*nie* nominalisations as there are diminutives with -*ko* in the real lexicon. Thus, type frequency does matter, although it does not seem to matter as much as phonological coherence: the class of neuter nouns is necessarily larger than the class of neuter nouns ending in -*nie*, yet speakers apparently have a well-entrenched rule for the latter but not the former. Notice, too, that although the masculine ending applies to more than twice as many nouns as the feminine -*e*, performance on masculines was actually slightly worse than on feminines. This suggests that the effects of type frequency are non-linear: robust generalisations require a relatively large number of exemplars; but beyond a certain threshold, further exemplars do not affect productivity.

8. Interim conclusions

Earlier in this chapter, we saw that research on the English past-tense and plural marking systems appears to support the dual-mechanism theory. In both of these systems, a single, phonologically unrestricted affix applies in a variety of circumstances in which memory cannot be accessed, and there is convincing psycholinguistic and neurolinguistic evidence that regular and irregular inflections are processed differently by the healthy brain and differently affected in neurological disorders. However, it is not clear whether these differences reflect the properties of two different mental mechanisms, or whether they are simply an artefact of the idiosyncratic properties of the English system of marking tense and plurality. We also saw that in the German plural, the distinction between regular and irregular endings is much less clear-cut. One of the endings, -*s*, does have a special status, but it is not always used in default circumstances, and, more importantly, speakers do not treat it as a default: German-speaking children overgeneralise -*en* or -*e* more frequently than -*s*, and both children and adults prefer these two 'irregular' endings with nonce words.

The Polish results cast further doubt on the idea that there is a clear-cut distinction between regular and irregular inflections. We have seen that irregular inflections can appear in default circumstances, and that at least some regular inflections (e.g. the dative feminine endings) are sensitive to phonological properties. Furthermore, regularity is a poor predictor of productivity: some irregular inflections (e.g. the two genitive masculine endings) are freely generalised to new words, while some regular ones (e.g. the genitive neuter and dative neuter endings) are not.

The dative experiment also revealed very strong similarity effects on neuter nouns, in spite of the fact that the dative neuter inflection is regular. This is important in the context of the debate between the connectionists and proponents of the dual-mechanism theory, since it undermines one of the strongest arguments against connectionist approaches to language. As noted by Pinker (1999) and Marcus (1998), connectionist models are, by their very nature, highly reliant on local similarities, and consequently have problems generalising to novel patterns which do not resemble items they have encountered in the training set. Research on the Polish case system suggests that this is also a feature of linguistic generalisation in humans, so this property of connectionist models is an argument in their favour, not against them.

Polish speakers' restricted productivity with neuter inflections also has important implications for linguistic theory. Most linguists take it as self-evident that speakers extract the most general rule compatible with the language they hear. The results reported here show that this is not necessarily the case. Although speakers probably have general rules as well, the most robust linguistic generalisations appear to be local. There is also evidence that people store the inflected forms of many familiar words as well as the citation forms (see Chapter 2, section 3.1.4; for evidence that Polish speakers store ready-made dative forms of neuter nouns, see Dąbrowska 2004: study 4). Thus, our mental grammars appear to be quite messy, with the same information represented redundantly at different levels of abstraction.

The research on the Polish genitive affords us yet another perspective on these issues. As shown in section 6.2, neither of the two genitive masculine endings is regular in the technical sense of the dual-mechanism theory. The mere existence of an inflectional system without a default, though awkward for the dual-mechanism theory, does not constitute definitive evidence that it is incorrect. Although the theory implies that inflectional systems normally have a default mechanism, it does not require that every inflectional category in every language have one: it is perfectly possible that some systems in some languages lack a default. In such cases, speakers would be forced to fall back on associative memory. There are two problems with this scenario, however.

First, the dual-mechanism theory does not explain how learners discover that a system does *not* have a default. Marcus, Pinker and their collaborators argue that children are programmed to look for the default inflection and identify it either by noting that it is phonologically unrestricted or by observing that it is used in 'one or two' of the circumstances listed in Table 8.1 (Marcus et al. 1995: 245; cf. also Clahsen 1999; Marcus et al. 1992: 133ff). Since both -*a* and -*u* are phonologically unrestricted, and both are found in a number of default contexts, Polish children could easily conclude that one or the other of the two endings is the default; and it is unclear how they could recover from this incorrect conclusion.

Another problem with this defence of the dual-mechanism theory is that it amounts to saying that children resort to symbolic rules when they are learning a relatively neat and tidy system such as the English past tense, but have to rely on associative memory when confronted with a more complex system such as the Polish genitive. Although such a position is logically consistent, it is not very attractive, particularly in view of the fact that English-speaking children learning the past tense appear to make more errors than Polish children learning the genitive (Dąbrowska 2001). It would seem, then, that the default system does not do very much, and that English-speaking children would do better to ignore it and rely simply on memory.

Another important lesson to be drawn from the work on the acquisition of the genitive is that children are extremely good learners. They master the Byzantine rules of Polish morphology early and almost without error (Dąbrowska 2001; Smoczyńska 1985). They seem to have no great difficulty in restricting each inflection to a particular subset of words belonging to a larger class, even if this subset is essentially arbitrary, at least with very frequent inflections such as the genitive. And they also learn which inflection to use in each of the special circumstances enumerated in Table 8.2. We do not know when or how they accomplish this, but learn it they must, since different circumstances call for different endings.

Marcus and Pinker repeatedly stress that some of the circumstances in which the default inflection applies in English are 'exotic', and although they do not explicitly say that they are unlearnable, there is a strong suggestion to this effect: verbs derived via nouns, bahuvrihi compounds with an irregular noun in the rightmost position etc., are so rare that children might not encounter enough examples in the input to learn which inflection they require. The dual-mechanism theory provides a simple explanation of how they come to know that the default inflection applies in each of these circumstances: children do not have to learn this, because the whole list falls out automatically from the architecture of the language-processing system.

Proponents of the dual mechanism theory are probably right when they argue that English-speaking children do not need to learn which inflection to use in these 'default' circumstances. They whole list does fall out automatically – not from the architecture of the language-processing system, but from the fact that the regular past-tense and plural endings are the only ones which are truly productive. Polish children, however, do have to deduce which ending to use in each circumstance, and the fact that they are able to do this shows that such contingencies are learnable, however exotic they may be.

9. Challenges for connectionism

The connectionist approach to language and language acquisition has much to recommend it. To implement their models on a computer, the designers are obliged to offer fully explicit accounts of the development of a particular aspect of a speaker's linguistic knowledge – an account in which all details of the network architecture, input and output representations, and training regime have to be spelled out fully. Computer simulations also make it possible to study the effects of using different architectures and different training regimes and to explore the consequences of 'lesioning' the network at different stages of development – experiments we cannot perform on human beings. Although connectionist nets are very different from real brains, they are neurologically much more plausible than models inspired by the serial computer, so prevalent in computer science. Most importantly, nets can learn: they are able to represent recurrent patterns and generalise them to novel situations – and they do this using relatively 'low-tech', general-purpose mechanisms. Furthermore, like humans, they are highly sensitive to frequency, extract patterns at varying degrees of abstraction, and are particularly good at learning local regularities.

These similarities suggest that the manner in which networks generalise – by capturing shared properties by means of partially overlapping representations – may be a good model of how humans extract linguistic generalisations.

In spite of these undeniable advantages, the connectionist approach to language has come under severe criticism (see, for example, Lachter and Bever 1988; Marcus 1998; Marcus et al. 1995; Pinker 1999; Pinker and Prince 1988). While much of the criticism applies to specific models (cf. section 3 above), other problems are of a more general nature. In this section, I discuss some of these general problems, possible solutions, and lessons that can be drawn from them.

One fairly obvious problem with many network models stems from the way their designers conceptualise the task facing the child. Most modellers assume, either explicitly or implicitly, that learning to supply the correct inflected form involves learning to relate the phonological representation of the stem and the phonological representation of the derived form (e.g. the past tense). In line with this view, networks are trained on stem–past pairs like *drink–drank*, *sleep–slept, like–liked.* This assumption, of course, is extremely implausible when taken at face value: the input available to children obviously does not consist of stems followed by the correct past tense form. It is possible that on hearing the past tense form of a verb they already know, children retrieve the stem from memory and compare the two – but there is no evidence that they do this. Furthermore, as pointed out earlier, past-tense forms cannot always be predicted from the phonological form of the stem, since some identical stems have different past-tense forms. Therefore, any network which only represents phonological form will be unable to learn certain mappings.

Inflectional properties such as the choice of a particular ending are associated with words, not phonological forms; so to be able to deal with homophones, the processing system must be able to identify unique words. Words are not just strings of phonemes: they are pairings of a phonological form and a semantic representation. It would seem, then, that the problem could be solved simply by giving the system access to semantic information. Such a solution was actually implemented (on a limited scale) by MacWhinney and Leinbach (1991; see also Cottrell and Plunkett 1994), who trained their model on input representations which contained semantic features in addition to phonological representations. The semantic features allowed the network to distinguish homophonous stems and to associate them with different past-tense forms. Thus, the network was able to supply *rang, ringed* and *wrung* as the past tense forms of $ring_1$ 'make a ringing sound', $ring_2$ 'put a ring around' and *wring*, respectively.

The critics, however, were not impressed with this solution. Pinker and Prince (1988: 175ff), Kim et al. (1994), and others have pointed out that the choice of past-tense form does not actually depend on semantic properties: all that matters, as far as the inflectional system is concerned, is that $ring_1$, $ring_2$ and *wring* are different words. The rule-inducing mechanism, they argue, cannot be sensitive to actual meanings, or it would extract incorrect meaning-based generalisations:

> Adding semantic features to a distributed representation has the effect of defining semantic subtypes of verbs that one would expect to have similar past-tense forms, just as overlap in phonological features defines clusters of verbs with similar past-tense forms – but this prediction, in the case of semantic features, is not true. For instance, though *slap, hit* and *strike* have similar meanings, they have different past-tense forms – *slap* has the regular past tense form *slapped, hit* has the no-change past-tense form *hit*, and *strike* has the stem-changing past-tense form *struck*. Conversely, though *sting, sing, swing*, and so forth form their past tenses in similar ways, they do not comprise a semantically coherent set of verbs. This is true not just of these examples, but throughout the verb lexicon. (Kim et al. 1994: 202)

It is true that the semantic features of the verb are not relevant in English. But the pattern-extraction mechanism cannot be blind to semantics because some inflectional endings in some languages *are* associated with classes of stems sharing certain semantic properties. The choice of the genitive inflection of masculine nouns in Polish, for example, to the extent that it is predictable at all, depends primarily on semantic factors. Thus, the learning system cannot simply ignore semantics: it must be able to identify which (if any) semantic features are relevant to a particular inflection.

But will giving the network access to semantic representations do the trick? According to Pinker and Prince (1988) and Kim et al. (1994), the answer to this question is an emphatic no. They point out that the choice of inflection depends not on the presence or absence of a particular semantic property, but on the grammatical structure of the word. As explained earlier, denominal verbs, deverbal nouns, bahuvrihi compounds, nouns derived from names and so on take regular inflections in English, even when they are homophonous with irregulars. Thus, the past tense of *spit* 'put on a spit' is *spitted*, not *spat*, and the plural forms of *sabre-tooth* and *Mickey Mouse* are *sabre-tooths* and *Mickey Mouses*, respectively, not *sabre-teeth* and *Mickey Mice*. The reason for this, according to the dual-mechanism theory, is that these words are exocentric (headless), and so information about irregular inflections cannot be passed on to the derived word. This generalisation, however, cannot be captured using semantic features, since headlessness is not a semantic property: no aspect of meaning is shared by *spit* 'put on a spit', *sabre-tooth, Mickey Mouse* and all other exocentric words. Endocentric compounds, on the other hand, always take the same inflections as their heads, regardless of their meaning. For example, *chessman* and *strawman* pluralise like *man*, even though they do not refer to adult male human beings; and *become, overcome, come about, come down with, come on* and so on share the same irregularity as *come* (their past-tense forms are *became, overcame, came down with, came on*) in spite of the fact that they designate very different types of events.

Semantic extensions also tend to take the same inflection as the basic sense on which they are based, however tenuous the link between the senses. This is particularly dramatic in the case of verbs like *come, go, have* and *get*, which, as Pinker and Prince put it, are 'magnificently polysemous . . . yet they march in lockstep through the same non-regular paradigms in central and extended senses – regardless of how strained or opaque the metaphor' (1988: 112–13). Consider the verb *get*. The *Collins COBUILD English Language Dictionary* lists 43 senses for the verb itself and 94 additional senses for various verb–particle combinations such as *get off, get out* and *get up*. All these senses have the same past-tense form, *got*, because they all share the same head.

Kim et al. (1991, 1994) provide experimental evidence suggesting that English speakers, including young children, are sensitive to the subtle difference between exocentric and endocentric words. In one experiment, they presented 3–5-year-olds with novel verbs homophonous with existing irregular verbs. Some of the novel verbs were denominal (for example, the experimenter announced that he was going to *fly this board*, and proceeded to put flies all over the board), and some were semantic extensions (the experimenter said that Mickey was going to *fly down the road* and then had him drive very fast down the road). Subsequently, the children were asked to complete a sentence describing what had just happened (*Mickey just . . .*). The general finding was that children were more likely to use the regular inflection with denominal verbs than with semantic extensions – in other words, they were more likely to say *You flied the board* than *Mickey just flied down the road*. However, the results were very noisy. The children gave the expected regular response to denominal verbs only 64 per cent of the time, and the expected irregular with semantic extensions only 23 per cent of the time. They also inappropriately regularised 47 per cent of the semantic extensions (e.g. *Mickey just flied down the road*), and used the irregular form with 6 per cent of the denominal verbs (e.g. *You just flew the board*, meaning 'You just put flies all over the board').

In another experiment, Kim et al. presented nouns with irregular roots as names (e.g. *Mr Tooth*), as exocentric compounds (e.g. *snaggletooth*, a stuffed toy with large teeth) or as ordinary nouns (*purple tooth*), and elicited plural forms from slightly older children (7- and 8-year-olds). The children used the expected irregular plural with 94 per cent of the ordinary nouns. Rather unexpectedly, however, they also used it with 70 per cent of the names and exocentric compounds. The difference in frequency of irregular responses is significant, showing that the children were sensitive to the distinction between ordinary nouns and the same roots used as names or in exocentric compounds; but the high proportion of irregular responses in the latter case is problematic for the dual-mechanism theory.

Kim and colleagues argue that these results show that speakers base their decision whether to use the regular or the irregular inflection on purely grammatical properties such as headedness – not on semantics. For example, speakers use the regular inflection with exocentric compounds like *sabre-tooth* because they know they are headless, and the irregular form with extended senses of irregular words because they know that semantic extensions share the same head. This solution, however, raises an obvious problem – namely, how speakers determine whether two words share the same head. For example, how can they tell that *tooth* is the head in the compound *wisdom tooth*, but not in *sabre-tooth*, or that all the senses of *get* share the same head? It is clear that the single most important clue (apart from identical phonological form) is meaning. A *wisdom tooth* is a kind of tooth, but a *sabre-tooth* is a very different kind of thing: a tiger. The use of the verb *fly* to mean 'drive fast' is clearly related to the basic sense ('move rapidly through the air'), while the novel denominal sense ('to put flies on') is not. With 'magnificently polysemous' verbs like *get*, things are slightly more complicated. Pinker and Prince are right to point out that the various senses of such verbs do not share any semantic properties (apart from the fact that, like other verbs, they designate relationships that unfold in time). However, there are many local similarities between the various senses. For example, the 'obtain' sense (as in *He's trying to get an antique lawnmower*) and the 'receive' sense (*He thinks he will get an antique lawnmower for Christmas*) share the element of coming to possess; the 'become' sense (*She got pregnant*) and the 'cause' sense (*He got her pregnant*) both designate events which involve a change of state; and so on. Presumably learners use such local similarities to make connections between the individual senses, and eventually integrate them into a single semantic network. The fact that the various senses share certain grammatical properties (including the past-tense form) might provide an additional clue.

Thus the decision to use the regular or the irregular inflection ultimately depends on a combination of phonological and semantic factors. A form used to express a new meaning will inherit the past-tense form from an established form–meaning pairing if the new use is perceived by speakers to be 'the same word' as the latter. If it is not, the usual conventions of the language apply. In English, which has only one truly productive pattern for both the past tense and plural, this almost always means that the regular endings are used.

As pointed out earlier, a word is neither a phonological form nor a semantic representation, but a pairing of the two. For speakers to judge a new form–meaning pairing to be 'the same word' as an existing irregular, it must have the same phonological form as the irregular word and share enough *relevant* semantic properties to be subsumed under the same superordinate category as at least one established sense of the word. This explains why words derived from another category (e.g. a noun derived from a verb or vice versa) are generally inflected regularly in English even if they are homophonous with existing irregulars. Such a derivation necessarily involves a dramatic change in meaning, and the derived form and the base cannot be subsumed under the same semantic category (for example, *ring* 'a circular object' refers to an object, while *ring* 'to put a ring around' designates a kind of action). Because of this, the new form tends to be perceived as a different word and cannot inherit the grammatical properties of the base; hence, speakers apply whatever inflection would normally apply to the new word.

The above proposal is quite similar to that put forward by proponents of the dual-mechanism theory. The main difference is that it explains grammatical behaviour without appealing to an autonomous level of grammatical representation. It also has an additional advantage, in that it can explain why semantic extensions sometimes lose the grammatical properties of the motivating sense and take a different inflection, and why some irregular-sounding words derived from another category are inflected irregularly.

Situations of the first kind arise when the extended sense is so different from the motivating sense that the two are no longer perceived as the same word. It was noted earlier (cf. example (2)) that the genitive form of *tenor* in Polish is *tenoru* when it refers to a singing voice and *tenora* when it refers to a singer with that voice. The contrast is quite systematic: words designating other singing voices also take *-u*, while words designating singers take *-a*. In English, the plural of *louse*, when used to refer to a group of particularly unpleasant people, is *louses*, not *lice*; and the past tense of *hang* 'to execute by hanging' is *hanged*, not *hung*. Occasionally, when the link between the basic sense and the extended sense is not very salient, speakers may be unsure whether or not they are the same word. When the word *mouse* refers to a small grey rodent, its plural form is *mice.* Many English speakers, however, hesitate to use the irregular plural when talking about more than one computer mouse, although they tend to prefer it to *mouses*. It seems that the reason why they are so squeamish about *mice* is that the two concepts are perceived as very distant. The computer device and the rodent do share certain properties – they are both small and grey – but they are very different kinds of things, so many speakers judge such superficial similarities to be irrelevant. Because the link between the two concepts is so tenuous, speakers are not sure whether they should be regarded as the same word, and, consequently, they are not sure which plural form they should use when talking about several pointing devices.[12]

Evidence that words derived from another category are not invariably given regular inflections can be found in a series of experiments conducted by Ramscar (2002). In one experiment, participants were introduced to the nonce noun *frink*, which was defined as 'the Muscovite equivalent of the Spanish tapas; it is served in bars, and usually comprises chilled vodka and some salted or pickled fish'. They were then presented with a homophonous verb meaning 'to consume a frink', and were asked to supply the past-tense form. A substantial majority (73 per cent) produced an irregular form such as *frank* or *frunk*. In another experiment, Ramscar had speakers rate the acceptability of past-tense forms of real verbs which were either denominal (e.g. *sink* meaning 'to hide in a sink') or semantic extensions of an irregular verb (e.g. the metaphorical sense of *sink*, as in *My hopes sank*). Two other groups of participants rated the same verbs for denominal status and semantic similarity to the prototypical sense of an existing irregular. Ramscar found that semantic similarity and grammatical status were highly correlated, and that speakers' intuitions about semantic similarity to the basic sense were a better predictor of the acceptability of irregular past-tense forms than their intuitions about denominal status.[13]

Thus the data discussed by Pinker, Marcus, Kim and their colleagues does not necessarily imply that an abstract autonomous level of grammatical structure is necessary to explain speakers' abilities. On the other hand, the facts need to be accommodated in some way, and it is clear that they cannot be accommodated in any existing connectionist network. Existing connectionist models of the past tense do not represent words; and although they are good at categorising, it is doubtful that they could learn to make the kind of categorisation judgements required in this task. To deal with the more complex problems discussed in this section, more sophisticated models will be required which have access to various types of linguistic and extralinguistic knowledge.

This brings us to the most serious problem yet. All existing connectionist models are quite restricted in application. The models discussed in this chapter produce past-tense forms of English verbs. Regier's network, briefly described in Chapter 7, learned to output terms corresponding to various locative relationships. Other networks had been trained, with varying degrees of success, to identify word boundaries, assign words to grammatical categories, or predict the next word in a sentence (Elman 1990, 1993; Gasser and Smith 1998). Thus, each of these models learned to carry out a specific – and fairly simple – operation on a particular kind of input. It is not clear, however, whether such models will 'scale up' – that is to say, whether they will be able to perform more complex linguistic tasks.

More complex types of processing would obviously require more complex networks. But a more complex network isn't simply a network with more units. Merely adding units to existing networks is unlikely to solve the problem, for several reasons. First, as new nodes are added, the number of connections between them grows exponentially. This means that there are more and more weights to be set, and as a result, adjusting the weights soon becomes computationally intractable. Therefore, larger networks will need to show more selective patterns of interconnectivity, more like the patterns found in the brain, where there are assemblies of units richly connected with each other, but with fairly sparse connections with units belonging to other assemblies.

More importantly, the various subtasks involved in language processing – inflecting words, identifying word boundaries, accessing phonological forms, parsing – rely on different kinds of knowledge, and hence, in network terms, require different connection strengths. A network trained to produce past-tense forms cannot identify word boundaries, and vice versa. Training it to perform the second task would involve altering connection weights, which would interfere with performance on the first task. Thus, if a network is to be able to perform a number of different tasks, various subparts will have to specialise. Complex problems may also require decomposition into smaller tasks, and these, too, would have to be assigned to different subnetworks.

It follows that a more realistic model of human linguistic abilities will require a certain degree of functional specialisation or 'modularisation'.[14] Unfortunately, it is not clear how such functional specialisation could be achieved in networks. Presumably some architectural features will have to be built in (as in Regier's model), but many leading figures in the field believe that functional specialisation could arise *as a result of learning* – in other words, that future models will be able to self-organise (see Elman et al. 1996).

All these problems notwithstanding, it is undeniable that connectionist models have stimulated research and helped us to develop new ways of thinking about language development and language processing. It is important to realise, however, that connectionism is not a theory of language processing or development: it is an approach to modelling these and other phenomena. Connectionist networks can be used to model learning in a variety of frameworks, empiricist, nativist or constructivist. Specific models, of course, do embody assumptions about how language is represented in the brain; however, the theories embodied in existing networks are very simple, almost trivially simple. The networks developed so far are useful research tools, but they are grossly inadequate as models of human linguistic abilities.

This does not mean that more realistic models are impossible in principle. Connectionism is a relatively young endeavour, and much of the emphasis so far has been on the mechanics of modelling – developing suitable algorithms, architectures, training regimes, and methods of analysing network behaviour. Future models, it is to be hoped, will implement more sophisticated theories of language and language acquisition.

Notes

1. Although applicability and frequency often co-vary, they are logically independent. One can envisage a system in which some inflections have narrow applicability (e.g. apply only to stems with specific phonological properties) but have high type frequency because these phonological properties are typical of most stems in the language.
2. The frequency of -*s* overgeneralisations appears to increase with age, however. They accounted for 58.5 per cent of all errors in an elicited production study with 3–9-year-olds conducted by Clahsen (1999).
3. Clahsen et al. assume a model of morphology proposed by Kiparsky (1985), according to which the morphological component is divided into several ordered levels, and processes that apply at later levels cannot alter units assembled earlier. According to the model, irregular inflections apply at level 1, compounding at level 2, and regular inflections at level 3.

Because irregular inflections are added at level 1, before compounding, they can occur inside compounds; but regular inflections, which apply after compounding, can only be added to the compound as a whole, not to an element inside a compound.

4. For an explanation in an optimality theory framework, see Wegener (1999).

5. The distribution of the two variants is determined by very general phonotactic rules, and some linguists (e.g. Nagórko 1998) even consider them allophones of the same phoneme. This decision, however, depends on assumptions about the phonemic status of preceding consonants which are somewhat controversial.

6. Feminine nouns usually end in -*a*, masculines in a consonant, and neuters in -*o*, -*e* or -*ę*.

7. These morphological effects are not independent of semantics. Nouns derived using the '*a*-friendly' suffixes -*acz*, -*arz*, -*ak*, -*nik*, -*ec* typically designate animate beings. The -*a* ending is also preferred with nouns designating small objects, and hence diminutives take -*a*. On the other hand, -*izm* and -*ot*, two of the suffixes which are associated with -*u*, are used to derive nouns designating ideologies and noises, i.e. abstract concepts. The phonological associations between affixes and stem-final consonants may result from a similar trickle-down effect (see Janda 1996; Kottum 1981).

8. Some masculine nouns (e.g. *syk* 'hiss', *pisk* 'squeak', *plusk* 'splash', *klekot* 'rattle', *stukot* 'clatter') might be regarded as onomatopoeic in that their phonological form resembles the noises they designate. These, like other masculine nouns designating sounds and abstract concepts in general, require -*u*. However, they are ordinary noun roots rather than actual renditions of sound, which is what Marcus et al. seem to have in mind, so they are not considered here.

9. The gender of the nonce words used in the experiment could be predicted from the phonological form of the nominative as well as from morphological cues such as agreeing adjectives and/or demonstratives.

10. The acquisition of the genitive by these children is described in more detail in Dąbrowska (2001, 2004). For further details about the corpus from which the data was drawn, see Smoczyńska (1998).

11. Note that this problem did not arise in the genitive study, for similar reasons: in the genitive, the masculine class is split up between -*a* and -*u*.

12. Actually, usage is somewhat variable in all four cases. For example, some English speakers use the irregular inflection with both senses of *hang* ('suspend in the air' and 'execute by hanging'), presumably because both refer to an act of suspending something so that it does not touch the ground.

13. This finding contradicts earlier research by Kim et al. (1991); however, there are some serious methodological problems with this study. See Ramscar (2002) for a discussion.

14. Note that the term 'modularisation' is used here to refer to functional specialisation. The resulting modules, or subnetworks, are not necessarily anatomically distinct. Moreover, they receive input from other subnetworks, so they are not informationally encapsulated.

9 Syntactic constructions

We saw in the previous chapter that there is no evidence for a strong dissociation between grammar and the lexicon in morphology: in principle, the same mental mechanism can account for speakers' ability to supply both regular and irregular inflections. It was also suggested that speakers extract patterns of varying degrees of abstraction and that associative memory plays a prominent role in this process.

In this chapter, I will argue that the same may also be true of syntax. This is seen most clearly in acquisition, so the main body of the chapter will be devoted to discussing developmental data. We will begin with a summary of studies showing that there is a very close relationship between lexical and grammatical development, at least in the early stages of language acquisition. We will then look at research which might explain this relationship, and examine converging evidence from a variety of sources suggesting that the starting point of syntactic development is the acquisition of a repertoire of rote-learned formulas, or multi-word phrases paired with meaning. Finally, we will look in considerable detail at the development of a particular construction (or rather family of constructions) – English interrogatives – in order to see how more creative patterns develop from such formulas, and conclude with some observations about lexically specific units in adult language.

1. Ties between lexical and grammatical knowledge

A series of large-scale studies conducted by Elizabeth Bates and her team have revealed the existence of close ties between expressive vocabulary size and grammatical development. Bates et al. (1988), in a longitudinal study of 27 children who were followed from the age of 10 months to 28 months, showed that there was a very high positive correlation (+.83) between expressive vocabulary size at 20 months and MLU (mean length of utterance) at 28 months. Indeed, the correlation coefficient is as high as the correlations between MLU measures obtained from different samples taken from the same child at 28 months: in other words, vocabulary at 20 months and MLU at 28 months are statistically indistinguishable.

These findings were confirmed by a second, much larger cross-sectional study of 1,800 children aged from 16 months to 30 months (Bates, Dale and Thal 1995; Fenson et al. 1994) which used the MacArthur Communicative Development Inventory (an extensive questionnaire completed by the parents). Although this study used a different measure of grammatical development (a 'grammatical complexity score' derived from parental report about the structures used by their children), the relationship between vocabulary size and sentence complexity was virtually identical (+.84). The same relationship was also found in various atypical populations, including early and late talkers, children with focal brain injury, and individuals with Williams's syndrome (WS) (Bates and Goodman 1999), as well as in normally developing Italian children (Caselli et al. 1999).

Such correlations cannot be explained simply in terms of maturation. Although both vocabulary size and grammatical complexity increase with age, age is a poor predictor of grammatical development. In the large cross-sectional study referred to above, age and vocabulary size together accounted for 71.4 per cent of the variance in grammatical complexity; when age was controlled for, vocabulary size accounted for 32.3 per cent of the variance; but when vocabulary size was controlled for, age accounted for only 0.8 per cent of the variance (Bates and Goodman 1999: 46).

Bates and Goodman (1997, 1999) also note there is evidence of close ties between lexical and grammatical knowledge in language impairment, including impairments acquired in maturity, which suggests that these ties are not restricted to the early stages of language acquisition. All aphasic patients, they point out, whatever other problems they might have, also have lexical deficits: in other words, there are no impairments which involve grammar and grammar only. Moreover, there are parallels between patients' lexical and grammatical difficulties. In some deficits (Broca's aphasia, Down's syndrome, some forms of SLI), the underlying problem seems to be in accessing linguistic representations, and it manifests itself in word-finding difficulties and omission of obligatory function words and inflections. Other groups (Wernicke's aphasics, people with Williams' Syndrome) make errors of commission rather than omission: they use both grammatical morphemes and words inappropriately. Still others (e.g. anomic aphasics and patients with Alzheimer's dementia) do not make outright errors, but have very restricted linguistic repertoires: that is to say, they are overly dependent on pronouns and other semantically 'light' forms and the most basic grammatical forms and constructions (see Chapter 4 for further discussion).

How can we explain these close ties between lexical and grammatical knowledge? The key to understanding this relationship, I will argue in this chapter, is formulas or multi-word prefabs: stored phrases associated with a specific meaning. Such prefabs are like words, in that they are form–meaning pairings.

On the other hand, they are *also* grammatical constructions: they have internal structure, and they may be partly underspecified and hence allow some variation. We saw in Chapter 2 that the use of prefabs is one of the processing shortcuts that help adults produce and understand complex utterances in real time. I will now review evidence that children learn such chunks, and that they play an important role in acquisition.

2. Multi-word units in acquisition

2.1 Premature usage

Most children occasionally say things which appear to be well in advance of their productive abilities. Nelson reports that the children she studied used invariant formulas such as *want a drink of water*, *how are you?*, *you're kidding*, containing the correct grammatical morphemes, long before they used these morphemes in any other contexts (1973: 107–8). Braine's (1976) subject David repeatedly used the phrase *Can I (have) X?* to make requests when he was still in the two-word stage, before he used other auxiliaries or learned how to form yes/no questions. Many children ask formulaic WH questions such as *What's this?*, *Where's X?*, *Whatchadoing?*, often in highly stereotypical contexts, months before they produce any other interrogative constructions (see below; also Brown 1968; Pinker 1984; Radford 1990).

Richards (1990) provides an even more striking example. Two children in his study produced well-formed tag questions at a very early stage, before they had learned to form yes/no questions or to use auxiliaries as pro-forms. In some cases, the tag was the first attested usage of a particular auxiliary. Since tags are one of the most complex syntactic contexts for auxiliaries, their early appearance suggests that these two children had learned them as unanalysed units. This is confirmed by errors such as *They swimming intit?* (109), *I know him aren't I?* (77), where the auxiliaries (and in the first example, also the subject) in the tag don't match the corresponding units in the main clause.

2.2 Developmental U-curves

In some cases, early correct but restricted usage is followed by periods of apparent regression, during which the form in question is either absent from the child's speech or is used inappropriately, before it reappears again, more reliably and in a wider range of contexts. For example, Bates et al. (1988), Hickey (1993), Peters (1983) and others have observed that some children produce functors in their early speech, then leave them out, and then begin to supply them again more reliably and in a wider range of contexts. In the development of WH questions, early correct forms with a contracted copula (*What's this?*, *Where's Daddy?*) may be followed by 'uninverted' forms (*What this is?*, *Where Daddy is?*) and then questions with the full form of the copula in the correct position (*What is this?*, *Where is Daddy?*) and eventually questions with both the contracted and the uncontracted form. Richards (1979) and MacWhinney (1985) note that while 3-year-old children produce correctly ordered strings of adjectives before nouns, performance often dips around the age of 5 before improving again in the school years. The early correct performance is attributable to the use of memorised strings such as *great big* and *nice little*.

2.3 Inappropriate and ungrammatical usage

Ungrammatical utterances produced by children are often regarded as evidence that they are relying on their own rules rather than merely imitating adult models. However, ungrammatical utterances are just as likely to arise when the child attempts to combine rote-learned chunks, as in the following examples:

(1)   a. *I don't wanna don't throw.* (Iwamura 1979, cited in Peters 1983)
         b. *Can I have break it?* [wants to break up a tinkertoy construction] (Braine 1976)
         c. *I don't know where's Emma gone.* (Clark 1974)
         d. *I want I eat apple.* (Clark 1974)
         e. *Where's the boy brought the milk?* [looking for the milk the boy had brought] (Clark 1974)

In (1a), the child simply incorporated the previous speaker's utterance (*don't throw*) into the frame *I don't wanna X*. The next two utterances are constructed by combining two phrase-sized units from the child's own repertoire. In (1b), the general-purpose request formula *Can I have X?* is combined with what is probably an unanalysed chunk (at the stage when the utterance was produced, the child used the verb *break* only in the expression *break it*). In (1c), the noun *Emma* is used to fill the slot in a well-established formula (*Where's X gone?*), and the resulting expression is combined with another formula *I don't know X*. Utterances (1d) and (1e) were probably assembled by embedding a simple constructed utterance (*I eat apple*, *the boy brought the milk*) inside a formulaic frame (*I want X*, *Where's X?*).

   In other cases, an utterance may be grammatical and its formulaic status is only revealed when it is used in inappropriate circumstances. One of the first plural forms used by Clark's son Adam occurred in the sentence *Take the cups away*, which he heard in the day nursery. He subsequently used it at home even when there was only one cup. Her other son Ivan produced the utterance *It will hurt me* after a door had slammed in front of him (Clark 1977). Clearly, he was not using *will* to signal the future, but simply 'recycling' an expression he had heard earlier in a similar context. What is noteworthy about this particular example is that the recycling did involve a certain amount of modification of the original utterance: he changed the pronoun to reflect the change of speaker.

2.4 Pronoun reversals

This brings us to a particularly interesting usage error in early child language: pronoun reversals, where the child uses the second person pronoun to refer to himself, or, less frequently, the first person pronoun to refer to the interlocutor, as in the following examples:

(2)   a. *I carry you.* [wants to be carried by his father] (Clark 1974)
        b. *Sit my knee*. [wants to sit on the adult's knee] (Clark 1974)
        c. *Let's see you climb up on this one.* [said while climbing a low wall] (Snow 1983)
        d. *The pj's you got on are slippery.* [referring to his own pyjamas] (Snow 1983)

Such errors have been reported quite frequently in the literature (Chiat 1986; Clark 1974; Dale and Crain-Thoreson 1993; MacWhinney 1985; Petitto 1987; Snow 1981), and there is no shortage of theories attempting to explain them. One popular explanation is that reversals are a result of young children's inability to assume the point of view of another person; others have attributed such errors to the unusual nature of deictic pronouns (unlike most other linguistic expressions, they refer to roles, not categories or individuals), characteristics of the input (in speech addressed to the child, *you* always refers to the child and *me* to the caretaker, so unless the child is exposed to language addressed to third parties, she has no evidence that pronouns refer to roles rather than individuals), and to processing complexity (pronoun reversal is a performance phenomenon, particularly likely when processing demands are high).

All four factors probably play a role, and their relative importance may vary over time and from child to child. However, I would like to suggest that the single most important cause of pronoun reversals is the child's use of preconstructed phrases.

Several lines of evidence point in this direction. First, cases of consistent reversals are rare. Most children who reverse pronouns produce correct forms most of the time, and comprehension tends to be good even in children who make errors in production (Chiat 1982). This argues against the first three hypotheses. Secondly, reversals are particularly frequent in imitations. All the utterances in (2) above are (deferred) imitations of parental utterances. (2a) and (2b) are reduced renditions of the parent's *I'll carry you* and *sit on my knee*; (2c) is an exact repetition of an utterance used on a number of similar occasions by the child's father; and (2d), an exact imitation of an utterance the child heard in a very similar context the previous day (he was standing at the top of the stairs in the morning in pyjamas with fabric feet; he reproduced the utterance the following morning while walking down the stairs, wearing the same pyjamas). In a study of deictic pronoun use in linguistically precocious children, Dale and Crain-Thoreson (1993) found that 52 per cent of all reversals occurred in imitations, in spite of the fact that imitations made up only 5 per cent of the children's utterances. Many of the remaining utterances with reversals could well be delayed imitations which weren't recognised as such because the original parental utterance was not captured on tape. For example, it is likely that the children whose utterances are reproduced in (3) below heard a parent say something like *Do you want mummy to help you now?/Should mummy help you now?* and *Do you want me to help you with this?*

(3)   a. *Mama help you now.*
            'Mama help me now.'
         b. *Want help you with screwdriver.*
            'I want you to help me with the screwdriver.'

Dale and Crain-Thoreson argue that reversals result from processing overload (the child fails to perform deictic shift in cognitively demanding situations), and note that they are particularly likely to occur in syntactically complex sentences. But if cognitive overload were the problem, reversals should be less frequent in imitations, which require less processing capacity than productive usage. A more plausible explanation, therefore, is that reversals occur when children 'recycle' an adult utterance, or parts of it. This often enables them to produce more complex utterances, but may lead to reversal errors when the adult utterance contains pronouns.[1]

It is worth noting that pronoun reversals are especially common in the speech of two clinical groups – blind and autistic children. Autistic children are well-known for their use of unanalysed formulas, and so this aspect of their speech supports the claim that pronoun errors are a tell-tale sign of holistic processing. In the case of blind children, inappropriate use of pronouns may be a consequence of a delayed development of a sense of self (see Fraiberg 1977) or of limited access to contextual information.[2] On the other hand, there is also evidence that blind children rely on formulaic phrases to a greater extent than seeing children (Dunlea 1989; Mulford 1988; Pérez-Pereira 1994; Urwin 1984; see also Chapter 3), so this could also contribute to the higher incidence of pronoun errors.

2.5 Filler syllables

Another characteristic feature of formulaic usage is the occurrence of phonological 'fillers' – unstressed syllables (usually a schwa, a nasalised schwa, or a nasal consonant) which usually occur in those positions where function words would appear in adult speech (in English, before open-class words). The following utterances produced by Seth, a child studied by Ann Peters (Peters 1995; Peters and Menn 1993), are a good example (the upper-case 'F' in the glosses marks the position of the filler):

(4)   a. /n si   zə hætʃ/ 'F see   F hedge.'
       b. /ən si   sons/ 'F see   stones?'
       c. /n si   ə bak/   'F see   F bark (of tree)?'
       d. /m pɪk ə fawis/ 'F pick F flowers?' (Peters 1995: 472)

Seth began using filler syllables while still in the one-word stage. During the period from 19 months to 21 months, they comprised about 30 per cent of the 'morphs' in his speech (Peters and Menn 1993: 748). It is often difficult to identify a specific target for these fillers, but their presence lent the entire utterance a more adult-like prosodic contour. Gradually, the fillers gained more phonetic substance and became more and more differentiated and eventually they evolved into various adult forms.

Peters's interpretation of the data was that Seth was unable to reproduce the adult utterance in full phonetic detail and attempted to approximate it at the prosodic level:

> In English closed-class morphemes tend to be (parts of) unstressed syllables whereas open-class words generally contain at least one stressed syllable . . . These two kinds of constituents therefore participate in complementary ways in the rhythm of language, with the open-class items providing the strong beats and the closed-class items contributing to the weak ones. Formulaic children seem to be sensitive to both rhythm and intonation, making noticeable efforts to reproduce them even in their early utterances. (Peters 1995: 476)

Another possibility is that fillers are a kind of all-purpose function word which is the 'common denominator' of all the function words that occur in a particular position.[3] For example, the prenominal filler occurs in the slot which is occupied by determiners in adult language and its phonetic indistinctness could be a result of the fact that it captures properties shared by several different words: *a, an, the* etc. Seth knows that he should use one of these words, but he is not sure which one – so he uses a time-honoured strategy by no means confined to children learning language: when in doubt, mumble.

Whatever the reason for the underspecification of filler syllables, they suggest that Seth is working with units larger than a single word – formulas such as NF-*see*-F-THING or possibly even NF-PROCESS-F-THING (where NF = nasal filler and F = filler), each associated with a specific intonational contour. The fillers are not nonsense syllables inserted between content words: they actually help to define the frame in which other items occur. They also act as placeholders for grammatical morphemes which will emerge later, and the frame itself embodies the child's emergent knowledge about the distribution of these morphemes.

How typical (or untypical) was Seth? Is there any evidence that other children use this strategy as well? The use of filler syllables has been reported by quite a few researchers working on the acquisition of a variety of languages (Peters 2001); but it is likely that most cases go unnoticed, partly because fillers are most characteristic of holistic children (and holistic children tend to be underrepresented in language-acquisition research), and partly because researchers often ignore syllables which have no discernible function. For example, Braine (1976: 43) notes that one of his subjects inserted short unstressed syllables (usually [ə] or [də]) before words, both utterance initially and medially. These syllables didn't seem to make any semantic contribution to the utterance and occurred before verbs as well as before nouns, so they could not be determiners. Because of this, Braine decided to ignore them. Presumably others have done likewise. Since many researchers working on grammatical development use orthographic transcriptions, they may not even be aware of the presence of fillers in the speech of the children they study unless they have transcribed it themselves.[4]

2.6 Lexically based patterns

Young children's grammatical knowledge can be surprisingly specific – in many cases, it is restricted to the combinatorial possibilities of a particular word or a narrow class of words. Some of the best-known evidence for this comes from studies of first word combinations by Braine (1963, 1976), who observed that his 2-year-old subjects reliably put some words in the correct positions in the utterance, but positioned other words belonging to the same grammatical category inconsistently. For example, one child consistently put colour words and the adjectives *big, little, hot* before the noun, but positioned (*all*) *wet* sometimes before and sometimes after the noun. This suggests that he was working with fairly specific 'positional patterns', or formulaic frames, such as *little* + *X*, *hot* + *X*, COLOUR WORD + *X*, rather than a fully general rule stating that adjectives come before nouns. Likewise, Braine found no evidence that 2-year-olds had a general rule for ordering the verb and the direct object: both VO and OV orders occurred, though with different verbs. Thus, the children seemed to be using very specific patterns like *want* + *X*, *see* + *X*, *eat* + *X*, *drink* + *X* and so on.

Similar findings were reported by Bowerman (1976), Tomasello (1992) and others. Between the ages of 16 months and 18 months, Tomasello's daughter Travis used 23 verbs and verb-like words (out of a total repertoire of 45) in combination with other words. Of these, 21 were consistently ordered. For example, Travis always put the object looked for after the amalgam *find-it*, producing utterances such as *find-it bird, find-it chess, find-it brick, find-it ball* etc. On the other hand, the object of *get-it* occurred both before and after the verb: *block get-it*, *bottle get-it*, *get-it hat*, *get-it birds*.

The existence of such lexically specific patterns in the speech of young children is well documented. What is less well known is that they persist for a long time after the child has advanced beyond the two-word stage, and seem to play an important role in the transition to multi-word speech. Thus, when Travis began to produce utterances containing three or more words, they were nearly always constructed by adding a single element to an existing formula or embedding one formula inside another. For example, adding an actor nominal to her *ride X* formula allowed her to produce utterances such as *Big Bird ride horsie*; embedding *Daddy's X* in *see X* resulted in novel expressions such as *see Daddy's car*; *big X* plus *X stuck* yielded *big rock stuck*; and so on.

Several facts about Travis's usage at this time suggest that her grammatical knowledge remained verb-specific at least until age 2;0. She tended to use different combinations of arguments with different verbs. Many verbs were combined with one argument only: some only with an agent, others only with a patient or only with a location. This cannot be explained away as a processing limitation, since other verbs occurred in frames with two or more arguments: for example, she consistently expressed all three arguments with the verb *gave* (but, interestingly, not with *give*, suggesting that the past- and present-tense forms were independent constructions). What is more, she explicitly marked locative relations in utterances with some verbs but not others: for example, she would say *Travis sit down chair* (without a locative preposition) but *Dana push me real high in a bagswing*. Her use of verbal inflections was also restricted to specific verbs. She used 24 verbs in the past-tense form and 23 in the progressive, but only four verbs were used with both endings. Her total verb vocabulary at the time was over 150, so over two-thirds of her verbs were never inflected (Tomasello 1992: 254). Likewise, explicit agreement marking was restricted to the copula and a few other verbs.

Tomasello's diary method allowed him to chart the emergence and gradual development of his daughter's formulas in fine detail, but it is difficult to draw general conclusions from a single case study. How typical was Travis? Are other children equally restrained in their generalisations, or do they form abstract rules right from the beginning? Fortunately, we do have similar data from other children which allow us to answer these questions.

Lieven et al. (1997) studied the distributional regularities in the speech of 11 children. They recorded all multi-word utterances until the child reached 25 word-based patterns. At this point, the children's ages ranged from 1;7 to 2;9 and their MLUs from 1.41 to 3.75 (mean 2.41). The researchers then divided all multi-word utterances into three categories: constructed (lexical formulas which had occurred at least twice before), intermediate (the second occurrence of a particular positional pattern, or the first if both words had been attested in single-word utterances), and frozen phrases (utterances which contained at least one word which did not occur in any other expression). They found that lexical formulas accounted for 60.3 per cent of all utterances (range 51.3–71.9 per cent). A further 31.2 per cent were frozen phrases. Of the remaining 8.4 per cent, about half showed no positional consistency, and the other half did (and hence could be instantiations of emerging lexical frames).

The more complex sentences that children produce also tend to be quite formulaic. A detailed analysis of utterances with finite complement clauses produced by children aged from 2 to 5 conducted by Diessel and Tomasello (2001) revealed that the main clauses in such sentences are usually very short. Typically, they consist only of a pronoun (*I* or sometimes *you*) and a present-tense verb, with no auxiliaries or adverbials; and even the subject is sometimes omitted. Diessel and Tomasello point out that the proposition in such utterances is typically expressed by the complement clause, while the main clause functions as an epistemic marker (*I think*, *I bet*), a deontic modality marker (*I hope*, *I wish*) or an attention getter (*see*, *look*), so the structures are, in effect, monoclausal, and can be paraphrased with a simple sentence:

(5)   a. *I think it's in here.* [= 'Maybe it's in here.']
        b. *I hope he won't bother you.* [= 'Hopefully he won't bother you.']

This analysis is supported by the fact that what appears to be the subordinate clause is virtually never introduced by a complementiser, and that the 'main clause' sometimes comes after the complement clause (as in *It's in here, I think*).

The children in the study also produced some sentences which do appear to involve true subordination. These sentences were much less formulaic: the main clauses contained a variety of subjects and verb forms as well as modifiers and expressed an independent proposition, and the subordinate clauses were sometimes introduced by complementisers. It is noteworthy, however, that the vast majority of them had one of just three verbs – *say, tell, pretend* – as the main predicate. This, argue Diessel and Tomasello, suggests that they were licensed by fairly specific schemas like *I'm just pretending S*, *NP SAY S*, *NP TELL NP S* (where *SAY* and *TELL* stand for various forms of these two verbs) rather than a fully general subordination rule, since if children had a general rule, they would apply it to sentences containing other verbs as well.

Lexically specific units, then, are a ubiquitous feature of early production, which strongly suggests that young children's knowledge may be described in lexically specific terms. However, it is also possible that children do, in fact, have fully general, adult-like rules but for some reason do not use them in production. In order to rule out this alternative possibility, Tomasello and colleagues have conducted a series of experiments in which they investigated children's ability to use unfamiliar words in novel ways. They found that even children as young as 1;6 to 1;11 freely assimilate novel *nouns* to a variety of constructions. Thus, if they are taught the nonce word *wug* referring to an unfamiliar animal, they spontaneously use it in combination with items which are already part of their repertoire, producing utterances such as *where's the wug?*, *I want my wug*, *wug did it* and so on (Tomasello et al. 1997). However, children's performance in experiments involving novel verbs is dramatically different: the under-threes tend to use novel verbs only in the construction in which they heard them. For example, Brooks and Tomasello (1999) taught children aged about 2;11 two novel verbs designating highly transitive actions. One of the verbs was presented in the transitive construction (*Big Bird tammed the car*) and the other in a passive construction (*The car got meeked by Big Bird*). They then attempted to elicit transitive sentences by asking what the agent was doing. They found that only 25 per cent of the children who heard passive models were able to use the novel verb in an active transitive sentence describing the same action with a different set of participants. However, when tested on the verb they heard in the transitive construction, all of the children succeeded in this task.

In other experiments, Tomasello's team attempted to elicit a full transitive with a novel verb modelled in intransitive (*The lion is gorping*), imperative (*Gorp, lion!*) and presentative constructions (*Look, this is called gorping*). The results are very consistent: children aged 2;0 and below virtually never produce full transitives with a novel verb modelled in another construction; the proportion of children who succeed in such tasks increases steadily with age until it reaches 80 per cent by about 4;0; after 4, progress levels off slightly, but by about 8 years of age, virtually all children are able to use a novel verb in the transitive (see Tomasello 2000). Berman (1993) obtained comparable results with Hebrew-speaking children. In her experiment, the novel verb was modelled in the intransitive construction and elicited in the transitive. In Hebrew, this transformation is more complex, as it requires morphological changes to the verb as well as a rearrangement of the arguments, and so, not surprisingly, the task turned out to be even more difficult for children: only 9 per cent of the youngest participants (2;9) were successful; the proportion rose to 38 per cent by 3;9 and to 69 per cent by 8;0.

While most of the work with novel verbs focused on the transitive construction, the same methodology has also been used to study children's productivity with other structures, with similar results. Brooks and Tomasello (1999), for example, also attempted to elicit passives, and found that 85 per cent of the children in the youngest group they tested (age 2;11) were able to produce a full passive with a novel verb if the verb had been modelled in the passive (with different NPs expressing the agent and patient roles). However, if they had only heard the verb in active sentences, none of the children produced a full passive, and only 12 per cent were able to produce a truncated passive (a passive clause without the *by*-phrase).

The Brooks and Tomasello study also provides evidence bearing on another acquisition issue. English-speaking children begin to produce full passives fairly late – typically between 4 and 5 years of age. One explanation for their late appearance, often put forward by researchers working in the generative tradition (e.g. Borer and Wexler 1987), is that passives are difficult because they involve movement, which is a late-maturing syntactic ability. An alternative account, preferred in usage-based approaches, attributes children's difficulties to the fact that full passives are very rare in the input: Gordon and Chafetz (1990), for example, found only four tokens of this construction in over 86,000 child-directed utterances. The fact that most of the under-threes in the Brooks and Tomasello study were able to use full passives productively after brief but intensive training (two 30-minute sessions containing about 100 models) suggests that the latter explanation is correct: that is to say, that frequency in the input is the determining factor.

Further support for the idea that young children's knowledge about word order is lexically specific rather than general comes from comprehension studies involving nonce words. In one such study (Akhtar and Tomasello 1997), children were taught a new activity involving two characters and an apparatus; then they were given two new characters and the apparatus and asked to *make Cookie Monster dack Big Bird*. The main finding was that while older children (mean age 3;8) did very well, only three out of ten 2;9-year-olds performed above chance.

But perhaps the most striking evidence for lexical specificity comes from two studies in which novel words were presented in constructions with non-canonical (i.e. non-English) word order. In the first of these, conducted by Nameera Akhtar (1999), children were taught novel verbs designating highly transitive actions in syntactic frames with SOV or VSO word order (e.g. *Elmo the car dacking, Gopping Elmo the car*) and then encouraged to describe scenes involving different participants using the newly learned verbs. The question was whether they would correct to the canonical SVO pattern (thus demonstrating verb-general knowledge of word order) or use the unusual word order they heard in the model sentences. Akhtar found that the oldest children (mean age 4;4) virtually always used the SVO pattern, no matter what word order was used in the model sentences, while the younger children (ages 2;8 and 3;6) corrected to the canonical word order or used the unusual constructions they had been to exposed to during the experiment equally frequently. However, all age groups consistently corrected to the canonical word order when a familiar verb was presented in an SOV or VSO pattern (for example, they would never say *He the car pushing*). Thus, the younger children's use of the unusual word order cannot be explained by appealing to irrelevant factors such as reluctance to correct an adult. Another interesting finding was that in nearly all the utterances with non-canonical orders, the agent and patient arguments were expressed by lexical NPs rather than pronouns, whereas half of the utterances that were corrected contained pronouns: that is to say, the younger children would happily say *Ernie the spoon dacking* but not *He it dacking*. This suggests that the 'corrected' utterances may have been produced using lexically specific schemas based on pronouns (such as *He's VERBing it*).

The second study, by Abbot-Smith et al. (2001), involved slightly younger children (aged 2;4 and 3;9) and used intransitive action verbs (i.e. unergatives) rather than transitives. The verbs were presented in three conditions:

1. Novel SV: novel verb in the canonical order, e.g. *The cow baffing*;
2. Novel VS: novel verb in a non-canonical order, e.g. *Baffing the cow* (meaning 'The cow is wobbling out');
3. Familiar VS: familiar verb in non-canonical order, e.g. *Jumping the cow* ('The cow is jumping').

The results were broadly compatible with those of the previous study: the 3-year-olds consistently used SV order in all three conditions, while the 2-year-olds generally corrected to the canonical word order with familiar verbs (72 per cent of the time), but not with novel verbs (only 21 per cent of the time), showing that they lacked a general SV schema they could rely on in production. As in the Akhtar study, the non-canonical word order was virtually never used with pronouns (i.e. children did not produce utterances such as *Baffed she*), while the majority of the utterances with corrected word order contained pronouns; the 2-year-olds, in fact, were almost five times more likely to correct to the canonical word order when the subject was a pronoun. Also, when using the non-canonical VS order the children never added the missing auxiliary, but they did tend to add it when using the SV order. Interestingly, they were more likely to add it after a pronominal subject than after a lexical subject (70 per cent v. 26 per cent of the time in the 2-year-old group). These asymmetries suggest that they have learned multi-word units such as *He's VERBing* and *She's VERBing*.

There is, however, an interesting twist to these 'weird word order' studies. In both experiments, children were considerably more likely to reproduce the word order they heard with a particular nonce word if it was compatible with the canonical word order in English. Akhtar's children produced approximately four times as many sentences with novel verbs in the control SVO condition as in the experimental conditions. Abbot-Smith et al. also recorded about four times as many productive uses of the nonce verb in the Novel SV condition as in the Novel VS condition. One explanation for this pattern of results is that the children were actively avoiding the strange word order used by the experimenter, which would suggest that they had some nascent verb-general knowledge, even if it was too weak to be reliably used in production. Another possibility is that knowing a large number of verbs associated with a particular construction makes it easier to acquire new verbs occurring in the same construction. This would entail that children make connections between their lexically specific patterns from the very beginning, although they may need time and/or a 'critical mass' of exemplars before they extract a general rule.

Further evidence about the nature of young children's syntactic representations comes from studies which used the preferential looking paradigm. This

method involves presenting the child simultaneously with two videos depicting two different scenes (e.g. a causative action such as a duck lifting a rabbit's
leg and a non-causative action such as a duck and a rabbit each covering its
own eyes) and a test sentence which describes one of them (e.g. *The duck is
gorping the bunny*). The experimenter then measures how long the children
look at each screen. If they spend more time looking at the matching video, it
is concluded that they are able to extract some information from the syntactic
form of the construction. The greatest advantage of this method is that it can
be used with very young children (13–14 months); the main disadvantage is
that it is not clear what kind of information children extract from the linguistic stimuli (cf. Naigles 1990; Tomasello and Abbot-Smith 2002).

Using the preferential looking procedure, Hirsh-Pasek and Golinkoff (1996:
experiments 5 and 6) found that the oldest children in their study (mean age
28–9 months) looked longer at the video showing a causative event when presented with a novel verb in a transitive sentence, but performed at chance when
presented with intransitive sentence; the middle group (24 months) showed a
preference for the matching video with familiar verbs only, thus demonstrating
verb-specific knowledge; and the youngest group (19 months) showed no evidence of understanding the sentential context with either familiar or novel
verbs. Kidd et al. (2001), who tested slightly older children (mean age 30
months), found that they performed above chance on both transitive and
intransitive sentences with nonce words. Another study (Naigles 1990) suggests
that the relevant knowledge may appear somewhat earlier, around 25 months.

Thus, the preferential looking findings are broadly compatible with the production studies described earlier, in that they suggest that lexically specific
knowledge precedes verb-general knowledge; they do, however, suggest that
verb-general knowledge emerges considerably earlier. It is important, however,
not to overinterpret these findings. The fact that the children were influenced
by the linguistic form of the sentences accompanying the video presentation
shows that they were picking up on *some* property or properties of the sentences and linking them to the display – but it is by no means clear what exactly
they were attending to. Specifically, there is no strong evidence that they were
using word order to assign agent and patient roles: it is possible that they associated the experimental sentences with fairly holistic representations of the corresponding visual displays. For instance, they could have linked transitive
utterances such as *The duck is gorping the bunny* to scenes involving two participants doing different things, and intransitive sentences such as *The duck and
the bunny are gorping* to scenes in which the two participants do the same thing;
note that in the latter case, the relevant cue might not be word order but the
word *and*.

Further evidence suggesting that young children's constructions are lexically specific while older children have more abstract representations comes
from an experiment by Savage et al. (submitted). In this study, children were
shown pairs of pictures. The experimenter described the first picture using a

particular construction (for example, a passive such as *The car got smashed by the tree*), and then the child was asked to describe the second picture, which showed different characters performing different actions. Children aged 4 and above showed evidence of priming (they were more likely to produce a passive sentence when describing the second picture if the had just heard this structure), but younger children did not. However, there was priming even in the younger children in another condition, when there was lexical overlap between the two sentences – that is to say, when the experimenter's sentence contained lexical material that the child could use in her own sentence (e.g. *He got VERBed by it*).

Thus, experimental research confirms that early grammatical knowledge is lexically specific. It also shows that the emergence of general word-order schemas is a very gradual process. The preferential looking studies suggest that some form of verb-general knowledge of the transitive construction begins to develop about age 2;6, but it takes another year or so before children's representations are strong enough to support production. Verb-general knowledge about less frequent structures such as the passives takes even longer to develop.

2.7 'Mosaic' acquisition

Even if early multi-word utterances are constructed using formulaic frames of the kind described in the preceding subsection, such frames can only account for certain aspects of language development. Acquiring the full adult system requires much more than learning the positional requirements of individual lexical items. The child will eventually be able to add various inflections to thousands of stems and command a wide range of complex syntactic constructions. Underlying these, as every linguistics undergraduate knows, are some rather abstract rules, which she must learn at some stage. Conventional linguistic wisdom has it that children are able to infer these rules with ease and after relatively little exposure. Moreover, once a rule is learned, it is immediately applied in all the contexts that require it. 'It is striking,' Chomsky tells us, 'that advances are generally "across the board"' (1964: 39; see also Chomsky 1999).

Or are they? This claim doesn't appear to be corroborated by longitudinal research, which suggests that grammatical development is typically slow and piecemeal. For example, research on the acquisition of grammatical morphemes shows that children initially learn to add the present-participle and past-tense endings to one verb at a time and that it can take quite a long time for the endings to penetrate the entire linguistic system (Brown 1973; Cazden 1968):

A considerable period of time elapses between the first appearances of a morpheme and the point where it is almost always supplied where required. The progressive ending, for example, is first supplied 100 percent of the time in obligatory contexts in sample 16. This comes 16 months later than sample 1 when -*ing* was supplied 50 percent of the time. We can be sure that there were some progressives and some plurals in Sarah's speech before we began to transcribe it, so that the time elapsing between first occurrences and a perfect performance is even longer . . . It is true of all the grammatical morphemes in all three children that performance does not abruptly pass from total absence to reliable presence. There is always a considerable period, varying in length with the particular morpheme, in which production-where-required is probabilistic. This is a fact that does not accord well with the notion that the acquisition of grammar is a matter of the acquisition of rules, since the rules in a generative grammar either apply or do not apply. One would expect rule acquisition to be sudden. (Brown 1973: 298)

Later research has tended to corroborate Brown's suggestion that the acquisition of grammatical inflections is a process of piecemeal addition rather than sudden revelation. Bloom et al. (1980) reported that the irregular-past, present-participle and third-person-singular inflections tend to be used with different populations of verbs: -*ing* predominantly with durative non-completive verbs such as *eat*, *play* and *write*; the irregular past with non-durative completive verbs such as *find*, *get* and *come*; and -*s* predominantly with *go* and *fit* (as in *This goes/fits in here*). More recently, similar findings have been reported by Tomasello (1992: see above), Pizzuto and Caselli (1992), Caselli et al. (1993) and Rubino and Pine (1998).

Rubino and Pine's work is particularly interesting since it shows that verb-specific learning can occur even at a time when the child already has general rules. They studied the acquisition of subject–verb agreement by a 3-year-old child learning Brazilian Portuguese. By this stage, the child appeared to have mastered the agreement system of his language, since the overwhelming majority of his verb forms had the correct inflections: the error rate was only 3 per cent. However, Rubino and Pine were able to show that this low overall rate was due to very good performance on a few very frequent categories (specifically, the singular inflections) and masked much higher error rates in other parts of the system. Plural forms accounted for only 3.4 per cent of the verb forms used by the child (which suggests that he avoided using the plural), and had much higher error rates: 23 per cent for the first person plural *a gente* and 43 per cent for the third person plural. (Second person plural forms did not occur at all in their corpus of almost 1,500 utterances.) Moreover, seven out of the twelve utterances exhibiting correct 3PL agreement contained one of two very frequent verb forms. Thus, there is little evidence for the mastery of plural inflections: the child appeared to be learning the system piecemeal.

But perhaps the most convincing evidence for such 'mosaic' acquisition comes from studies of the development of rules for auxiliary verb placement in English. Early studies of the development of interrogatives and negatives (Bellugi 1971; Klima and Bellugi 1966) reported that progress is across the board: that is to say, auxiliaries appear in all the syntactic contexts that require them at more or less the same time; and, moreover, once the child learns the rule of subject–auxiliary inversion, she applies it to all the auxiliaries she knows. However, these early studies were more concerned with writing grammars for early stages of language development than with documenting transitions from one stage to the next, and so simultaneous development was asserted rather than demonstrated. More recent research on auxiliaries shows a very different picture.

The first chink in the argument for across-the-board acquisition of English auxiliaries was an observation made by Bellugi and Klima themselves that subject–auxiliary inversion seemed to appear in yes/no questions first and spread to WH questions only later in development (Bellugi 1971; Klima and Bellugi 1966). However, Bellugi had a good story to tell about why this should happen: children at this stage, she argued, know both the subject–auxiliary inversion and the WH fronting rule, but due to limited processing power are unable to apply both in a single derivation. Hence, we get correctly placed auxiliaries in yes/no questions, which require inversion only, and 'uninverted' auxiliaries in WH questions, which require WH fronting as well as inversion. Bellugi's explanation, though elegant, is far from water-tight, as she herself acknowledges. If limited processing resources prevent children from performing both transformations at the same time, they should produce not only questions with WH fronting but no inversion (*Where you will go?*), but also inverted questions without WH fronting (*Will you go where?*). Such structures, however, do not occur.

Moreover, new evidence soon began to accumulate that the acquisition of the rules for auxiliary placement in questions is disturbingly piecemeal. In their study of auxiliary placement in yes/no questions, Kuczaj and Maratsos (1983) found that children preposed some auxiliaries but not others. The study was prompted by the observation that Kuczaj's son Abe first began using *would* and *could* in declaratives at 2;9 and 2;11 respectively, but did not use them in questions until 3;5, although he did produce interrogatives with other modals, including *will* and *can*. Kuczaj and Maratsos then looked at a larger cross-sectional sample of 14 children between the ages of 2;6 and 5;6. They found the same pattern for *could* in the speech of seven children and for *would* in the speech of three children. They also noted that none of the children overgeneralised the inversion rule to auxiliary-like predicates such as *better*, *gotta*, *hafta* and *wanna*, which also suggested that they did not have a general rule involving auxiliaries as a class.

Similar findings from a study that used experimental methods with older children (5–8-year-olds) were reported by Major (1974). Major asked children to imitate sentences with modal verbs, to transform declaratives into negatives and interrogatives, and to add tags to model sentences. Her general conclusion was that although all of the children were familiar with some of the uses of all modals and semi-modals, knowledge about the constructions in which a particular word could occur was not generalised from one member of the class to another. The children generally performed well on high-frequency modals (*will, would, can, could, should*) but error rates on *may, might, shall* and *must* were very high: for example, they were 25–60 per cent correct on negatives with *may*, depending on age group, and 0–20 per cent correct on questions with the same verb. When faced with the task of transforming *You may go home* into a question, most of the children (20) simply substituted a more familiar modal with a similar meaning – that is to say, they produced well-formed questions with *will, would, can* or *could*. Six children produced the target structure (*May you go home?*); one simply repeated the stimulus sentence using a rising intonation. Most revealing, however, were the ungrammatical sentences produced by some of the children. Two children responded with *Do you may go?* and 11 added another modal at the beginning of the sentence, producing *Can you may go? Could you may go?*, *Will you may go?*, or *Would you may go?* Differences between the modals showed up even on the imitation task. For example, 83 per cent of the 5-year-olds imitated *He should have finished his breakfast* and *We could have gone to the show*, but only 8 per cent were able to reproduce faithfully an analogous sentence with the auxiliary *can* (*Sally can have chased the dog*). Even more patchy was the children's command of tag questions. Every child produced at least one acceptable tag, but error rates were very high, and no child produced tags with *may, might, shall* or *ought to*. Moreover, some added the same tag to nearly all sentences, which also suggests that they had not fully mastered the structure.

Modals in WH questions show a similar pattern of development. An elicited imitation experiment conducted by Kuczaj and Brannick (1979) showed that children learn to place modals correctly first after one or two WH words (usually *what* and *where*), then after another word, and so on: in other words, they learn the rule piecemeal. Similar results have been reported by Labov and Labov (1978) and Ingram and Tyack (1979).

However, Kuczaj and Brannick also found that the children did eventually generalise, or at least some did. Fifteen of their subjects (out of 60) overgeneralised the rule to questions with *how come*, which resulted in ungrammatical utterances such as **How come will the wolf howl at the moon?* However, six of the children who overgeneralised failed to use modals at all with *how long*; and ten correctly repeated questions with *how come* + past verb (*How come the turtle fell on the ground?*) – in other words, the overgeneralised rule was not fully general!

There is also evidence suggesting that the knowledge that children acquire is not only lexically specific but also construction-specific: that is to say, children learn about specific words in specific constructions. Rowland and Pine's (2000) detailed analysis of WH questions produced by a single child revealed that he tended to prepose some auxiliaries after some WH words and use declarative word order with other WH+AUX combinations, and that the combinations that were preposed were more frequent in the input than the non-preposed ones. Fletcher, Rowland and Jackson (2003), using an elicited production task, showed that 3-year-olds performed very well on WH questions with the copula (which are very frequent in the input), but were unable to produce structurally identical questions with the auxiliary *should*. However, when the specific structure (i.e. WH questions with *should*) was modelled for the children in the course of the experiment, performance improved dramatically. In another experiment, the children were trained with inverted Y/N questions with *is*, *can* or *should* and tested on WH questions with the same auxiliary. In this case, the training did not improve performance: in other words, the children were not able to generalise knowledge about auxiliary placement in Y/N questions to WH questions.

Another telling example of piecemeal learning is provided by Todd's (1982) study of the acquisition of tag questions by his daughter Audrey. Audrey first began to use tags at 3;2, but except for two frozen forms which occurred very early on, all her tags were affirmative. This resulted in ungrammatical utter ances when the tagged sentence was also affirmative: *I look funny, do I?, We're going home, are we?* (both said with a rising intonation).[5] She began to use negative tags productively at 4;2, but only with two verb forms, *is* and *will*. At 4;11, she added *wasn't NP?* to her repertoire of negative tags. Finally, about 5;3, negation spread to all auxiliaries used in tags and was overgeneralised to negative sentences, where she had previously supplied the correct form (**There isn't very much people here, isn't there?*).

Taken together, the studies reviewed here provide very strong evidence that the development of auxiliary placement rules in English is a step-by-step, bottom-up process involving the gradual accumulation of specific bits of knowledge which are only later integrated into a system. Children do not acquire an abstract rule of subject–auxiliary inversion: they learn about specific forms in specific constructions. They may subsequently develop broader rules by generalising over these low-level patterns, but the early rules are highly specific.

This conclusion is corroborated by a more comprehensive study of the English auxiliary system by Richards (1990). Richards's monograph surveys the development of auxiliary verbs in seven children over a period of some eight months. Using recordings of spontaneous speech as well as an elicited imitation task, he charts the emergence of all allomorphs of the core auxiliary verbs in all syntactic contexts in which the auxiliary occurs: declaratives, negatives, Y/N questions, WH questions, and emphatic and elliptical uses, including tags. The study revealed wide-ranging individual differences and a great deal of piecemeal learning:

'Across the board' developments did not occur, though there were periods of rapid development for some children. Instead, progress was typified by piecemeal additions to the range of forms and the range of linguistic contexts and syntactic frames in which they were used. (Richards 1990: 214)

3. A case study: questions

We saw in the preceding section that children's early use is dominated by fixed phrases and low-scope patterns. There is considerable disagreement, however, about the relationship between these early formulas and the more general patterns which emerge later. Some researchers (e.g. Bates et al. 1988; Brown and Hanlon 1970; Krashen and Scarcella 1978) have argued that formulas are a developmental dead-end, or at best a side street, a kind of linguistic crutch which allows children to get by in the early stages of development, but which is eventually superseded by 'real' syntax with standard combinatorial rules. Others (e.g. Lieven et al. 1992; Pine and Lieven 1993; Tomasello 2000, 2003) have suggested that rote-learned phrases play a critical role in the development of productive use. On this account, the transition to adult syntax is quite gradual and does not involve qualitative shifts.

In this section, I will address this issue by examining in some detail the acquisition of a particular construction, or rather family of constructions, namely, English questions. Question constructions can provide more conclusive evidence about the role of lexically specific learning in development than argument structure constructions. It makes sense for children to be conservative when acquiring the latter, since different verbs have different subcategorisation requirements. Questions, on the other hand, share some very general structural properties (often captured by means of two abstract rules: WH fronting and subject–auxiliary inversion), so if children acquire fully general knowledge from the start, this is where we would expect to find evidence of it. The acquisition of question constructions is also interesting from a theoretical point of view, since the two movement rules have played a very important role in the development of generative linguistics.

I have already noted that children sometimes acquire interrogative formulas such as *What's that?* and *Where's X?* in early stages of development, long before there is any evidence of 'true' syntax. We will now examine children's questions more systematically in order to determine how prevalent such formulaic uses are, how long they persist, and whether there is any evidence of developmental discontinuities in the transition to more productive usage which might signal the acquisition of rules.

3.1 Early interrogative utterances

Lieven (2003) studied syntactic questions (multi-word utterances containing a preposed auxiliary and/or a preposed WH word) in the speech of four 2-year-olds recorded for five hours a week over a six-week period. This recording regime produced samples which are five to ten times denser than those used in most studies and comprise 7 to 10 per cent of each child's linguistic experience during this period. With such relatively large samples, it is possible to identify recurrent word combinations which are likely to be retrieved from memory as ready-made units.

Lieven was interested in two types of preconstructed units, or formulas: lexically fixed phrases (e.g. *What's that?*) and frames with a slot which can be filled by a variety of expressions (e.g. *Where's X?*). For the purposes of the study, Lieven assumed that an utterance was formulaic if the corpus contained at least three tokens of the same combination of words produced on three different occasions. A frequency of three or more might not seem like very much; however, extrapolating from the sample, we can estimate that the child is likely to have produced 30–40 tokens of the utterance in question during the six-week period covered by the study, so the assumption does not seem unreasonable.[6]

Lieven's findings are presented in Table 9.1. As we can see, the children had from 6 to 19 different interrogative formulas, and these accounted for between 78 per cent and 98 per cent of their syntactic questions (mean 92 per cent). The table also contains the results of an analysis of a comparable corpus of data from a Polish-speaking child, Marysia (Dąbrowska and Lieven 2003). The figures are very similar, thus providing some cross-linguistic validation for Lieven's findings.

Table 9.1 Formulaic questions in the speech of five 2-year-olds

	Brian	**Chris**	**Annie**	**Delia**	**Marysia**
MLU (words)	1.72	1.98	2.12	2.23	1.87
Number of formulas	6	17	11	19	18
Total syntactic questions	346	434	409	300	695
Of which:					
Fixed phrase	70%	45%	17%	17%	80%
Frame with slot	28%	49%	77%	61%	14%
Non-formulaic	2%	6%	5%	21%	6%

Note: The figures for the English-speaking children (Brian, Chris, Annie and Delia) are based on Lieven (2003). The figures for the Polish-speaking child, Marysia, are based on Dąbrowska and Lieven (2003).

The data for the four English-speaking children is arranged from least advanced to most advanced, as measured by MLU. This reveals an interesting pattern: the longer the MLU, the lower the proportion of fixed formulas and the higher the proportion of frames with slots. The most advanced child, Delia, also has a relatively high proportion of non-formulaic utterances. This could mean that Delia had acquired some more general knowledge about interrogative utterances. However, Lieven notes that all but two of Delia's 'non-formulaic' questions could be traced back to utterances in the input in a relatively straightforward way: that is to say, they were either exact repetitions of things the mother had repeatedly said before, or were based on frames which could have been derived from the input (for example, the utterance *What's Mama making?* may be based on a *What's Mama V-ing?* frame, derived from parental utterances such as *What's Mama doing?*, *What's Mama cooking?* etc.).

3.2 From formula to schema

Lieven's study confirms that early questions are highly formulaic. Furthermore, the fact that the least advanced child used primarily invariant formulas, while more advanced children relied more on formulaic frames and also produced a higher proportion of non-formulaic utterances, suggests that development at this stage may involve a progression from invariant formulas to more schematic templates. However, it is also possible that the more formulaic children were relying on more holistic learning strategies, which, according to some researchers (e.g. Bates et al. 1988), may be less effective. Thus, to determine whether development indeed proceeds from formula to schema, we need to look at longitudinal data.

In this section we examine the development of questions in three children from the CHILDES database (MacWhinney 1995): Naomi, Sarah and Shem (Table 9.2). Because the corpora for these children are larger (though less dense) than those used by Lieven, I will adopt a slightly more stringent criterion for formulaicity: a question type will be considered formulaic if there are at least five instances of it in the child's speech. As in Lieven's study, the term 'formula' will subsume frames with a single slot as well as lexically fixed phrases.

Figure 9.1 shows the proportion of the two types of formulas as well as non-formulaic questions in the speech of the three children during the period covered by the study. As we can see from the graphs, virtually all of the questions produced by the 2-year-olds are formulaic by our criterion: these findings thus replicate the results of Lieven's study. As the children's linguistic systems develop we see a steady decrease in the proportion of fixed formulas

Table 9.2 Data for the longitudinal study

Corpus	Corpus size (child words)	Age range	Number of syntactic questions
Naomi (Sachs 1983)	38,729	1;8–3;8	1,439
Shem (Clark 1982)	65,651	2;2–3;2	1,173
Sarah (Brown 1973)	89,086	2;3–5;1	2,006

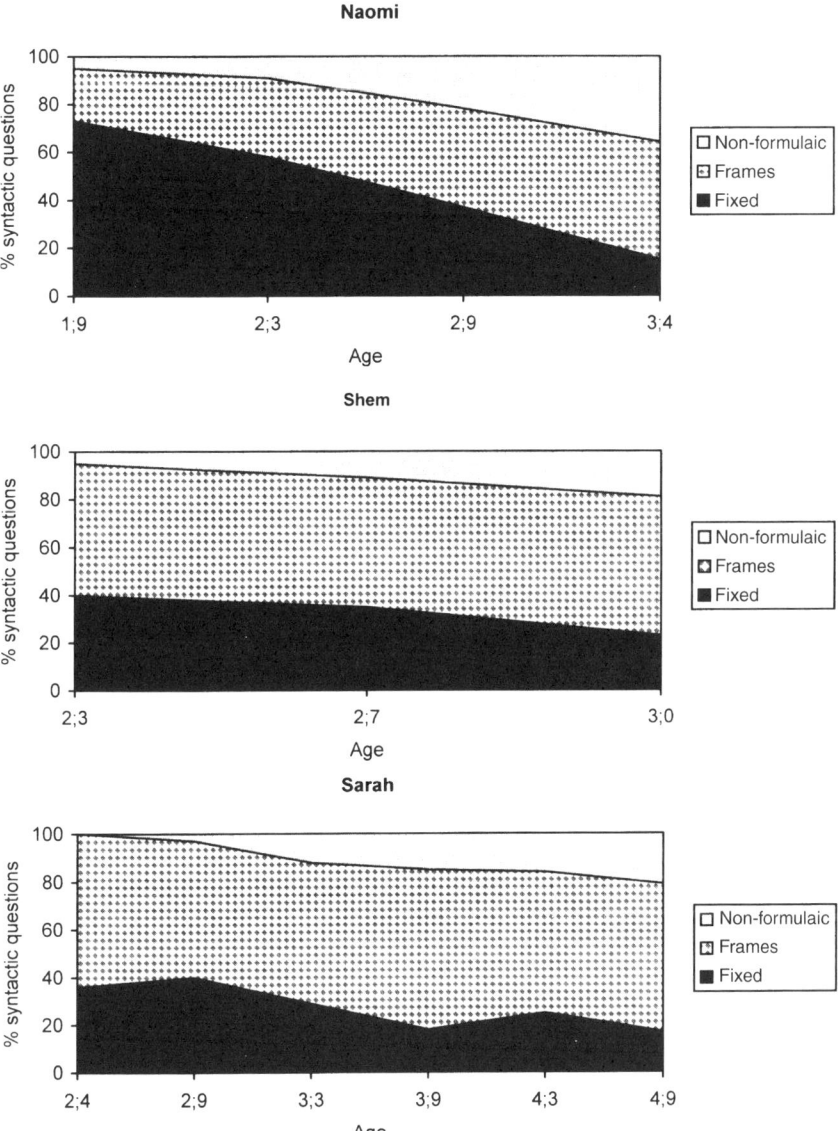

Figure 9.1 Formulaic and non-formulaic questions in the three children
Note: The ages on the Y axis represent the midpoint of each period.

and a corresponding increase in the proportion of more creative utterances. This pattern is most clearly visible in Naomi and Sarah, where we have data spanning longer periods, but it is also discernible in Shem.

Several further observations are in order. First, each child acquired a different set of question formulas (cf. Table 9.3), although, not surprisingly, some

Table 9.3 The children's 10 earliest formulas (in order of emergence)

Naomi (1;8–1;11) MLU 1.4–2.6	Shem (2;2) MLU 2.8	Sarah (2;3–2;8) MLU 1.6–2.4
what's this/that?	*what's this/that?*	*where NP?*
what do you VP? (VP = *see*)	*where's NP?*	*what's this/that?*
where's NP?	*what are (you) doing?*	*are you AP?* (AP = *bad*)
who VP? (VP = *did that*)	*what (is) NP doing?*	*who V it/that?*
where is NP? (NP = *it*)	*what's LOC?*	*where S?* (S = *gone*)
where did it go?	*what's NP?*	*where NP go?*
is this NP?	*what is that?*	*what VP?* (VP = *happen*)
is it AP?	*what happened to NP?*	*where is it?*
where's NP go? (NP = *it*)	*what S?*	*why S?* (S = *need them*)
is NP going to work?	*where NP go?*	*who('s) this?*

Note: The figures in the column headings indicate the time span during which the first 10 formulas emerged and the child's MLU at the beginning and the end of this period. If there was no variation in a particular slot during this early period, the only attested filler is given in parentheses after the formula. The very first recording in the Shem corpus already contains 10 formulas, suggesting that they developed earlier.

(e.g. *what's this/that?*, *where's NP?*) show up in all three. Secondly, there are marked differences in the rate of development. Naomi acquired her tenth question formula at age 1;11, while Sarah needed another nine months to reach the same milestone. Finally, and most importantly, formulaic utterances also feature very prominently in later development: even at age 3 and 4, a substantial majority of the children's utterances can still be accounted for in terms of a relatively small number of lexically specific units.

Thus the longitudinal data appears to support the scenario proposed earlier, namely, that development proceeds from fixed phrases through formulaic frames to more abstract patterns. Furthermore, there are no abrupt changes in behaviour which might signal the acquisition of a general rule. What we see instead is a slow but steady increase in the proportion of creative utterances, suggesting a series of small changes. To understand what such small changes might involve, it will be helpful to examine the development of a few formulas in more detail.

3.2.1 *Sarah's* who VP?

Sarah's earliest *who* questions were *who did it?* (produced at 2;4.26) and *who did that?* (produced two weeks later). During the next four weeks, she produced another six tokens of this formula, and a further 10 were attested in later recordings. (Note that *it*, *that* and *this* are frequently substituted for each other, but not for other forms, in a variety of constructions. Because the variation is very limited, it is not regarded as defining a slot, so *who did it/that?* was treated as a single fixed formula.) A related lexically fixed phrase appeared at 2;6.20:

(6)   a. *Who broke it?*   (2;6.20)
        b. *Who broke that?*   (2;7.5)

The corpus contains seven tokens of this formula in total. Two months later, Sarah began using other verbs in this construction:

(7)   a. *Who rip that?*   (2;8.25)
        b. *Who bought that?*   (2;8.25)
        c. *Who done this?*   (3;0.18)
        d. *Who drop this?*   (3;3.20)
        e. *Who lost it?*   (3;6.6)

Meanwhile, four other formulas with *who* appeared in Sarah's speech: *who this?*, *who is it?*, *who's that?* (all attested for the first time between 2;8 and 2;11; note that different pronouns were used with different forms of the copula), and, a little later, *who('s) goin(g to) VP?*, first attested at age 3;6. Finally, almost a year and a half after the emergence of the earliest formula, we get subject questions with *who* in sentences containing non-pronominal objects and non-transitive verbs, e.g.:

(8)   a. *Who didn't work?*   (3;9.26)
        b. *Who said can't?*   (3;10.16)
        c. *Who put the bandaid on?*   (4;1.11)
        d. *Who scribbled on it?*   (4;3.19)

Thus, development seems to have begun with two fixed formulas, *who did it/that?* and *who broke it/that?* The formulaic frame *who TRANS.V it/that?* which emerged somewhat later seems to be a generalisation over the two lexically fixed phrases (and possibly others which have not been captured in the sample). The fully general template for producing questions with *who* in the subject slot (*who VP?*) appeared considerably later, after Sarah had mastered a number of more specific *who*-subject formulas.

3.2.2 *Naomi's* what's NP doing?
Naomi's first recorded attempt at such questions was a telegraphic *What doing?* produced at 1;11.11. Ten days later she imitated a complete question with both a subject and a contracted auxiliary, *What's Mommy doing?* The transcripts for the next four weeks contain nine further occurrences of this utterance in exactly the same form. Then, at 2;0.18, she began producing similar questions with subjects other than *Mommy*:

(9)   a. *What's donkey doing?*   (2;0.18)
        b. *What's toy doing?*   (2;0.18)
        c. *What's Nomi doing?*   (2;0.18)

After this, there are many questions with the names of various people and toys in the subject slot. A week later, Naomi began substituting other verbs for *doing*:

(10)   a. *What's Mommy holding?*   (2;0.26)
        b. *What's Georgie saying?*   (2;1.9)

At this point, she could be said to have acquired a template with two slots (*What's NP TRANS.V-ing?*). Finally, just before her third birthday, she began to use the uncontracted form of the auxiliary, which suggests that she had analysed *what's* into its component morphemes:

(11)   a. *What is the boy making?*   (2;11.17)
        b. *What is Andy doing?*   (2;11.18)

Thus, we see a similar progression from a rote-learned lexical chunk (*What's Mommy doing?*) through increasingly general schemas (*What's NP doing?*, *What's NP TRANS.V-ing?*) to a fairly general template (*What BE NP TRANS.V-ing?*) which can be used to produce a wide variety of interrogative utterances.

3.2.3 Naomi's can I VP? *and* could I VP?
Questions with the modal auxiliary *can* appeared in Naomi's speech shortly before her second birthday.

(12)   a. *Can I get down?*   (1;11.9)
        b. *Can I get up?*   (1;11.9)
        c. *Can lie down?*   (1;11.16)

These early questions were quite stereotypical: the auxiliary was always placed at the beginning of the sentence, and the subject, if present, was always the first person pronoun *I*; when the subject was left out, it is clear from the context that the agent of the action was Naomi herself. This suggests that at this stage, she did not have a general auxiliary placement rule, but merely a formula for requesting permission.

With time Naomi's usage gradually became more flexible. First she acquired a variant of the permission-seeking formula with the auxiliary *could* instead of *can*. Like the canonical form of the formula, this variant was produced sometimes with and sometimes without an explicit subject.

(13)   a. *Could do this?*   (1;11.21)
       b. *Could eat that?*   (1;11.21)
       c. *Could I throw that?*   (2;0.3)

Then, at 2;0.28 – seven weeks after the first recorded use of the formula – we find the first question with a subject other than *I*.

(14)   a. *Can you draw eyes?*   (2;0.28)
       b. *Please can we do that?*   (2;8.14)

So, as in the previous two examples, early usage was highly stereotypical and gradually became more flexible as new slots opened up inside the formula.

3.3 Where do 'non-formulaic' utterances come from?

We have seen that questions produced by 2-year-olds are extremely stereotypical, in that virtually all are instances of one of a relatively small number of formulas. Older children continue to use such stereotypical phrases, but also produce increasingly high proportions of apparently more creative utterances. Where do these non-formulaic questions come from, and what do they tell us about the children's grammatical abilities?

It is important to realise that many of the utterances which were classified as 'non-formulaic' according to the frequency criterion (five or more child tokens in the corpus) could actually be instances of well-practised routines. The transcripts analysed here contain a tiny sample of the children's linguistic experience – somewhere between 1 per cent and 2 per cent of what they said and heard – so even utterances that the child had produced hundreds of times may only occur once in the sample, or not be found at all. Furthermore, 30–50 per cent of the non-formulaic utterances, though rare in the child, occur five or more times in the input, so there is a good chance that they have been memorised. (Note that the *mean* frequency of utterances which occur five times in a 1 per cent sample of the input is 500, assuming the sample to be representative.)

On the other hand, some non-formulaic questions are without doubt creative. This is evident from the fact that they contain relatively high proportions of errors of commission (cf. Table 9.4).[7] What is more, in contrast to the errors found in formulaic utterances (see below), these tend to be quite unsystematic, which suggests that they are one-off innovations produced when the child attempts to go beyond the well-practised formulas and say something he or she had not yet learned to say.

The most interesting subcategory of non-formulaic utterances is those which are grammatical yet cannot be regarded as delayed imitations of phrases which occur frequently in the input. Such utterances *do* indicate that the child is moving beyond lexically specific formulas. However, as we saw in

Table 9.4 Errors of commission in formulaic and non-formulaic questions

Child	Number of questions		% errors of commission	
	Formulaic	Non-formulaic	Formulaic	Non-formulaic
Naomi	1,271	168	2	12
Shem	1,058	115	14	27
Sarah	1,681	325	7	16

the preceding subsection, they don't necessarily require abstract movement rules, since they could be produced by substituting new material into more abstract templates with two or even three slots. For example, *can we do that?* could be constructed by inserting *we* and *do that* into the NP and VP slots in *can NP VP?*; *what's Georgie saying?* could be constructed by inserting *Georgie* and *say* into the appropriate slots in *what's NP TRANS.V-ing?*; and so on.

3.4 Evidence for piecemeal learning

On the other hand, the fact that the children's questions can be described in terms of lexically specific formulas and templates does not entail that they should be so described, since the same data could also be accounted for (more economically) in terms of general rules. In order to determine how abstract or concrete children's syntactic representations really are, we need to turn to other sources of information. As indicated earlier, there are several experimental studies suggesting that knowledge about particular auxiliaries and WH words is indeed acquired piecemeal. There are also some interesting patterns in the longitudinal data examined here which support this interpretation (see also Dąbrowska 2000 for a more detailed discussion of the Naomi data).

3.4.1 Auxiliary placement
Y/N questions in English are normally marked by a preposed auxiliary (*Can I do that?*), with rising intonation acting as a secondary marker. Another option is to use only rising intonation (*I can do that?*). Young children often rely on this simpler method; then, as they acquire the adult system, the proportion of inverted questions (i.e. questions with a preposed auxiliary) increases (see Figure 9.2).

It is noteworthy that the course of development is different in different children. In Shem, we see a steady increase in the proportion of inverted questions during the entire period of observation. Sarah shows a similar pattern, except that progress levels off after age 4;0. Naomi's development, in contrast, follows a very clear U-shaped curve. In the early stages (before age 2), the number of questions with preposed auxiliaries was relatively high, but they were very stereotypical. As she became more adventurous and started asking questions about a wider variety of situations, the proportion of inverted questions

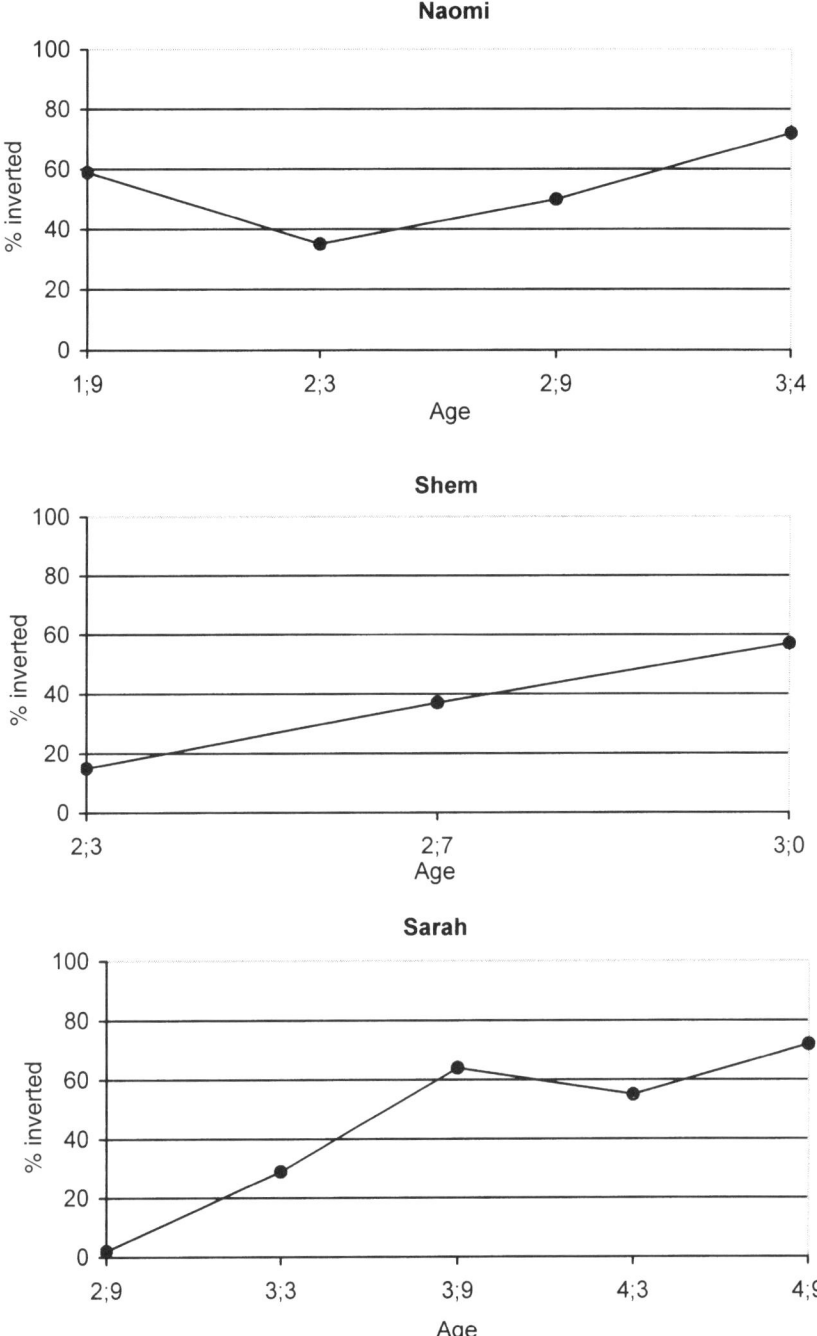

Figure 9.2 Proportion of inverted Y/N questions

dropped. Then, from about 2;6 onwards, it started rising again until, towards the end of the period covered by this study, it reached levels similar to those found in the input.[8]

The overall inversion rates in Figure 9.2 mask some interesting low-level patterns suggesting that the children acquired knowledge about specific combinations of words rather than general rules. To show such effects, one would ideally want to compare the proportions of inverted and uninverted questions for each auxiliary + subject combination at different stages of development. However, such an analysis would require a corpus containing a much larger sample of each child's speech for each developmental period. Fortunately, some patterns are discernible even if we collapse figures across auxiliaries or subjects; and it is also possible to conduct a more fine-grained analysis of questions with the most frequent auxiliary, namely *do*.

Table 9.5 shows the proportions of inverted yes/no questions with the most frequent auxiliaries in the three children, and, for comparison, in one of the mothers.[9] To avoid collapsing across very long periods, and also to give some sense of development, the Sarah corpus has been split into two parts: Sarah1 covers the period from 2;3 to 3;7, and Sarah2, from 3;8 to 5;1.

Table 9.5 Inverted Y/N questions according to auxiliary

Auxiliary	Naomi N	Naomi %	Shem N	Shem %	Sarah1 N	Sarah1 %	Sarah2 N	Sarah2 %	Naomi's input N	Naomi's input %
can	32	100	36	80	21	88	138	91	68	97
will	6	86	3	–	10	78	38	83	0	–
would	11	100	1	–	0	–	3	–	40	100
aux-*be*[a]	21	54	12	43	2	–	40	68	93	72
copula[a]	78	76	34	44	22	59	227	75	90	68
do/does	36	39	55	37	4	3	169	40	207	62
did	8	53	5	31	10	67	88	77	93	72

Note: Percentages are provided only when there were at least eight questions with a given auxiliary (inverted and uninverted).
[a] Present-tense forms only

It is clear from the figures in the table that the children preposed some auxiliaries considerably more often than others. All three used the inverted form by far the most frequently with *can*. This is also true of the mother, so the children's behaviour may be simply a direct reflection of the input: they heard both inverted and uninverted questions with the other auxiliaries, so they produced both types; with *can*, they virtually never heard uninverted questions, so they rarely produced them themselves. The remaining differences are partly attributable to order of acquisition (since the data was collected over a period of time, if a child acquired the inverted pattern for a particular auxiliary fairly late, the overall inversion rate for that auxiliary will be low) and partly to the fact that different auxiliaries follow different developmental trajectories (for example, although questions with *do* and *did* appeared in Sarah's speech at about the same time, she used the latter much more consistently than the former).

Such differences between inversion rates for individual auxiliaries can be accommodated in a rules-based approach: even if children acquire a general rule, they still need to learn about the lexical properties of each auxiliary, and it is perfectly possible that they acquire such knowledge at different times for different auxiliaries. Much more problematic for such approaches is the fact that there are also substantial differences in the frequency of inversion with different subjects.

Consider first questions with *do*. *Do* is used when there is no other auxiliary in the sentence, so the uninverted (i.e. intonation-only) analogues of such questions normally lack an auxiliary (*You want some?*), except when they are emphatic (*You do want some?*). Table 9.6 shows frequency of inversion with

Table 9.6 Inverted Y/N questions with present-tense forms of the auxiliary *do*

Person and number	Naomi		Shem		Sarah2		Naomi's input	
	N	%	N	%	N	%	N	%
1sg	0	0	0	0	21	44	0	–
2sg	29	52	53	54	92	35	153	61
3sg	7	23	1	5	45	52	43	67
Plural	0	–	1	7	11	48	11	55
	36	38	55	38	169	40	207	62

Note: Percentages are provided only when there were at least eight questions with a given subject (inverted and uninverted).

first, second and third person singular and with plural subjects in the three children and, for comparison, in one of the mothers.[10] (The figures for plural subjects have been collapsed to allow meaningful comparisons, as such questions are relatively rare.) As we can see, the mother's inversion rates are very similar for all person/number combinations. The children, on the other hand, put *do* before some subjects considerably more often than before others, which is precisely what one would expect if they initially acquired knowledge about particular combinations of subjects and auxiliaries.[11]

Moreover, there are differences between the children in this regard. Naomi and Shem invert by far the most frequently with second person subjects – in fact, Shem almost never uses *do* with any subject other than *you*. The most plausible explanation for this early proficiency with second person subjects is frequency in the input: children hear a great many questions of the form *do you VP?*, so they have plenty of opportunity to pick up the pattern. Questions with third person subjects are also quite frequent, but considerably more varied (*does it VP?*, *does he VP?*, *does she VP?*, as well as some with lexical subjects), so there are fewer opportunities to learn any particular pattern. *Do* questions with first person and plural subjects, on the other hand, are rare in the input; and it is also these combinations that Naomi and Shem have most difficulty with.

Sarah, however, shows a very different pattern: she is *least* likely to invert with second person subjects. It seems that several factors have conspired to produce this effect. First, as is evident from Figures 9.1 and 9.2, Sarah's early development was quite slow compared to the other children. She appeared to have particular problems with the auxiliary *do* (cf. Table 9.5), possibly because it was often contracted to [d] or [dʒ] in the input (as in *d'you want an apple?*), and hence not very salient acoustically. Consequently, by the time she learned her first *do*-frames, she already had several well-entrenched intonation-only formulas such as *you want NP?* and *you know what?* which often pre-empted the emerging templates with auxiliaries. We see this very clearly when we compare the frequencies of lexical verbs in inverted and uninverted questions. The latter are dominated by high-frequency verbs: 52 per cent have either *want* or *know* as the main verb, and 73 per cent contain one of just six verbs; the corresponding figures for inverted questions are 29 per cent and 56 per cent respectively. Thus Sarah's development, although it followed a different course from that of the other two children, also shows evidence of lexically specific learning.

Similar differences in the proportion of inverted and uninverted questions, depending on the subject, are found with other auxiliaries (cf. Table 9.7); and

Table 9.7 Inverted Y/N questions according to person and number in questions with auxiliaries other than *do*

Auxiliary	Naomi		Shem		Sarah1		Sarah2		Naomi's input	
	N	%	N	%	N	%	N	%	N	%
1sg	28	85	31	74	25	81	129	87	20	65
2sg	32	67	20	53	23	61	177	80	268	79
3sg	69	45	33	29	22	43	298	75	176	76
Plural	7	54	4	–	3	–	22	50	20	69
Total	136	55	88	44	73	59	626	77	484	77

Note: Percentages are provided only when there were at least eight questions with a given subject (inverted and uninverted).

again, the differences are small and not statistically significant in the mother, and highly significant in the children.[12] It is interesting to note that the relative proportions of inverted and uninverted questions with different subjects are different than with *do*: all three children invert most often in questions with *I*, and least often with third person singular and plural subjects.

The pattern of inversion/uninversion with the pronoun *I* is particularly interesting, and merits a more detailed discussion. Questions with first person subjects are relatively rare in the input. Only 3 per cent of the Y/N questions addressed to Naomi had first person subjects, and almost half of these had the form *can I VP?* Children, on the other hand, ask such questions quite often, thus offering the analyst an excellent opportunity to determine to what extent they have generalised the patterns in the speech addressed to them. If inversion rates with *I* are as high as with other subjects, this would suggest that children have fairly general rules; and conversely, low inversion rates would entail failure to generalise. As we saw earlier, children rarely produce syntactic questions with first person subjects and the auxiliary *do*; but inversion rates for *I* with other auxiliaries are quite high (cf. Table 9.7). However, a closer analysis reveals some striking patterns. The high inversion rates that we see in Table 9.7 are due to the fact that the vast majority of the children's questions with first person subjects are *can I VP?* questions – the only frequent first person pattern in the input – which all three children consistently invert (see Table 9.8). If we exclude questions with *can*, inversion rates with first person subjects will be very low, except for the second half of the Sarah corpus, which covers data for a relatively late period (3;8–5;1). Moreover, if we scrutinise the constructions in Table 9.8 more closely, we will see that there is very little overlap in the inverted and uninverted combinations of first person subject and auxiliary: that is to say, for any particular combination, each child either consistently inverts (e.g. *can I . . . ?*) or consistently uses declarative word order (*I'm . . . ?*). (The only exception to this pattern is, again, the second part of the Sarah corpus: but it is not surprising to find evidence of more general knowledge in a child of this age.) Thus, the pattern of inversion/uninversion with *I* provides particularly clear evidence for piecemeal learning: children acquire knowledge about particular subject–auxiliary combinations rather than general rules which apply 'across the board'.

3.4.2 Contraction

In addition to their canonical or full forms, the English copula and some auxiliaries have contracted forms (e.g. *'s, 're*) which cliticise to the preceding word. The contracted forms predominate in informal adult speech, and are also quite frequent in children's earliest questions. Many children, however, go through a stage when they prefer the full forms, sometimes after a period of fairly consistent use of contracted forms. This marks a departure from the adult pattern which is usually interpreted as indicating that the child has segmented previously unanalysed forms (e.g. *whats, wheres*) into their component

Table 9.8 Inverted and uninverted questions with first person singular subjects

Corpus	Inverted questions	Tokens	Uninverted questions	Tokens
Naomi	*can I . . . ?*	25		
	could I . . . ?	3		
			I/me V-PRES . . . ?	8
			I'm . . . ? (copula)	1
			I'm . . . ? (auxiliary)	1
			I can't . . . ?	1
Shem	*can I . . . ?*	27		
	could I . . . ?	2		
	is I . . . ?	1		
	should I . . . ?	1		
			I V-PAST . . . ?	1
			I V-PRES . . . ?	12
			I'm . . . ? (auxiliary)	3
			I'll . . . ?	1
			I can't . . . ?	1
			I was . . . ? (copula)	1
			I was . . . ? (auxiliary)	1
Sarah1	*will I . . . ?*	2		
	shall I . . . ?	1		
	can I . . . ?	18	*I can . . . ?*	1
	did I . . . ?	4	*I* V-PAST . . . ?	2
	do I . . . ?	1	*I* V-PRES . . . ?	33
			I can't . . . ?	1
			I didn't . . . ?	1
			I be . . . ? (copula)	1
Sarah2	*could I . . . ?*	11		
	shall I . . . ?	1		
	am I . . . ? (copula)	7		
	was I . . . ? (copula)	1		
	can I . . . ?	77	*I can . . . ?*	2
	should I . . . ?	5	*I should . . . ?*	1
	did I . . . ?	21	*I* V-PAST . . . ?	6
	am I . . . ? (auxiliary)	5	*I'm . . . ?* (auxiliary)	4
	do I . . . ?	21	*I* V-PRES . . . ?	27
	don't I . . . ?	1	*I don't . . . ?*	1
			I was . . . ? (auxiliary)	1
			I can't . . . ?	1
			I didn't . . . ?	1
			I will . . . ?	1
Naomi's mother	*didn't I . . . ?*	3		
	shall I . . . ?	1		
	did I . . . ?	1		
	would I . . . ?	1		
	can I . . . ?	9	*I can . . . ?*	1
	am I . . . ? (copula)	1	*I am . . . ?* (copula)	3
	am I . . . ? (auxiliary)	1	*I am . . . ?* (auxiliary)	1
	should I . . . ?	3	*I should . . . ?*	3
			I shouldn't . . . ?	1
			I can't . . . ?	2

morphemes (*what* + *is*, *where* + *is*). What is particularly interesting from our point of view is that this development appears to occur at different times in different constructions.

We can see this when we compare contraction rates in different contexts at different points in time. Ideally, one would want to follow changes in contraction rates in each question construction (e.g. *what* object questions with the auxiliary *is*, *what* subject questions with the copula, etc.) – but this would require much larger corpora. With the data available, we can only follow the combination of the most frequent WH words with the most frequent contracted form, *'s*. However, even when we collapse across different construction types in this way, some patterns are clearly discernible. Figure 9.3 shows the percentage of contracted forms after *what* and *where* in all three children and after *who* in Naomi and Sarah (there is not enough data on *who* in Shem). The ages on the X axis represent the midpoints of each period; and the final point represents the proportion of contracted forms in the input (i.e. the hypothetical end result of development).

As we can see from the figure, adults used contracted forms equally frequently after all question words, which suggests that any differences in the children's levels of provision of such forms are not attributable simply to phonological factors. There was some variation in the parents' overall levels of contraction, which may reflect dialect differences; however, within the input to individual children, the levels of provision with different WH words were very similar. Also, all three children, as well as their parents, contracted after the pronoun *that* at the same levels (93 per cent or more of the opportunities) throughout the entire period of observation. (This is not shown in the figure to avoid cluttering it up.) On the other hand, the children used contracted forms with different frequencies after different WH words, and, what is more, the use of such forms developed along different trajectories in different constructions.

The children's questions with *what* follow a very similar developmental pattern. All three initially preferred the contracted form in this context, and supplied it about as frequently as their parents. This was followed by a period of relatively frequent use of the full form, and later still, one presumes, by a return to adult-like levels of provision, although we do not see this in the data (except in Shem, where there is a slight rise at the last data point). Note, however, that while the overall pattern of development is similar in all three children, there are considerable differences in the timing: the trough in the frequency of contracted forms occurred about 2;9 in Shem and about 4;9 (or perhaps even later, since this is the last data point) in Sarah.

Contraction after *where*, on the other hand, follows a different course of development in each child. Sarah supplied contracted forms at about the same rate throughout the entire period of observation. In Shem, we see a slow but steady decrease in the frequency of such forms which continued even when the frequency of contracted forms after *what* began to rise. Finally, the

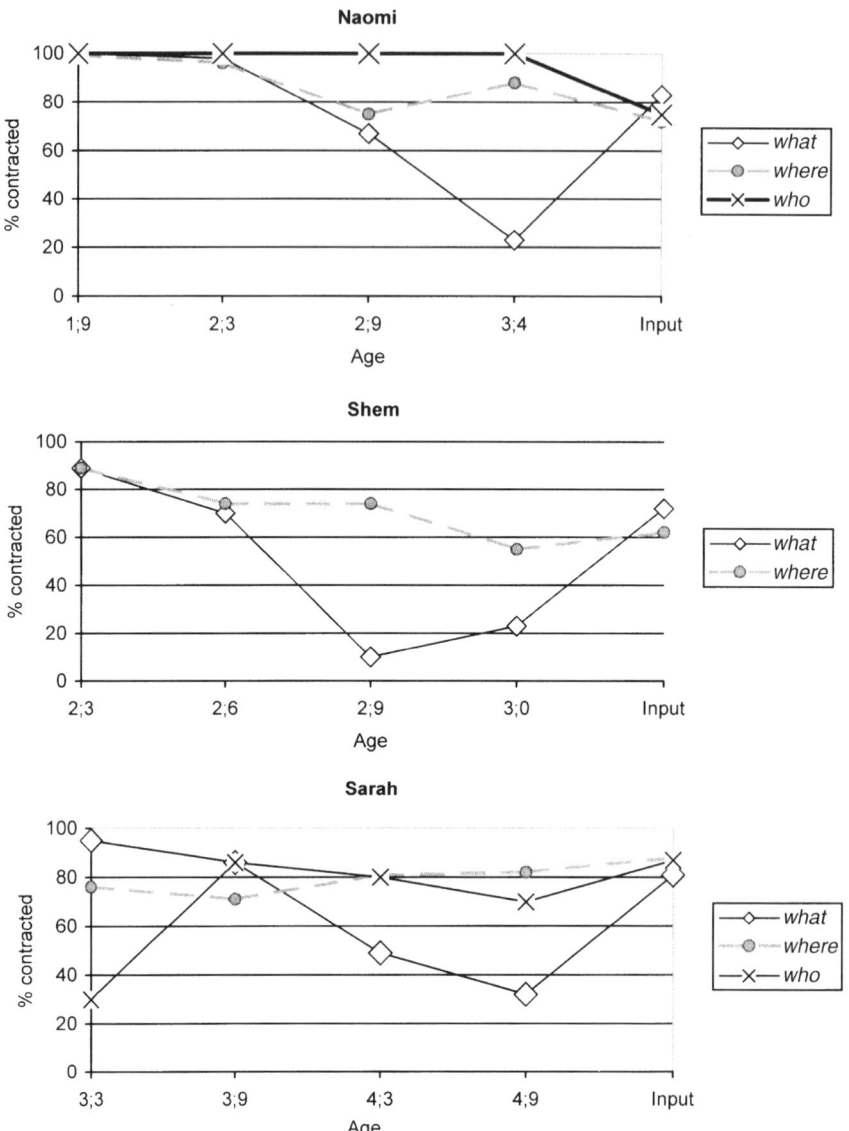

Figure 9.3 Contraction of auxiliary/copula *is* after *what*, *where* and *who*

Naomi data shows a small decrease about 2;6, followed by a rise; note that the frequency of contracted forms after *what* fell steeply during the same period.

Contraction after *who* also follows a strikingly different pattern in the two children for whom enough data is available. There are few questions with the contracted form in Sarah's earlier transcripts; but after 3;6, her use of this variant rose sharply to adult-like levels. Naomi, in contrast, consistently used the contracted form during the entire period of observation.

Thus, we find differences in the pattern of use or non-use of contraction in different constructions in the same children, as well as considerable differences between children. This supports the hypothesis that knowledge about auxiliaries develops independently in different constructions.

3.4.3 Errors

Further evidence for piecemeal learning is to be found in the children's errors. Errors – specifically, errors of commission – are of course prime evidence for productive language use, since they involve the production of structures that, by definition, do not occur in the input. However, this productivity is for the most part very restricted. Most errors of commission involve agreement or auxiliary placement. The former kind arise most often when a plural NP is inserted into a frame containing a singular verb (e.g. *where's X? + deir feets = where's deir feets?*). Auxiliary placement errors occur when a WH word is combined with a clause containing an auxiliary (e.g. *where X? + he's taking it? = where he's taking it?*).

Most other errors are very restricted in scope. The Shem corpus, for example, contains 20 'double-auxiliary errors', in which the auxiliary verb is placed both before and after the verb. Twelve of these are one-off innovations involving a variety of different combinations of auxiliaries, e.g. *did . . . is* (*what did he's showing?*), *does . . . be* (*where does these pictures be taken?*), *is . . . are* (*why is dese clothes are blowing by?*). The remaining eight, however, involve exactly the same combination of words: *what i(s) he's doing?* All of these questions have *he* as subject and *doing* as the main verb, the first auxiliary is rendered as [ɪ] or [ɪz] and the second is always contracted. Such questions are productive in the sense that they are extremely unlikely to be imitations of an adult utterance; but the fact that the same mistake recurs again and again in the same combination of words, but not with other subjects and other verbs, suggests that they are formulaic – in other words, it seems that Shem memorised his own creative utterance and reproduced it on subsequent occasions.[13]

A similar example can be found in the Naomi corpus. Between the ages of 2;0 and 2;3, Naomi produced 15 WH questions in which the contracted form of the auxiliary *is* was followed by a bare infinitive. All of these had the form *What's Nomi do?* With all subjects other than *Naomi*, she consistently used the correct form of the verb: *What's Mummy doing?*, *What's fish doing?*, *What's recorder doing?* and so on.

Even more striking is Naomi's use of forms of self-reference. Like many children, she sometimes referred to herself using the first person pronoun and sometimes used her name (which she pronounced *Nomi*). These two forms, however, occurred in different contexts. Naomi consistently used *I* in declaratives (99 per cent of the time) and intonation questions (100 per cent) as well as questions with the modal auxiliaries *can* and *could* (also 100 per cent). On the other hand, all but one of her 43 WH questions about herself contain her name. They are all instantiations of three lexically specific formulas: *What's Naomi do?*, *What's Nomi doing?* and *Where's Nomi?* It is difficult to see how such very specific restrictions in distribution could be explained without appealing to preconstructed phrases.

3.5 Questions with long-distance dependencies

The schematic templates hypothesised above can account for Y/N questions of arbitrary complexity and for WH questions about any element of a simple clause. What is potentially problematic for such an account, however, is questions involving long-distance dependencies (LDDs), i.e. those in which the questioned element is in a subordinate clause, as in the following examples:

(15)   a. *What did you say Chris needed?*
       b. *What did you say they thought Chris needed?*
       c. *What did you say they thought Maria believed Chris needed?*

Here *what* is construed as 'belonging' with the last verb in the sentence, namely *needed.* Because there can be any number of clauses between the question word and the place where it logically belongs, it is difficult to account for such sentences using schematic templates: indeed, sentences with LDDs were the main motivation for postulating WH movement in the first place.

Not surprisingly, questions involving LDDs are acquired late. As far as we can tell from the transcripts, only one of the three children whose linguistic development was discussed earlier in this chapter, Sarah, produced any such structures – only three in total, all recorded at age 4;4 or later. Given that such questions are relatively infrequent, their absence in the transcripts of the other two children could be an accident of sampling. However, Table 9.9, which contains the relevant figures for five other developmental corpora, suggests that this is not the case. As we can see from the table, only two of these additional children produced the relevant structure, and in both cases it appeared fairly late: at 3;8 in the case of Abe, who was a rather precocious child,[14] and at 4;3 in Adam's case. The late emergence of questions involving LDDs is confirmed by experimental research. In a series of production studies, Crain and Thornton (Crain and Thornton 1991; Thornton and Crain 1994) were able to elicit this structure from most 4-year-olds, but only a few younger children succeeded on the task.

It is also worth noting that the questions with LDDs were quite formulaic. Of the 49 tokens produced by the children (44 by Abe, 2 by Adam and 3 by Sarah), all but two had the form *WH do you think S?* There was some variety within this schema, in that the children used different WH words to ask about different parts of the subordinate clause:

Table 9.9 Child questions with long-distance dependencies (LDDs) in five other CHILDES corpora

Corpus	Corpus size (child words)	Age range	LDD questions	Age of emergence
Manchester (Theakston et al. 2000)	538,000	1;8–3;0	0	–
Hall (Hall et al. 1984)	295,000	4;6–5;0	0	–
Gleason (Belliger and Gleason 1982)	60,000	2;1–5;2	0	–
Adam (Brown 1973)	164,000	2;3–4;10	2	4;3
Abe (Kuczaj 1976)	163,000	2;4–5;0	44	3;8

Note: The first three corpora contain samples from a number of children; the last two from individual children. The figures include only questions containing a WH word followed by an auxiliary and subject and a finite subordinate clause.

(16)   a. subject: *What do you think's under here?* (Abe, 3;10)
        b. locative complement: *Where do you think they're going?* (Abe, 3;11)
        c. adjunct: *How do you think she made that train?* (Abe, 4;11)
        d. subject predicative: *What do you think it was?* (Abe, 4;0)

All but two of the questions, however, had *think* as the main verb, *you* as the main verb subject, and *do* as the auxiliary. The same is true of the questions elicited in the Crain and Thornton studies. Thus, by about age 4, children have some knowledge about questions with LDDs; but it is not clear how general such knowledge is.

Interestingly, adult LDD questions are also highly stereotypical. There are 325 tokens of this construction in the adult input in the Manchester corpus. None of these contains more than one finite subordinate clause – that is to say, there are no sentences such as examples (14b) and (14c) above – and only one has an overt complementiser. In 96 per cent of the questions, the main verb is either *think* or *say*; 91 per cent have *you* as subject (and 6 per cent have other pronominal subjects); and 99 per cent have some form of *do* in the auxiliary position. Moreover, specific main verbs appear to be associated with specific auxiliary forms: *think* with *do* (276 out of 280 tokens), *say* and *tell* with *did* (31 out of 33 and six out of six tokens respectively), and *pretend* with *shall* (three out of three tokens). The remaining four verbs (*see, hope, reckon, suppose*) occurred only once in LDD questions, and hence could not occur with different auxiliaries. In fact, even the verbs in the subordinate clauses are fairly stereotypical, so that the following eight templates account for 50 per cent of all LDD questions in the entire corpus (CAPITALS indicate that a particular verb occurred in several different forms: for example, BE stands for *is, was, are, could be* etc.):

(17)   a. *What do you think NP BE?*
        b. *What do you think NP DO?*
        c. *What do you think NP EAT?*
        d. *What do you think NP LIKE?*
        e. *What do you think NP NEED?*
        f. *Where do you think NP BE?*
        g. *Where do you think NP GO?*
        h. *What did NP say NP was?*

Arguably, child-directed speech is not the most representative example of adult linguistic abilities, so it is important to obtain comparable statistics about other genres. The relevant evidence is offered by Verhagen (forthcoming), who studied LDD questions in the Brown corpus (which includes a wide variety of written texts) as well as two Dutch corpora. The Brown corpus contains 11 instances of questions involving LDDs. In 10 of these, the matrix verb is *think*, and in one, *say*; in nine, the subject is *do*, while the remaining two take third person pronouns as subjects; and 10 contain some form of *do*. The Dutch results are very similar: the overwhelming majority of LDD questions have second person subjects and *denken* 'think' as main verb. Verhagen also notes that when an LDD question deviates from the prototype, it does so in only one respect: that is to say, it either takes a different matrix verb *or* a different subject, but (in his data) never both.

Similar observations can be made about the Manchester corpus. Of the questions with LDDs, 89 per cent instantiate the *WH DO you think/say S* prototype; 9 per cent deviate from prototype in one respect (they contain a different matrix verb *or* a different auxiliary *or* a different subject); and only 2 per cent deviate from the prototype in more than one way. This clustering around a prototypical pattern suggests that speakers may produce such utterances by inserting novel material into a ready-made template and modifying it when necessary (e.g. by substituting a full NP for *you*) rather than assembling them from scratch. This possibility will be discussed more fully in the next chapter; for now, we will examine some independent evidence that adult speakers store partially lexically specific templates of long-distance WH questions.

The evidence comes from a grammaticality judgement study involving prototypical and unprototypical LDD questions. The former had the form *WH do you think S-WH?* or *WH did you say S-WH?*, where S-WH stands for a subordinate clause with a gap. Unprototypical questions contained a different auxiliary (*will, should, would, might* or *have*), a lexical subject (e.g. *the customers, your sister*), and a different main clause verb (e.g. *claim, reveal, believe, remember*), followed by the same subordinate clause. Interspersed with these 20 test sentences were 20 declarative control sentences containing the same lexical material and 10 ungrammatical fillers (five interrogatives and five declaratives; see Table 9.10 for examples). The participants (10 adult native

Table 9.10 Examples of sentences used in the grammaticality judgement study

Condition	Example
Prototypical interrogative	*Where do you think they sent the documents?*
Unprototypical interrogative	*Where will the customers remember they sent the documents?*
Prototypical declarative	*You think they sent the documents to the Head Office.*
Unprototypical declarative	*The customers will remember they sent the documents to the Head Office.*
Ungrammatical	**Who do you think that left?*
	*He left in the office and had to go back.

Table 9.11 Acceptability ratings

Condition	Mean	SD
Prototypical interrogative	4.5	0.4
Unprototypical interrogative	3.3	0.6
Prototypical declarative	4.0	0.5
Unprototypical declarative	3.7	0.5
Ungrammatical	1.9	0.6

speakers of English) were asked to rate the acceptability of the 50 sentences on a scale from 1 (completely unacceptable) to 5 (fully acceptable).

If people rely on fully general rules, there should be no differences between prototypical and unprototypical questions, provided that the corresponding declaratives are equally acceptable. If, however, they use lexically specific templates, they should rate the prototypical questions as more acceptable than the unprototypical ones. The mean acceptability ratings and standard deviations for each type of sentence are given in Table 9.11. As we can see, prototypical questions were indeed given higher ratings than unprototypical questions. The effect is quite robust and highly significant ($t(9) = 7.54$, $p < 0.001$). The difference in the acceptability of the corresponding declaratives, in contrast, was not significant ($t(9) = 1.57$, $p = 0.15$), showing that the effect cannot be attributed to the combination of the lexical properties of the auxiliary, subject and verb in the unprototypical sentences. Thus, the results support the hypothesis that people store lexically specific templates for long-distance questions. It should be noted, however, that the ratings for unprototypical questions were considerably higher than those for the ungrammatical controls ($t(9) = 5.93$, $p < 0.001$), which suggests that speakers also have some more general knowledge about such structures.

3.6 Conclusion

On the standard generative account, the acquisition of questions involves learning to apply two rules, WH fronting and subject–auxiliary inversion. Both of these rules are very general, but subject to certain constraints. Such constraints are thought to be unlearnable, and hence the fact that humans apparently obey them is sometimes regarded as providing the clinching evidence for the existence of innate Universal Grammar (cf. chapter 6, section 4.1).

The evidence reviewed in this chapter, however, suggests a very different view of development. We saw that early usage is highly stereotypical and that development proceeds from invariant formulas through increasingly general formulaic frames to abstract templates. Furthermore, development is piecemeal, in the sense that children learn the correct word order independently for each construction,[15] and 'the same' changes occur at different times in different constructions. We also found no evidence of abrupt changes in behaviour which might indicate a shift to a different productive mechanism: instead, we see slow, steady progress. This suggests that the endpoint of development – that is to say, adult grammar – might be rather similar to the kinds of representations that children use; in other words, that adult knowledge comprises not constraints on movement and suchlike, but rather fairly general templates like *Can NP VP?*, *Who VP?* and *What BE NP TRANS.V-ing?* These would also allow speakers to produce and understand a wide variety of different question types, thus accounting for the observed flexibility of adult behaviour. However, they do not involve movement, and hence do not require innate constraints or an abstract level of syntactic representation distinct from surface structure.

Some linguists have argued that speakers' ability to produce and understand questions involving LDDs constitutes evidence against schematic templates, since such dependencies are 'unbounded': that is to say, there is no limit (in principle) on the number of clauses intervening between the WH word and the place where it logically belongs. Clearly, an adequate account of LDD questions must explain how such structures are produced and understood. However, our examination of adult use of such structures revealed that they are in fact highly formulaic, so the data actually supports the hypothesis that even adults rely on lexically specific templates.

It should be stressed that the use of such frames requires grammatical knowledge. Speakers must know that certain slots can only be filled with items which have certain grammatical properties (for example, the VP in *who VP?* must be tensed, while the VP in *can NP VP?* cannot); and there are often relationships between items in different grammatical slots (for example, in *What BE NP TRANS.V-ing?* the auxiliary must agree with the subject in person and number). The challenge for linguistics, then, is to develop a theory of grammar which will capture such knowledge in psychologically realistic terms. The next chapter introduces one such theory.

Notes

1. The 'processing complexity' and 'formulaic' explanations of pronoun reversals, and the other proposals mentioned earlier, are not mutually exclusive. The use of prefabricated patterns does not preclude tinkering with them to adapt them to one's present communicative goals; and such tinkering is less likely to occur in cognitively demanding situations.

2. To discover the shifting nature of deictic pronouns, children need to observe speech events involving third parties, since in speech addressed to them, *you* always refers to the child and *I* to the caretaker. Since blind children often do not know what these third parties are doing, discovering the deictic properties of the pronouns is much more difficult.

3. A similar case of a child developing a phonological form which does not occur in adult speech but which can be viewed as a 'phonological common denominator' of several adult forms expressing a similar meaning is provided by Mills (1985). The first definite article used by some German-speaking children is *de*, which is the nearest you can get to the 'common denominator' of the adult forms *der*, *die*, *das*, *dem*, *des* and *den*.

4. A researcher working in Menn's lab compared audio tapes of Berko Gleason's subject Patricia with transcriptions available on the CHILDES database. Patricia rendered the object pronoun *it* as /ɪt/, /ə/ or zero, forcing the transcribers either to underrepresent or overspecify Patricia's knowledge. They chose the latter (Peters and Menn 1993: 753, footnote). Such idealisations give a distorted picture of grammatical development, making it appear less continuous than it really is.

5. Sentences with tags of matching polarity (*He is coming, is he?*) are an instance of a different construction with a different pragmatic function and a distinct intonation.

6. Unless we have a full record of everything the child said, we have no way of knowing the actual frequency of any expression in his or her speech. It is possible that the three recorded occurrences were the only ones the child ever produced; and it is also possible that an utterance with a frequency of three in the corpus had actually been produced hundreds of times. However, assuming the sample to be representative, the *mean* actual frequency of expressions with a frequency of three in the sample is 30 if we have a 10 per cent sample, and 43 if we have a 7 per cent sample.

7. Errors of commission are errors involving incorrect use (e.g. wrong form or wrong word order), as opposed to errors of omission, which can be corrected simply by adding the omitted elements.

8. It is possible that Shem's development showed a U-shaped pattern similar to Naomi's, but we don't see this in the data because the recordings began fairly late. If this is the case, then the trough would be much deeper in Shem's case than in Naomi's (notice that he inverted less than 20 per cent

of the time at the beginning of the recording period, while Naomi's lowest rates were about 40 per cent).

9. Naomi's mother's questions were used for this comparison. The data analysed here consists of a corpus of the mother's questions matched in size to the child's corpus.

10. There are only four Y/N questions with *do* in the first half of the Sarah corpus, so this part of the data was not included in Table 9.6.

11. The differences are not statistically significant in the mother: $\chi^2 = 1.2$, $df = 2$, $p = 0.550$. However, they are significant in all three children: for Naomi $\chi^2 = 12.6$, $df = 2$, $p = 0.002$; for Shem, $\chi^2 = 31.7$, $df = 3$, $p < 0.001$; for Sarah2, $\chi^2 = 8.3$, $df = 3$, $p = 0.039$.

12. For the mother, $\chi^2 = 4.2$, $df = 3$, $p = 0.236$; for Naomi, $\chi^2 = 20.6$, $df = 3$, $p < 0.001$; for Shem, $\chi^2 = 27.3$, $df = 3$, $p < 0.001$; for Sarah1, $\chi^2 = 13.5$, $df = 3$, $p = 0.004$; for Sarah2, $\chi^2 = 28.0$, $df = 3$, $p < 0.001$.

13. Note that *he's* was not an unanalysed chunk. Shem did not use it in contexts which did not require an auxiliary or copula or in combination with an auxiliary in declaratives.

14. Abe's first recorded use of a question with an LDD occurred at age 2;10, but this was an imitation of the immediately preceding adult utterance.

15. It remains to be seen whether this is also true of later stages of language acquisition. Development does speed up noticeably at about age 3, suggesting that there may be transfer of knowledge between constructions during this period.

10 The cognitive enterprise

1. Towards a psychologically realistic grammar

In the first part of this book, we looked at some general properties of human language that must be accommodated in any model of language that purports to be psychologically realistic. Language processing is flexible (we are able to make use of whatever information is available and integrate various sources of information as required) and very fast. It is also remarkably robust, in that it develops even in very inauspicious circumstances and is difficult to destroy completely, so that some linguistic abilities are preserved even after damage to the parts of the brain which normally play a central role in language processing. Last but not least, it relies to a large extent on relatively low-tech, general-purpose mental mechanisms shared with other species, including the ability to perceive, categorise and store information, form cross-modal associations, and plan hierarchically organised action sequences.

In Part II, we have examined specific aspects of linguistic organisation in more detail, considering developmental evidence as well as research on adult knowledge. This has enabled us to glean some hints about how these properties are implemented in the 'language machine'. One of the reasons why language processing is so fast is because it relies to a considerable extent on prefabricated units which need to be modified only minimally in order to be used in communication. The flexibility and robustness of the system are due, in a large measure, to its redundancy: the fact that the same information is represented in different parts of the system, and hence there are typically different ways of assembling the same utterance or arriving at its meaning. These are tried out in parallel, which also makes for speed. We have also seen that memory plays a very important role in language acquisition and production. There is an intimate relationship between lexical and grammatical development, between rote learning and rule extraction; and grammatical phenomena, like words, are subject to frequency effects.

Much of the research discussed in Part II has focused on language-specific aspects of linguistic knowledge. We have seen that such knowledge can be quite subtle. It follows that we need a well-articulated descriptive framework to capture it, and a theory of acquisition which explains how humans are able to learn the idiosyncratic features of their language as well as the more general aspects which can be captured by means of universal principles.

This chapter is devoted to approaches to language which meet these requirements. While the requirements place strong constraints on linguistic theory, they still allow for a number of alternatives. Rather than surveying all the possible options, I will focus on one particular theory, Cognitive Grammar (Langacker 1987, 1991a, 1991b, 2000), which is the most fully elaborated of these, although the discussion will also incorporate some key ideas from related frameworks, notably Construction Grammar (Fillmore and Kay 1993; Fillmore et al. 2003; Goldberg 1995) and Radical Construction Grammar (Croft 2001). I will begin with an informal overview of this framework, and then show how the kinds of representations that it postulates might develop and be used in production. The chapter concludes with some general observations about the challenges facing cognitive linguistics.

2. A crash course in Cognitive Grammar

2.1 Linguistic expressions are symbolic units

The central idea of Cognitive Grammar (CG) is that language – including grammar – is essentially symbolic in nature, and thus linguistic knowledge can be captured by means of symbolic units, or pairings of a phonological form and a meaning. Figure 10.1a illustrates the usual conventions for representing symbolic units. The schematic diagram in the top panel stands for the meaning of the lexeme *cat* (or, in Langacker's terminology, its semantic pole) and the phonemic transcription in the bottom panel for its pronunciation, or phonological pole; the vertical line connecting the two panels corresponds to the symbolic relationship between the two. The caption underneath the figure

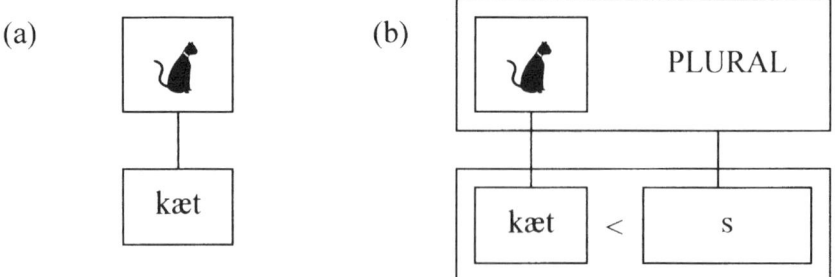

Figure 10.1 The symbolic units [CAT]/[kæt] (a) and [[CAT]-PLURAL]/[[kæt]<[s]] (b)
Note: Boxes indicate semantic and phonological units; vertical lines correspond to symbolic relationships. The '<' symbol indicates linear order.

shows an alternative way of representing the same unit: by convention, SMALL CAPITALS are used to abbreviate the meaning of an expression, and phonemic transcription its phonological form. The slash indicates that the latter symbolises the former.

Symbolic units can be simple, as in the above example, or complex. The latter include morphologically complex words (e.g. *cats*, *relationship*), phrases (*after school, in the long run, deep down*) and sentences (*All's well that ends well, Would you like a cup of coffee?*): all of these expressions, like simple lexemes, are pairings of a phonological form and a meaning. Such complex units consist of two or more components, each of which is a symbolic unit in its own right. For example, the symbolic unit *cats* is made up of two simpler units, the noun *cat* and the plural morpheme -*s* (Figure 10.1b). Symbolic units can also be partly or wholly schematic. As we shall see shortly, schematic symbolic units are used in the CG framework to capture grammatical knowledge.

2.2 Imagery

The *raison d'être* of linguistic forms is to express meaning. Cognitivists take a rather broad view of meaning as comprising not just 'content' but also 'imagery'. This refers to our ability to construe the same content in alternate ways by focusing on different aspects of a scene, viewing it from different perspectives, or conceptualising it at different levels of abstraction.

One of the most ubiquitous aspects of imagery is the imposition of a profile on a base. The **base** is the knowledge structure within which an expression is understood and defined; it is similar to Fillmore's notion of frame (Fillmore 1975, 1978) and Lakoff's idealised cognitive model (Lakoff 1987). The **profile** is a substructure within the base that an expression actually designates. For example, the expression *diameter* designates, or profiles, a line, but it also evokes a larger cognitive structure – a circle – which is its base: it is impossible to entertain the notion of DIAMETER without at the same time entertaining the notion of CIRCLE. Two linguistic expressions can have the same base but different profiles and hence contrast in meaning. For example, the terms *aunt* and *niece* designate different nodes in the kinship network which is their base; *win*, *lose* and *beat* profile different relationships in a knowledge structure we could describe as a COMPETITIVE EVENT; and *winner*, *loser* and *runner-up* profile individuals participating in these relationships. Conversely, two expressions can have the same profiles, but differ in meaning because the profiles are imposed on different bases. An example would be the adjective *dry* and the past participle *dried*: both profile the same property (lack of moisture), but only the latter has as its base a series of events in the course of which an object undergoes a change of state (from 'wet' to 'not wet').

Another dimension of imagery, crucial to the conceptualisation of relations, is trajector/landmark organisation. When we perceive relations, we tend to impose a certain perspective on the participating entities. Specifically, we tend to view one of the participants as the central element of a scene – a figure that stands out against a background of other entities. In CG, the most salient entity is called the **trajector** and the other salient participants are called **landmarks**. For instance, in (1), *the Toyota* is the trajector and *the Mercedes* the landmark; in (2), the roles are reversed. In this example, the relationship between the trajector and the landmark is spatial, but the terms are used to refer to the corresponding roles in other kinds of relations as well. Complex linguistic expressions usually have several levels of trajector/landmark organisation. In (3), *Chris* is the trajector of *put* and *the drink* its landmark; but the latter is also the trajector of *on*, while *the table* is its landmark.

(1)　　*The Toyota is in front of the Mercedes.*
(2)　　*The Mercedes is behind the Toyota.*
(3)　　*Chris put the drink on the table.*

In most cases, some element of the scene is inherently more salient than the others and hence the most natural choice for the trajector. For example, moving objects and agents are more likely to be construed as trajectors than stationary objects or patients. This prototypical alignment is reflected in (3), where the agent is the clausal trajector and the displaced object the trajector of the preposition. However, even when the relationship is inherently asymmetrical speakers enjoy a certain degree of freedom and may choose the less likely candidate as the figure. The humorous effect of (4), for example, is due largely to the fact that the displaced object (the Scotch and soda) is construed as landmark of *outside*, while the most natural choice for the landmark (the 'container' into which the Scotch is poured) becomes the trajector.

(4)　　*He was seated at the Savoy bar when he told me this, rather feverishly putting himself outside a Scotch and soda.* (P. G. Wodehouse, *The World of Mr Mulliner*)

Or consider a scene in which two cars, a Toyota and a Mercedes, crash into one another. Although all of the sentences in (5) could be used to describe this event, they are clearly not synonymous. Choosing one of the cars as the trajector has the effect of highlighting its causal role in the crash and downplaying the role played by the other car; construing both cars as trajectors results in a more neutral description.

(5)　　a. *The Toyota collided with the Mercedes.*
　　　　b. *The Mercedes collided with the Toyota.*
　　　　c. *The Toyota and the Mercedes collided.*

Similar observations can be made about the pairs of sentences given in (6) and (7). In both cases, the two sentences describe different construals of the same event and hence differ in meaning, although the differences are quite subtle. Since the content words are the same in both members of each pair, it is clear that the difference in meaning is part of the meaning of the construction and the grammatical functors that form an integral part of it.

(6)   a. *Lil decorated our wedding cake.*
        b. *Our wedding cake was decorated by Lil.*

(7)   a. *Andy sent Neil the new personal organiser.*
        b. *Andy sent the new personal organiser to Neil.*

Yet another aspect of imagery is our ability to conceive the same content at different levels of schematicity. For example, we can think of the same person as IMOGEN, GIRL, CHILD or PERSON, or of the same activity as PLANTING THREE DAFFODILS, PLANTING SOME FLOWERS or GARDENING. We are also able to make categorising judgements such as PERSON ⇒ CHILD (the concept PERSON is schematic for CHILD) and PLANTING SOME FLOWERS ⇒ PLANTING THREE DAFFODILS. The term **schema** refers to the superordinate term in such relationships; the subordinate term is called the schema's **instantiation**. These terms are more general than the traditional labels 'superordinate' and 'hyponym' in that they apply to all kinds of linguistic units, including phonological units (for example, CVC is schematic for [kæt], [niːd], [fɪʃ] and so on) and grammatical units (see below).

2.3 Things, processes and atemporal relations

The distinction between content and imagery is extremely useful in providing a semantically based account of grammatical distinctions which in other theories are dealt with by means of arbitrary syntactic features. Consider the expressions *investigate* and *investigation*. As far as actual semantic content is concerned, the two words are identical; but they contrast semantically because they impose different images on the same content. *Investigate* profiles a process, or a series of states occurring at different points in time; *investigation*, on the other hand, involves conceptual reification, or construing an event as a type of 'thing'. **Thing** in CG is a technical term defined as 'a region in some domain' (Langacker 1987: 189), where a region is 'a set of interconnected entities' (Langacker 1987:198). The term covers not just physical objects, but various abstract entities as well, including stretches of time, colours and qualities. Thus, *week* designates a region in the temporal domain; the noun *blue* designates a region in colour space; *beauty* designates a region in quality space; and so on. Even events can be construed as abstract 'things' in this technical sense. The component states of an event include the same participants and occur at adjacent points in time. Because of these interconnections, the component states constitute an implicit region. A nominalisation such as *investigation* profiles this region (and backgrounds the temporal dimension). Thus, the noun and the verb impose contrasting images on the same content: they have the same base, but different profiles (Langacker 1991b: 97ff).

Lexical categories such as nouns and verbs are also considered symbolic units in CG, albeit highly schematic ones. A noun is an expression which profiles a thing, with maximally underspecified phonological content (that is to say, it must have some content, but it can be any speech sound whatsoever). A verb is defined as a phonologically unspecified symbolic unit which profiles a **process**, or a temporal relation; and prepositions, adjectives and adverbs profile **atemporal relations** (Langacker 1991b: 78ff).

2.4 Constructional schemas

As indicated earlier, symbolic units can be simple or complex and concrete or schematic. A symbolic unit which is both complex and schematic is called a **constructional schema**. Constructional schemas are the CG equivalent of rules: they capture speakers' knowledge about the internal structure of complex expressions, and can be used to assemble novel expressions. However, unlike traditional rules, they are represented in the same format as their instantiations (that is to say, actual expressions of the language).

This is best explained by means of an example. Figure 10.2 shows simplified representations of the expression *The girl wants a cat* and two constructional schemas, *WANTER.NP want WANTED.NP* and *NP V NP*. The expression *The girl wants a cat* describes a process or temporal relationship involving two participants, a girl and a cat, represented in the diagram by simplified drawings. The relationship itself is represented by the horizontal line labelled WANT which connects the two participants. Although this relationship is stative (i.e. it doesn't change in time), it is nevertheless a temporal relation, in that it involves a series of configurations scanned sequentially (cf. Langacker 1987, 1991a, 1991b) – 'observed' at different points in time, as it were. Thus, the temporal dimension is part of its profile; this is represented by the arrow in the diagram. As in the previous figure, the lower panels represent phonological form, and the vertical lines the symbolic relationships between the *signifiant* and the *signifié*. Thus, the phonological units [ðə'gɜːl], ['wɒnts] and [ə'kæt] symbolise the semantic units GIRL, WANT and CAT, respectively; and the symbol '<' indicates the linear order of the three elements. (To simplify the discussion, I am ignoring the contribution of the determiners and the third person inflection on the verb.[1])

Figure 10.2b shows a low-level schema representing the same relationship at a more abstract level.[2] The schema captures the commonality in various sentences containing the relevant sense of *want* (*The girl wants a cat, Her brothers want three dogs and a rabbit, Their mother wants some peace* and so on), and hence the speaker's knowledge about the combinatorial possibilities of this verb. It can also be regarded as (part of) the lexical entry for *want*. The

(a)

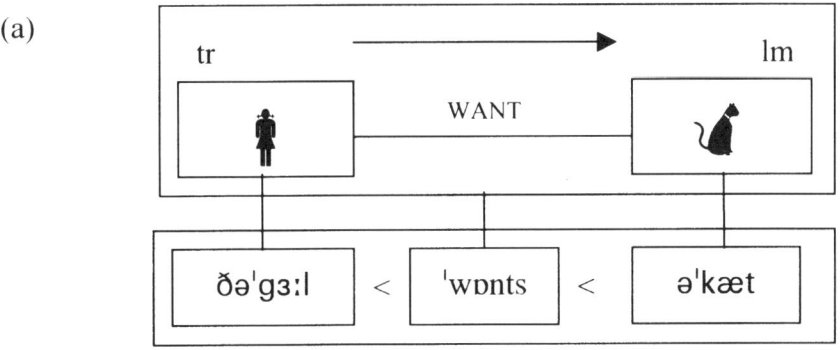

(b)

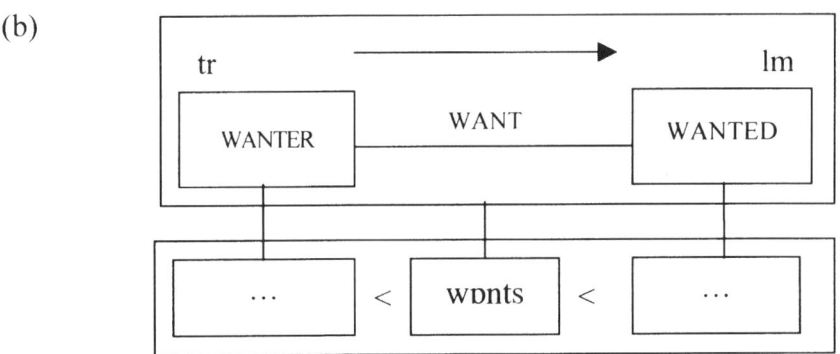

(c)

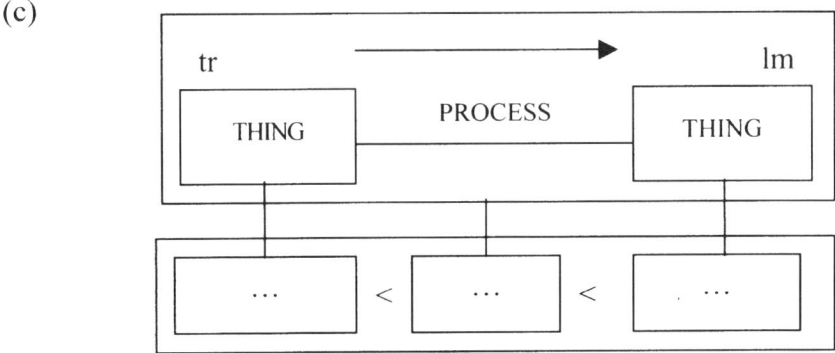

Figure 10.2 A simple clause (a), a low-level schema (b), and an abstract schema (c)

semantic pole of the schema, like that of the concrete expression, contains a subpart corresponding to the trajector (the 'wanter') and the landmark (the desired object), since they are part of the meaning of *want* (it is impossible to think of *wanting* without simultaneously thinking of an animate being experiencing this state and the object of their desire). Both of these participants are 'things' in the technical CG sense. The phonological pole spells out the segmental content of the predicate and the linear order of the expressions corresponding to the 'wanter' and the desired object in relation to the predicate; the actual segmental content of the expressions symbolising the trajector and landmark is unspecified (this is represented in the diagram by three dots, which act as place markers, or slots into which contentful expressions can be inserted).

Finally, Figure 10.2c represents the abstract transitive construction, which is highly schematic at both levels: the semantic representation indicates that the construction profiles a temporal relationship involving two 'things', and the phonological representation spells out the linear order of the three components. The actual segmental content of these component units is left unspecified.

The three diagrams in Figure 10.2 represent the same content at varying levels of abstraction: *WANTER.NP want WANTED.NP* is schematic for *The girl wants a cat*, and *NP V NP* is schematic for both of these units. The crucial point is that all three representations are symbolic units and have the same overall structure. In this respect, the CG approach is very different from most mainstream approaches to language, in which syntactic knowledge is represented in a different format from lexical knowledge, using constructs such as phrase structure rules, movement rules, and various abstract principles and constraints. In the CG framework, schemas and their instantiations are represented in the same format and differ only in the degree of specificity: the schema is specified in less detail than its instantiations. It follows that schema extraction involves reinforcement of shared properties and loss of detail, rather than translation into a different representational format (see below).

2.5 Language as a structured inventory of conventional linguistic units

In the CG framework, linguistic knowledge is seen as a complex, richly interconnected network (or 'structured inventory') of linguistic units. There are three types of units: phonological, semantic and symbolic, and three types of relationships between them: symbolisation, composition and schematicity. **Symbolisation**, as explained earlier, is the relationship between a chunk of semantic structure and the phonological form which can be used to evoke it. **Composition** relationships hold between component units and the composite unit which they form, and are found at all three levels of linguistic organisation. For example, the noun *cat* and the plural morpheme are components of the complex symbolic unit *cats*, which in turn is a component of higher-order units such as *it's raining cats and dogs.* Likewise, the phonological form [kæts] and the semantic unit [[CAT]-PLURAL] consist of simpler elements and can form parts of larger assemblies. **Schematicity** is the relation between the schema (the superordinate term in a taxonomic hierarchy) and its instantiation (the subordinate term). As in the case of composition, schematic relationship can hold between semantic units (e.g. ANIMAL is schematic for CAT, which in turn is schematic for PERSIAN), phonological units (CVC is schematic for the phonological form [kæt], which is schematic for actual phonetic realisations of the word), and symbolic units (the plural construction [[THING]-PLURAL]/[...S] is schematic for the expression *cats*, and the abstract symbolic unit [THING]/[...] is schematic for both *cat* and *cats*).

All the examples given above involve **full schematicity**: the instantiations are fully compatible with the properties of the schema, but are characterised in more detail. This is not always the case: a linguistic expression (or phonological form or conceptualisation) may not fully match the properties of the schema, but still be included in the category defined by the schema. In such cases, we speak of **partial schematicity** or extension. This is typically the relation between the different senses of a polysemous word. Consider, for example, one of the basic senses of the verb *fly* ('move through the air by flapping the wings') and an extended sense meaning 'flutter' (as in *Her hair was flying in the wind*). Both senses designate situations involving a particular kind of movement in the air, but in the extended sense, the moving object is attached to something and is not displaced.

We saw earlier that polysemy is rampant in language (see Chapter 2, section 1; Chapter 7, section 1.2; Chapter 8, section 9), so the semantic representations of most words are not single senses but families of related senses. This is illustrated in Figure 10.3, which shows some intransitive uses of the verb *fly* and the relationships between them. Note that each sense is related to at least one other sense, and that there are several schemas (represented by the three boxes in the upper part of the diagram) which capture some of the local similarities: 'move through the air', 'move quickly', 'resist the force of gravity'. However, there is no single superschema which would be compatible with all the uses of *fly*.

Most constructional schemas, too, are complex categories in which the various meanings are connected by relations of full or partial schematicity (cf. Goldberg 1995; Lakoff 1987). For example, the caused motion construction has at least five interrelated senses (Goldberg 1995):

(8)   a. X CAUSES Y TO MOVE TO/FROM Z: *Barbara dragged Michael out of the kitchen.*

        b. CONDITIONS OF SATISFACTION IMPLY X CAUSES Y TO MOVE TO/FROM Z: *Barbara ordered Michael out of the kitchen.*

        c. X ENABLES Y TO MOVE TO/FROM Z: *Barbara let Michael out of the kitchen.*

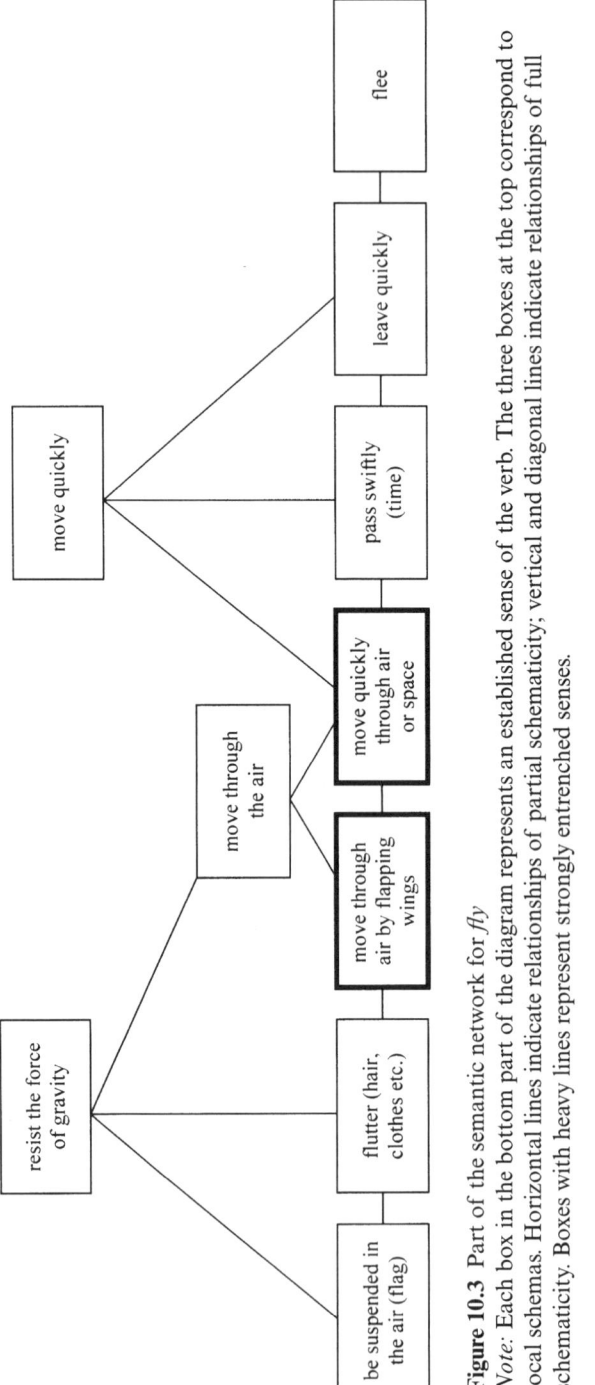

Figure 10.3 Part of the semantic network for *fly*

Note: Each box in the bottom part of the diagram represents an established sense of the verb. The three boxes at the top correspond to local schemas. Horizontal lines indicate relationships of partial schematicity; vertical and diagonal lines indicate relationships of full schematicity. Boxes with heavy lines represent strongly entrenched senses.

    d. X CAUSES Y NOT TO MOVE FROM TO/FROM Z: *Barbara locked Michael out of the kitchen.*

    e. X HELPS Y TO MOVE TO/FROM Z: *Barbara helped Michael out of the kitchen.*

Senses (b)–(e) share some similarities with the basic sense exemplified in (a) which can be captured by means of local schemas. However, there are no features common to all five senses (apart from the fact that they describe some kind of action; this, however, is a property shared with many other constructions).

Finally, many words have variant pronunciations which share most but not all features, and these form similar interconnected structures. Thus, most symbolic units are not simply pairings of a phonological form with a meaning, but rather pairings of a family of senses with one or more pronunciations – subnetworks within the larger network that constitutes the grammar of a language.

2.6 A usage-based model

Cognitive Grammar (CG) emphasises the importance of usage. Speakers' knowledge of their language is captured in phonological, semantic and symbolic units which are generalisations over actual usage events. It is also assumed that each usage event leaves a trace in the processing system. Every time a particular unit is accessed, its representation is strengthened, or **entrenched**, so units which are accessed frequently become easier to activate; conversely, units which are not accessed gradually decay, and become more difficult to activate. It follows that a person's mental grammar is a dynamic system constantly shaped by experience with language. Early in development, such changes are relatively rapid and large; later modifications involve smaller adjustments – 'fine-tuning' of the system.

The CG view of language is also maximalist in the sense that linguistic knowledge is represented at various levels of abstraction: concrete units exist alongside schemas of varying degrees of abstraction. Moreover, CG emphasises the importance of low-level schemas, since these are necessary to capture actual patterns of usage:

> Lower-level schemas, expressing regularities of only limited scope, may on balance be more essential to language structure than high-level schemas expressing the broadest generalizations. A higher-level schema implicitly defines a large 'space' of potential instantiations. Often, however, its actual instantiations cluster in certain regions of that space, leaving other regions sparsely inhabited or uninhabited altogether. An adequate description of linguistic convention must therefore provide the details of how the space has actually been colonized. (Langacker 2000: 29)

It follows that in ordinary language use, speakers rely preferentially on concrete lexical units and local schemas – that is to say, units which are relatively close to actual usage events. Our mental inventories also contain more abstract schemas capturing higher-level generalisations, but these, Langacker suggests, have 'an organizing function rather than an active computational one' (1991b: 265).

2.7 Meeting the specifications

It should be evident even from this brief introduction how CG meets the requirements outlined earlier. The CG conception of linguistic knowledge as a network of symbolic units of varying size and degree of schematicity can easily accommodate prefabs. The network is highly redundant and richly interconnected, so speakers can access the information represented in it in various ways. For example, a complex lexical expression such as *All's well that ends well* might be accessed in a single step as a ready-made unit. Alternatively, the speaker might first activate some salient components (e.g. the lexical units *end* and *well*), which in turn will activate the composite unit; and a speaker who has never heard the expression will have to construct it from scratch, without using any prefabs. These features help to explain the observed flexibility and robustness of language, and also allow for the possibility that individual speakers' mental grammars differ in many details. Furthermore, since the nodes in the network differ in entrenchment, the cognitive approach can easily accommodate frequency effects. Last but not least, CG relies whenever possible on cognitive mechanisms which are not specifically linguistic, that is to say, mechanisms involved in perception (e.g. perceptual primitives, figure–ground organisation), categorisation and memory. It does not rule out the possibility that humans are endowed with language-specific biological adaptations: however, it is assumed that these are likely to be fairly modest, and should only be postulated as a last resort, when there is no other way of explaining a given phenomenon.

Another attractive feature of the CG approach is the fact that lexical and grammatical knowledge is captured in the same representational format, with no sharp contrast between grammar and the lexicon. As pointed out earlier, constructional schemas differ from phrasal lexemes only in degree of specificity; and lexical entries for verbs and other relational expressions are, in effect, mini-grammars. Thus, the close links between grammatical and lexical knowledge observed in language acquisition and impairment fall out as a natural consequence of the organisation of the network.

3. Language production in a CG framework

Linguistic communication involves the use of symbolic expressions, which are pairings of a form and a meaning. Each participant begins with half of the expression (either the form or the meaning), and their task is to (re)construct the other half: thus, production basically involves finding a phonological form which matches one's communicative intentions, and comprehension, finding a conceptualisation which matches the sounds one is hearing. In the simplest case, a speaker's mental lexicon will contain a unit with the appropriate meaning, so all she needs to do is to access its phonological form and pronounce it. If the expression is also available to the listener as a unit, all he has to do after he has recognised it is access its semantic representation. On most occasions, however, a ready-made unit will not be available. In such cases, the speaker will have to find units which correspond as closely as possible to parts of her communicative intentions and combine them into a novel expression; and the listener will have to recognise the component units, access their semantic representations, and integrate them into a coherent conceptualisation. For the sake of simplicity, in the following discussion we will look at the processing of novel expressions from the perspective of the speaker; but many of the observations about the operations involved in symbolic integration also apply to comprehension.

New expressions can be assembled by juxtaposing or superimposing established units. Juxtaposition involves simply putting the two components next to each other (in either order). For example, juxtaposing *come here* and *now* yields *come here now* or *now come here*; juxtaposing *Kate* and *would you like another drink?* yields either *would you like another drink, Kate?* or *Kate, would you like another drink?* The relationship between the two components is paratactic rather than truly syntactic: the fact that they are placed next to each other signals that their meanings are to be integrated, but the grammar does not spell out how this is to be done, so it must be inferred by the listener. Furthermore, the grammar doesn't impose any requirements on the component expressions (other than the fact that they should be elements capable of functioning as utterances in their own right, given the right context). For example, *now* can combine with a clause or a verb phrase (as in the examples above), with a prepositional phrase (*in America now*) or just a noun phrase (*now the gravy*).

Superimposition, on the other hand, is a more constrained process in which one component (a **filler**) elaborates a schematically specified subpart of another component (the **frame**). For example, the expressions *want* and *my desk* can be superimposed to derive the composite expression *want my desk* (cf. Figure 10.4). Superimposition happens simultaneously at the phonological and the semantic poles of the two components. In Figure 10.4, this is shown by the dotted lines linking corresponding elements: MY DESK elaborates the landmark of the semantic structure [[WANTER] WANT [THING WANTED]], and the phonological form [maɪˈdesk] elaborates the second slot in [...wɒnt...]. (Again, the diagram is simplified: for example, it does not represent the internal structure of *my desk*.) Note that the filler must match the properties specified in the frame: in our example the frame requires a filler designating a thing (in the technical CG sense).

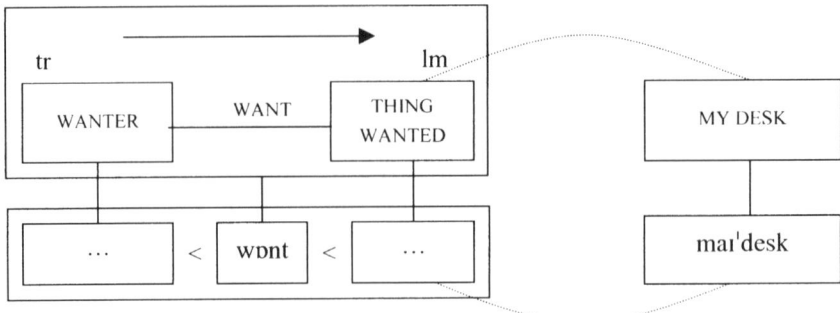

Figure 10.4 Superimposition of a typical frame and filler

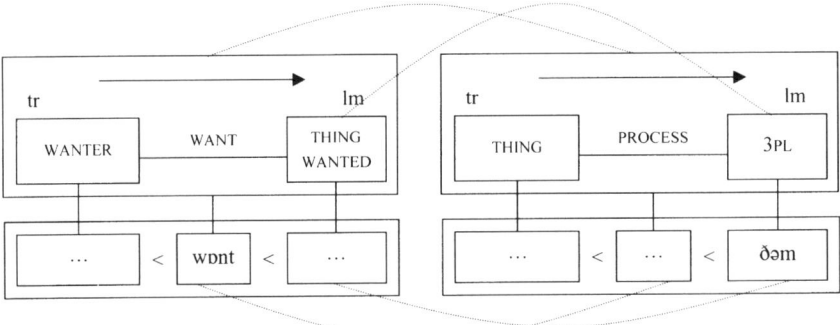

Figure 10.5 Superimposition with mutual elaboration

It is also possible for both units to be partially schematic and elaborate different parts of each other: in such cases each unit acts as a filler as well as a frame. This is illustrated in Figure 10.5, which depicts the superimposition of the symbolic units *want* and *them*. Again, integration takes place simultaneously at the semantic and the phonological poles of the expressions. At the semantic pole, 3PL (third person plural) elaborates the schematically specified landmark of [[WANTER] WANT [THING WANTED]], and WANT elaborates the schematically specified process in the semantic representation of [[THING] PROCESS [3PL]]. At the phonological pole [wɒnt] elaborates the second slot in [… … ðəm] and at the same time [ðəm] elaborates the second slot in [...wɒnt...].

In subsequent discussion, I will treat phonological and semantic superimposition as a single process of symbolic integration, and will use *italics* to indicate symbolic expressions, with traditional grammatical labels (NP, V etc.) representing phonologically underspecified components in symbolic units, or 'slots', which can be elaborated by more contentful units. For example, *WANTER.NP want WANTED.NP* and *NP V them* represent the symbolic units [[WANTER]-WANT-[THING WANTED]]/[...wɒnt...] and [[THING] PROCESS [3PL]]/ [... ... ðəm] respectively.

It was suggested earlier that speakers store units of various sizes and degrees of specificity: general templates such as *NP V NP*, low-level schemas such as *WANTER.NP want WANTED.NP*, as well as fully specified lexical units like *I want it*. When speakers construct novel expressions, they normally use the most specific (i.e. largest and most concrete) unit available. This is because more specific units share more properties with the speaker's conceptualisation, and hence are easier to access in a content-addressable memory. Furthermore, using more specific units allows the target utterance to be assembled more easily, that is to say, in fewer steps. (Of course, speakers cannot know in advance which method of assembling an utterance is the simplest; but if we assume that the various possibilities are tried out in parallel, the simplest one is the most likely to be used because it will deliver a pronounceable utterance first.)

This preference for specific units helps explain how speakers avoid overgeneralising the patterns found in their language to inappropriate contexts. The existence of the well-entrenched unit *ate* pre-empts the application of the general past-tense schema, which would produce **eated*; the existence of schematic units such us *NP V them* prevents speakers from producing expressions such as **want they*, in which the simple unit *they* is superimposed over the second slot in the schema *WANTER.NP want WANTED.NP*; in French, the availability of a subject + clitic pronoun + verb pattern (e.g. *je le dis* 'I say it') pre-empts the application of the general *NP V NP* pattern, preventing speakers from producing ungrammatical utterances such as **je dit le*.

Let us now consider how one might assemble a more complex utterance, such as this question:

(9)   *Where do you think they are going?*

For the sake of the following discussion, we will assume that the speaker has the following symbolic units at his or her disposal:

(10)   *Where AUX NONFINITE.S?*
(11)   *WH do you think S-WH?*
(12)   *they are going LOCATION*

The first unit, *Where AUX NONFINITE.S?*, is simply the lexical representation of the interrogative pronoun *where*. The construction represents the speaker's knowledge about how *where* is used in sentences, including the fact that it requires a preposed auxiliary. Note that this fact must be explicitly represented in the grammar, since not all question words impose this requirement. (*How come*, for example, does not: we say *How come she is coming?*, not **How come is she coming?*) Unit (11) is the prototypical LDD question construction discussed in Chapter 9 (section 3.4); the symbol S-WH stands for a tensed clause with a gap (i.e. an unfilled slot). Unit (12) is a prefab containing a single slot for a locative expression.

To derive the target question, the speaker must combine the three units. The combination of (10) and (11) is a straightforward case of superimposition with mutual elaboration:

1. *where* from (10) elaborates the schematic WH slot in (11);
2. *do* from (11) elaborates the AUX slot in (10); and
3. *you think S-WH* from (11) elaborates the *NONFINITE.S* slot in (10).

The result is this complex expression:

(13)   *where do you think S-WH?*

The next step involves the superimposition of (12) and (13). Note that these two components have partially incompatible specifications: both contain a location substructure, but (12) requires that the corresponding phonological unit come after *going*, whereas (13) specifies that it should come at the beginning of the sentence, before the auxiliary. To create a composite structure, the speaker must resolve the conflict, which can be done in two ways: either the specifications of (12) override those of (13), or vice versa. These two options correspond to two different constructions. In ordinary questions, the WH word is used as the framing unit and hence its requirements prevail: the resulting expression has interrogative word order and is used as a request for information (14). In echo questions, the verb provides the frame, resulting in a structure with declarative word order and a semi-declarative meaning: (15) can be used either as a request to repeat part of the preceding utterance or (with heavy stress on *where*) to express surprise, but not as a true question.

(14)   *where do you think they are going?*
(15)   *you think they are going where?*

Note that the approach outlined above allows for alternative ways of assembling the same expression. For example, the three components of *where do you think they are going?* can be combined in a different order: the speaker could begin by superimposing (11) and (12) to produce *WH do you think they are going LOCATION?*, and then superimpose this and (10) to derive the target utterance. And of course if *they are going LOCATION* is not available as a unit, it would have to be constructed (for example, by superimposing *they are V-ing* and *NP go LOCATION*).

As hinted in Chapter 9, it is likely that speakers also have some more general knowledge about LDD questions, which might be captured by this more abstract schema:

(16)   *WH AUX MENTAL.V (NP) S-WH?*

Here, *MENTAL.V* stands for an untensed verb designating a mental state or a communication event. When assembling questions such as (9), the use of this schema would normally be pre-empted by the more specific *WH do you think S-WH?* schema, but the more abstract unit can be used to produce non-prototypical LDD questions such as *where will my brother think they are going?* Alternatively, such questions could be produced by substituting *will* for *do* and *my brother* for *you* in (11): such use would involve extension rather than instantiation of the motivating schema.

Schemas (11) and (16) also sanction questions involving dependencies reaching over more than one clause, such as examples (17) and (18):

(17)   *What did you say Claire thought he did?*
(18)   *Where do you think Ben knew they were going?*

Such sentences, like the more prototypical LDD question discussed earlier, consist of a WH word followed by an auxiliary and an untensed clause with a gap, but in this case the missing element logically belongs in the doubly embedded clause (the clause that functions as the complement of *thought* in (17) and *knew* in (18)). To be able to form such questions, the speaker must extend the category S-WH to include expressions such as *Claire thought he did* and *Ben knew they were going.*

4. A cognitive view of language acquisition

According to CG, language is a structured inventory of conventional linguistic units. It follows that learning a language involves acquiring a repertoire of linguistic units and making the appropriate connections between them. To understand how language learners accomplish this, we must begin by considering the type of information that is available to them. The language addressed to children – even very young children – consists predominantly of multi-word utterances rather than simple expressions.[3] The utterances occur in a rich and fairly predictable context which enables the child to form some idea about their meaning. They are also quite stereotypical: that is to say, some forms repeatedly occur in similar contexts.

For example, let us suppose that during breakfast one day the child looks at a milk carton and the mother says *Do you want milk?* and pours him some. During the following weeks, the child hears *You want milk, D'you want milk?* or *Do you want milk?* while the mother is holding the milk carton and looking at him, walking towards the fridge (which the child knows contains the milk), and in other mealtime contexts. Eventually he learns that *you want milk* is used when he wants milk and is offered it – in other words, he acquires a fixed formula with a specific communicative function (Figure 10.6a).[4] The child's semantic representation is probably richer than the conventional adult meaning of the expression (for example, it might incorporate his knowledge that this is something that the mother frequently says at mealtimes and that it is an offer of milk). It might also be incomplete or inaccurate in certain respects. However, because humans are generally very good at guessing other people's communicative intentions (see Chapter 6, section 2.2), we can assume that the child's representation will capture at least some relevant aspects of the adult meaning.

Such formulaic phrases are the starting point of grammatical development. To acquire units which will enable them to produce and understand novel expressions, language learners must do three things:

1. segment the phonological representation, that is to say, identify chunks of phonological material that function as units ([juː‚wɒntˈmɪlk] = [juː]<[wɒnt] <[mɪlk]);
2. establish correspondences between phonological chunks and salient aspects of semantic structure (MILK=[mɪlk], WANT=[wɒnt] etc.); and
3. extract the component units of the formula, including constructional schemas (in our example, [[WANTER]-WANT-[THING WANTED]]/[[…]<[wɒnt] <[…]]).

We have a reasonably good idea of how children accomplish the first of these tasks. In principle, it is possible to identify word boundaries simply on the basis of statistical regularities in the phonotactic structure of texts (Cairns et al. 1997; Elman 1990). A variety of prosodic cues (intonation, rhythm, stress) are also available, and we know that children make use of these (Cutler and McQueen 1995; Mattys et al. 1999; Peters 1985).

The next stage – establishing correspondences between chunks of semantic and phonological structure – would be fairly straightforward *if* semantic representations were given *a priori*. The problem is that concepts are not available *a priori*: different languages partition the same scenes in radically different ways, so part of the learner's task is to determine which aspects of a scene are lexicalised in his or her language (cf. Chapter 7). This is especially true of the meanings of relational words, which tend to vary cross-linguistically much more than the meanings of concrete nouns. In addition, relational words tend to have more abstract meanings (you can see, feel and taste milk, but you can't see or taste wanting; you can point to milk but not to wanting) and are more difficult to isolate conceptually (wanting cannot exist independently of the individual who wants and the thing wanted).

So how can the child determine which semantic configurations are lexicalised in his language and perform the sound-to-meaning mapping? I would like to suggest that the way information is organised in memory plays a critical role in this process. Human memory is content-addressable, which means that:

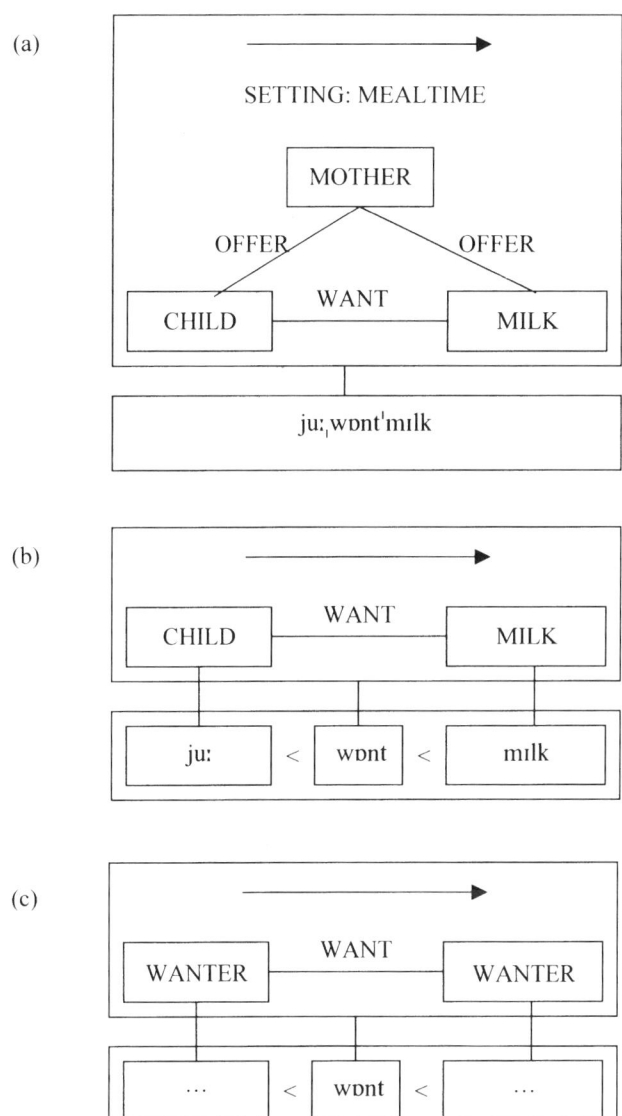

Figure 10.6 The emergence of a schema. (a) An unanalysed formula. The holistic representation is open to alternative semantic analyses and may contain irrelevant contextual detail. (b) Analysed formula. Aspects of semantic structure have been mapped onto chunks of phonological material. The schema is implicit in the formula, but not independently accessible. (c) A low-level schema, or the lexical representation of one sense of the verb *want*. Aspects of (b) shared with other *want*-formulas have been entrenched through repeated use and acquired independent status, making the schema available for production and interpretation of novel expressions.

1. expressions which share aspects of semantic structure have partly overlapping semantic representations;
2. expressions which sound similar (at either the segmental or the suprasegmental level) have partly overlapping phonological representations; and
3. expressions which share aspects of semantic structure and aspects of phonological structure have partially overlapping representations at both levels.

To see how this property can help in acquiring language, let us assume that our learner, who has already learned to associate the phonological form [ju:]<[wɒnt]<[mɪlk] with a holistic representation of the milk-offering situation, acquires a second formula with a similar function, e.g. *I want (the) ball*. The two formulas share some semantic substructures (they are both used in situations when someone wants something) and the phonological chunk [wɒnt], while other parts (e.g. the visual and motor images associated with *ball*, the phonological chunk [bɔ:l]) are not shared. Once the learner has acquired two (or more) formulas with partially overlapping representations, interesting things start happening. The parts shared by several formulas are activated, and hence entrenched, every time the learner hears (and later, produces) any formula that contains them. In our example, the learner's representations of the phonological chunk [wɒnt] and semantic relationship between the experiencer and the desired object become active every time either formula is used; and of course [mɪlk] and [bɔ:l] also occur in other expressions, not just as objects of the verb *want*, so they, too, are activated in a variety of situations. The elements making up the substructures shared by several formulas are frequently co-activated, and eventually become units in their own right. In this way, shared representation results in analysis: the internal structure of the formula becomes visible to the learner (Figure 10.6b). In other words, the component parts which are implicit in the unanalysed formula gradually become more salient because certain configurations of semantic and phonological material frequently co-occur. At this stage, the learner may be said to have a 'mini-grammar': a grammar of the expression *you want milk*.

This change has several important consequences. First, as the formula is analysed into its component units, meaning becomes more compositional. In our example, whatever meaning *You want milk* might have had above and beyond that contributed by its components is not strengthened as a result of sharing a representation with other formulas, and gradually becomes less salient; as a result, the meaning of the component units (notably the relational expression) is distilled from the formula. The contextual meaning may not disappear altogether: adult lexicons contain many multi-word units which are not fully compositional. These include not only idioms, but also 'regular' expressions whose meanings are more specific than the sum of the meanings of their parts, such as *I told you so* ('I told you this would happen and you should have listened to my advice/warning') or *forget it* ('forget it because it is not important'). It may also survive as knowledge about the kinds of situations in which it is appropriate to use a particular expression (e.g. formal v. informal, when speaking to a social superior, when speaking to a member of the opposite sex, and so on) and about what we call connotation (knowledge about the emotional associations of a particular expression).[5]

Another important consequence of analysis is that it is now easier for the learner to acquire new formulas, since part of their representation is already there. Analysis is basically a chunking process: complex configurations of substructures become units in their own right. The child might have needed 50 repetitions to learn *you want milk*, 30 repetitions to learn *I want (the) ball* and 10 repetitions to learn *you want yoghurt*; subsequently he will be able to reproduce other instantiations of this lexically based pattern after just one or two learning episodes (assuming he already knows the nominals).

Once a formula has been analysed into its component units, the learner has acquired some knowledge about *want* constructions which one might describe as an incipient schema. It is, however, a **passive generalisation**, not readily available for use in production of novel expressions: it has a similar status to the -*en* plural in English (which is found in only three nouns: *oxen*, *children*, *brethren*) or the patterns underlying the smaller classes of irregular verbs (e.g. the *buy–bought–bought* pattern, which applies to six or seven verbs only). There are good reasons for believing that such generalisations are captured in our mental grammars, but they are not normally applied to new nouns and verbs.

As observed earlier, high-frequency forms are more entrenched, and hence easier to access. Since components shared by several stored units are necessarily accessed more frequently than any of the units which contain them, it follows that they will become more entrenched than the larger units, and, after a time, they will become accessible as units in their own right (Figure 10.6c). This has little impact on high-frequency formulas, which are easy to access anyway, but has important consequences for other aspects of language use. First, the learner now has an alternative method of retrieving low-frequency formulas: they can be activated by accessing the component parts and allowing them to activate the whole. Secondly, and much more importantly, the schema can be combined with other established units in order to form novel expressions – in other words, it becomes productive.

It should be clear from the preceding discussion that the accessibility of a component unit, and therefore the potential to use it in novel expressions, is a matter of degree. The more accessible the schema, the easier it is to apply productively, and hence the greater the likelihood that it will be used productively. Schema accessibility depends on two main factors: specificity (as explained earlier, more specific units are easier to access) and entrenchment, which is a function of frequency (other things being equal, more frequent units are easier to access).

However, even schemas which are generalisations over a relatively small number of exemplars can be used productively. The irregular *-en* plural in English is occasionally applied to new nouns, mostly in word-play: computer hackers, for example, sometimes use the forms *VAXen* ('several VAX computers'), *faxen, boxen, Macintoshen* (Pinker 1999: 52). Even components which occur in a single lexicalised unit are sometimes extended to new items. For example, the pseudo-morpheme *-k* in *fork* can be used to produce novel words like *threek* (meaning 'fork with three tines'). This is sometimes found in humorous musings about language (there are a number of examples on the web); but it has also been spontaneously produced by a pre-school child (Kaplan 1998). It should be stressed, however, that such uses are rare and untypical in that they require extra effort on the part of both speaker and addressee. Normal language use, in contrast, relies on well-established units and is automatic and relatively effortless.

Thus, the capacity for grammatical productivity emerges gradually as a result of analysis of rote-learned phrases and is a by-product of the way symbolic units are stored in long-term memory. A schema is implicit in its instantiations; and schema extraction involves 'finding' it in the stored exemplars and strengthening it until it becomes accessible as a unit in its own right. For lexically specific patterns, this process is facilitated by the shared phonological material. Higher-level schemas (e.g. a verb–general transitive construction) are more difficult to 'find' because they have no shared phonological content and rather abstract meanings. However, as explained above, such general schemas have the same structure as their instantiations (i.e. low-level schemas and lexically fixed units), and therefore can be derived from lexically specific units by 'filtering out' irrelevant details while preserving the overall structure.

This account fits in very well with the developmental data discussed in the last chapter: the tight correlation between vocabulary size and grammatical development and the observed progression from highly stereotypical to more flexible usage. Since formulas are essentially big words, we would expect the acquisition of both types of units to be mediated by the same mental mechanism. More flexible use requires constructional schemas, but since these emerge from formulas with partially overlapping representations, the development of productivity depends on the prior acquisition of a repertoire of rote-learned phrases.

The above proposal also offers some insight into how learners discover the meanings of relational words. Unlike most nouns, which are conceptually relatively autonomous, the meanings of relational words such as verbs and prepositions presuppose the entities participating in the relation: one cannot conceptualise a relation without also conceptualising the entities involved in it, even if the latter are conceived only in very schematic terms. This is easiest to see with converse terms like *own* and *belong to*, *above* and *below*, *in front of* and *behind*, *before* and *after*, *give* and *receive*, *buy* and *sell* etc. Every act of giving is also an act of receiving: if you give me a lollipop, it's also necessarily true that I receive a lollipop from you. Therefore in order to learn the difference between *give* and *receive* children must match conceptualisations of events with entire clauses rather than with single words, and the units they extract must preserve information about which chunk of phonology corresponds to which aspect of semantic structure. In other words, the verb *give* is a linguistic unit consisting of four component units: *GIVER.NP give RECIPIENT.NP GIFT.NP*.

Learners also need to rely on information about the linguistic context to discover more subtle aspects of meaning. Take a set of near-synonyms like *shake, shiver, shudder, quake, quiver, tremble* and *vibrate*. These seven verbs all designate a similar type of movement, but they are not fully synonymous and cannot be used interchangeably: for instance, if you think of something terrible, you might shudder or tremble but you wouldn't vibrate. How do we learn these differences in meaning? Clearly not from definitions given by more experienced language users, since most people find the differences very difficult to verbalise. We also do not learn them by consulting a dictionary, as dictionary definitions are typically circular: according to the *Chambers English Dictionary*, for example, *quake* means 'quiver or vibrate', *vibrate* means 'shake or tremble', and so on.

Learners can glean some hints about the meaning of such near-synonyms by paying attention to the general context in which they are used: for instance, the kind of situation that might make a person shake or tremble. However, the single most useful and reliable source of information about such subtle semantic differences is the types of words that each verb collocates with. As shown in a corpus study by Atkins and Levin (1995), the seven shaking verbs tend to take different kinds of subjects: a voice can shake or tremble, but not shudder; a machine can vibrate, but it does not shiver; light or a shadow can quiver or tremble, but they do not shake. Thus, learning the semantic difference between *shake, shudder, tremble* etc. is (to a large extent) learning what classes of words they collocate with – in other words, acquiring schemas such as PERSON *tremble*, PERSON'S VOICE *tremble*, MACHINE *vibrate* and so on.[6] Note that apart from *shake,* all of these verbs are fairly literary, and hence are normally acquired relatively late. This suggests that partially underspecified phrase-sized units continue to play an important role in later language acquisition as well.

5. More on regularity

The account outlined above emphasises stored units and low-level patterns which are learned piecemeal. This seems to be at odds with a basic tenet of modern linguistics, namely, that languages are highly systematic: in each language, there are some broad regularities shared by many different elements, characteristic of the language as a whole: word-order patterns, agreement rules, structural parallels between different types of constructions (for example, interrogatives, relatives) etc. Where do such patterns come from, and what is their status? If each verb is a mini-grammar acquired independently of other verbs   ([[POSSESSOR]-HAVE-[POSSESSED]]/[[…]<[hæv]<[…]],   [[CONSUMER]-EAT-[FOOD]]/ [[…]<[iːt]<[…]], [[WRITER]-WRITE-[TEXT]]/[[…]<[raɪt]<[…]], etc.), why does English have a fixed word order (SVO) shared by all (transitive) verbs, and why do all verbs have to agree with their subjects? Why don't different verbs impose different word-order and agreement requirements?

Before we address this question, it is worth pointing out that modern linguistics has tended to overemphasise regularity. There is, in fact, a great deal of irregularity in language: very few rules are completely exceptionless. This is most evident in morphology, where the existence of minor patterns and outright exceptions is quite commonplace. What is more, many languages have classes of words to which the normal morphological rules do not apply, or apply only optionally. It was noted in Chapter 8, for example, that some Polish nouns are not inflected for case – in other words, the usual rules of grammar, which require inflected forms in certain contexts, do not apply to these nouns. One can, of course, say that the rules do apply, but their operation is invisible: the words are inflected for whatever case is required, but the inflections are realised as zero. This, however, is regularity by fiat: the linguist's grammar is regular – but it is not clear that the language itself is.

Similar observations apply to syntax. The English passive construction is sometimes described as a product of fully general rules which convert an underlying structure in which the direct object follows the verb into one with passive word order. Not all transitive verbs in English, however, can be used in the passive construction: cf. the unacceptability of *A book is had by her*, *You are suited by this dress*, *A good life was lived by Robin*. One could rescue the claim that the passive rule is fully general by stipulating that a transitive verb is a verb which passivises, and thus *have*, *suit* and *live* are not fully transitive – but this amounts to saying that the passive construction can apply to any verb which can be passivised: in other words, it makes the claim vacuous.

Word-order and agreement patterns may also be to some extent lexically specific. For example, in French, most adjectives come after the noun, but some precede it, and a few can occur in either position, depending on their meaning (cf. *femme ancienne* 'old woman/wife' and *ancienne femme* 'ex-wife'). Even English, with its relatively rigid word order, is not fully consistent: in addition to the normal adjective–noun order, we also have noun–adjective in expressions such as *secretary general, court martial, proof positive, sister-german, battle royal*. Or consider British Sign Language, which has three types of verbs: the so-called plain verbs are not marked for agreement and are strongly associated with SVO word order; agreement verbs, as their name suggests, do require agreement (with both subject and object), and normally appear in sentence-final position; and spatial verbs are marked for location and movement rather than subject and object (Sutton-Spence and Woll 1999).

Thus, in this case we have three different word-order and agreement patterns in the same language.

On the other hand, it is undeniable that there are many high-level regularities in all human languages, and these require an explanation. As noted in Chapter 6, grammars are to some degree shaped by external discourse pressures and processing constraints: some utterances are preferred by language users because they are easier to process or are less likely to lead to ambiguity, and hence their use spreads. Since the same pressures act on different constructions, the result is that individual constructions converge towards the same points. Such functional pressures still leave considerable variety (since there is generally more than one workable solution to a particular communication problem), but they do reduce it in that they eliminate some variants.

There are also pressures for systematicity. Systems in which there are several competing patterns are inherently unstable, as it is virtually inevitable that speakers will occasionally overgeneralise some of them, sometimes because of memory failure, and sometimes to achieve a special effect. Such innovations may be picked up by other speakers, which results in fluctuation in the frequency of the individual variants. However, once a particular variant gains a clear advantage over the other(s), whether by chance or as a result of a language fad, it will tend to spread (since, other things being equal, more entrenched patterns are easier to access) and may eventually monopolise the grammar. Of course, not all language change is regularising: processes which result in the emergence of irregular structures are also very common – otherwise all mature languages would be completely regular. However, research on the emergence of creole languages suggests that regularisation processes predominate in the early stages of the development of a language (Aitchison 1989; Mühlhäusler 1986).

6. Future directions

The approach to language outlined above has much to recommend it, and has been applied successfully to a variety of linguistic domains (see for example Casad 1996b; Casad and Palmer 2003; Cienki et al. 2001; Foolen and van der Leek 2000; Langacker 1991a; Rudzka-Ostyn 1988). However, Cognitive Grammar is a relatively young endeavour, and is only beginning to address certain issues, among them phenomena such as extraction, binding and control, which have been the mainstays of generative linguistics. While there is some promising work in these areas (see e.g. Deane 1993; Langacker 1995; van Hoek 1997), it remains to be seen whether CG can provide a workable alternative to generative accounts of these aspects of a speaker's linguistic knowledge.

Furthermore, although cognitive linguists are officially committed to developing an account of language that is usage-based and firmly grounded in human cognition, in practice, only a few have begun to go beyond the traditional introspective methods. It is to be hoped that more researchers will move in this direction in the future. A firm empirical basis is indispensable for work that purports to be psychologically realistic because, as stressed repeatedly throughout this book, speakers' knowledge about their language may be less abstract than is commonly believed, and may differ considerably from one individual to the next.

Another challenge for future research will be to develop CG accounts of language acquisition and processing. The approach to language production outlined above has been applied quite successfully to the speech of young children (Dąbrowska and Lieven submitted); it remains to be seen how well it will work with adult data. With respect to language acquisition, there is a large body of research either directly inspired by or compatible with CG (comprehensively reviewed in Tomasello 2003). Most of it has focused on early development: how children learn words and multi-word units and extract the first generalisations from them. There is much less work on later language development addressing such crucial issues as how early piecemeal knowledge is integrated into a system (although Tomasello has some interesting proposals), or how children learn about different construals of the same scene. However, now that cognitive linguists have begun to work with representatives of other language sciences, there are good prospects for progress in these areas in the future.

Notes

1. For a detailed discussion of determiners and tense/agreement marking in English from a CG perspective, see Langacker (1991a: chapters 3 and 6). A more accessible introduction can be found in Taylor (2002: chapters 18 and 20).
2. Readers familiar with the CG framework will note a significant departure from standard Langackerian notation: while the subparts of semantic structure representing the arguments of the verb are linked to their corresponding phonological structures (for example, [CAT] is connected to [ə'kæt]), there is no direct link between the semantic representation of the verb and the corresponding phonological unit – only between the whole relational predication with its arguments and the corresponding phonological structure. Likewise, in Figure 10.1b, there is no direct link between the semantic notion of plurality and its phonological exponent. This notation is meant to reflect the fact that these lexical units are not single words, but constructions: that is to say, their representations contain structures which must be elaborated by other units.
3. Only about 7–8 per cent of the input are single-word utterances (Tomasello 2003), and these are predominantly interjections such as *yeah, no, oh, OK*

– that is to say, words which do not enter into syntactic relationships with other words.

4. For the sake of the following discussion, I assume that the unit that the child extracts does not contain the initial auxiliary, since it is phonologically indistinct and often omitted in informal speech. It is also possible, of course, that the child does represent the full adult form (*do you want milk?*) or just *want milk*. This will obviously affect subsequent development: if the child extracts the larger unit, he will have more analysis to do, and if the original unit is *want milk*, he will have to learn some larger units at a later stage.

5. These non-compositional aspects of meaning are usually regarded as an extra that somehow gets added to the meanings contributed by the lexical items when utterances are interpreted in context. However, from a developmental point of view, it is the other way around: the contextual meaning is more basic, and the meanings of individual lexical items are carved out of it.

6. Gleitman makes a very similar point in her argument for syntactic bootstrapping (the hypothesis that children discover verb meanings by observing which syntactic frames verbs can occur in: see Gleitman 1990; Gleitman and Gillette 1995). However, the above discussion suggests that our knowledge about the distributional properties of words is much more specific than a purely syntactic subcategorisation frame.

Bibliography

Abbot-Smith, K., Lieven, E. V. and Tomasello, M. (2001), 'What preschool children do and do not do with ungrammatical word orders', *Cognitive Development*, 16, 679–92.

Aitchison, J. (1989), 'Spaghetti junctions and recurrent routes: some preferred pathways in language evolution', *Lingua*, 77, 151–71.

Akhtar, N. (1999), 'Acquiring basic word order: evidence for data-driven learning of syntactic structure', *Journal of Child Language*, 26, 339–56.

Akhtar, N. and Tomasello, M. (1997), 'Young children's productivity with word order and verb morphology', *Developmental Psychology*, 33, 952–65.

Albert, M. and Obler, L. (1978), *The Bilingual Brain: Neuropsychological and Neurolinguistic Aspects of Bilingualism*, New York: Academic Press.

Alegre, M. and Gordon, P. (1999), 'Frequency effects and the representational status of regular inflections', *Journal of Memory and Language*, 40, 41–61.

Altenberg, B. (1998), 'On the phraseology of spoken English: the evidence of recurrent word-combinations', in A. P. Cowie (ed.), *Phraseology: Theory, Analysis and Applications*, Oxford: Clarendon Press, pp. 101–22.

Altmann, G. T. M. and Kamide, Y. (1999), 'Incremental interpretation at verbs: restricting the domain of subsequent reference', *Cognition*, 73, 247–64.

Altmann, G. T. M., Garnham, A., van Nice, K. and Henstra, J. A. (1998), 'Late closure in context', *Journal of Memory and Language*, 38, 459–84.

Anderson, J. (1971), *The Grammar of Case: Towards a Localistic Theory*, Cambridge: Cambridge University Press.

Anderson, J. (1994), 'Localism', in R. E. Asher and J. M. Y. Simpson (eds), *The Encyclopedia of Language and Linguistics* (Vol. 4), Oxford: Pergamon Press, pp. 2276–82.

Anderson, S. R. and Lightfoot, D. W. (2002), *The Language Organ: Linguistics As Cognitive Physiology*, Cambridge: Cambridge University Press.

Aram, D. M. (1998), 'Acquired aphasia in children', in M. T. Sarno (ed.), *Acquired Aphasia* (3rd edn), San Diego: Academic Press, pp. 451–80.

Atkins, B. T. S. and Levin, B. (1995), 'Building a corpus: a linguistic and lexicographical look at some near-synonyms', *International Journal of Lexicography*, 8, 85–114.

Baayen, H., Dijkstra, T. and Schreuder, R. (1997), 'Singulars and plurals in Dutch: evidence for a parallel dual-route model', *Journal of Memory and Language*, 37, 94–117.

Baker, N. D. and Nelson, K. E. (1984), 'Recasting and related conversational techniques for triggering syntactic advances by young children', *First Language*, 5, 3–21.

Baldo, J. V., Elder, J. T., Larsen, J., Dronkers, N. F., Redfern, B. and Ludy, C. (2001), 'Is cognition intact in patients with aphasia?', *Brain and Language*, 79, 64–7.

Barsalou, L. W. (1992), *Cognitive Psychology: An Overview for Cognitive Scientists*, Hillsdale, NJ: Lawrence Erlbaum.

Barsalou, L. W. (1993), 'Flexibility, structure and linguistic vagary in concepts: manifestations of a compositional system of perceptual symbols', in A. C. Collins, S. E. Gathercole and M. A. Conway (eds), *Theories of Memories*, London: Lawrence Erlbaum, pp. 29–101.

Barsalou, L. W. (1999), 'Perceptual symbol systems', *Behavioral and Brain Sciences*, 22, 577–609.

Barsalou, L. W., Yeh, W., Luka, B. J., Olseth, K. L., Mix, K. S. and Wu, L. (1993), 'Concepts and meaning', *Papers from the Parasession on Conceptual Representations, Chicago Linguistic Society*, 29, 23–61.

Basso, A., Della Sala, S. and Fabrola, M. (1987), 'Aphasia arising from purely deep lesions', *Cortex*, 23, 29–44.

Bates, E. (1994), 'Modularity, domain specificity and the development of language', *Discussions in Neuroscience*, 10, 136–49.

Bates, E. (1997), 'On language savants and the structure of the mind', *International Journal of Bilingualism*, 1, 163–86.

Bates, E. (1999), 'Language and the infant brain', *Journal of Communication Disorders*, 32, 195–205.

Bates, E. and Goodman, J. (1997), 'On the inseparability of grammar and the lexicon: evidence from acquisition, aphasia, and real-time processing', *Language and Cognitive Processes*, 12, 507–84.

Bates, E. and Goodman, J. (1999), 'On the emergence of grammar from the lexicon', in B. MacWhinney (ed.), *The Emergence of Language*, Mahwah, NJ: Lawrence Erlbaum, pp. 29–79.

Bates, E., Bretherton, I. and Snyder, L. (1988), *From First Words to Grammar: Individual Differences and Dissociable Mechanisms*, Cambridge: Cambridge University Press.

Bates, E., Dale, P. S. and Thal, D. (1995), 'Individual differences and their implications for theories of language development', in P. Fletcher and B. MacWhinney (eds), *The Handbook of Child Language*, Oxford: Blackwell, pp. 96–151.

Bates, E., Wulfeck, B. and MacWhinney, B. (1991), 'Cross-linguistic research in aphasia: an overview', *Brain and Language*, 41, 123–48.

Bates, E., Harris, C., Marchman, V. and Wulfeck, B. (1995), 'Production of complex syntax in normal ageing and Alzheimer's disease', *Language and Cognitive Processes*, 10, 487–593.

Bates, E., Thal, D., Trauner, D., Fenson, J., Aram, D., Eisele, J. and Nass, R. (1997), 'From first words to grammar in children with focal brain injury', *Developmental Neuropsychology*, 13, 447–76.

Bavin, E. L. (1990), 'Locative terms and Warlpiri acquisition', *Journal of Child Language*, 17, 43–66.

Behrens, H. (2001), 'Learning multiple regularities: evidence from overgeneralization errors in the German plural', in A. H.-J. Do, L. Dominguez and A. Johansen (eds), *Proceedings of the 26th Annual Boston University Conference on Language Development*, Somerville, MA: Cascadilla Press, pp. 72–83.

Behrens, H. (submitted), 'How to learn a minority default: the acquisition of the German -s plural'.

Belliger, D. and Gleason, J. (1982), 'Sex differences in parental directives to young children', *Journal of Sex Roles*, 8, 1123–39.

Bellugi, U. (1971), 'Simplification in children's language', in R. Huxley and E. Ingram (eds), *Language Acquisition: Models and Methods*, London: Academic Press, pp. 95–119.

Bellugi, U., Wang, P. P. and Jernigan, T. L. (1994), 'Williams syndrome: an unusual neuropsychological profile', in S. H. Broman and J. Grafman (eds), *Atypical Cognitive Deficits in Developmental Disorders*, Hillsdale, NJ: Lawrence Erlbaum, pp. 23–56.

Bellugi, U., Marks, S., Bihrle, A. and Sabo, H. (1993), 'Dissociation between language and cognitive functions in Williams syndrome', in D. Bishop and K. Mogford (eds), *Language Development in Exceptional Circumstances*, Hove: Lawrence Erlbaum, pp. 177–89.

Bellugi, U., Lichtenberger, L., Jones, W., Lai, Z. and St George, M. (2000), 'The neurocognitive profile of Williams syndrome: a complex pattern of strengths and weaknesses', *Journal of Cognitive Neuroscience*, 12, 7–29.

Benedict, H. (1979), 'Early lexical development: comprehension and production', *Journal of Child Language*, 6, 183–200.

Berko, J. (1958), 'The child's learning of English morphology', *Word*, 14, 150–77.

Berman, R. (1993), 'Marking verb transitivity in Hebrew-speaking children', *Journal of Child Language*, 20, 641–70.

Bickerton, D. (1996), *Language and Human Behaviour*, London: UCL Press.

Bierwisch, M. (1970), 'Semantics', in J. Lyons (ed.), *New Horizons in Linguistics*, Harmondsworth: Penguin, pp. 166–84.

Bierwisch, M. and Schreuder, R. (1992), 'From concepts to lexical items', *Cognition*, 42, 23–60.

Bishop, D. (1993), 'Language development after focal brain damage', in D. Bishop and K. Mogford (eds), *Language Development in Exceptional Circumstances*, Hove: Lawrence Erlbaum, pp. 203–19.

Bishop, D. V. M. (1983), 'Linguistic impairment after left hemidecortication for infantile hemiplegia? A reappraisal', *Quarterly Journal of Experimental Psychology*, 35A, 199–207.

Bishop, D. V. M. (1992), 'The underlying nature of specific language impairment', *Journal of Child Psychology and Psychiatry*, 33, 3–66.

Bishop, D. V. M. (2002), 'Motor immaturity and specific speech and language impairment: evidence for a common genetic basis', *American Journal of Medical Genetics*, 114, 56–63.

Bishop, D. V. M., North, T. and Donlan, C. (1995), 'Genetic basis of specific language impairment: evidence from a twin study', *Developmental Medicine and Child Neurology*, 37, 56–71.

Blackwell, A. and Bates, E. (1995), 'Inducing agrammatic profiles in normals: evidence for the selective vulnerability of morphology under cognitive resource limitation', *Journal of Cognitive Neuroscience*, 7, 228–57.

Bloom, L., Lifter, K. and Hafitz, J. (1980), 'Semantics of verbs and the development of verb inflection in child language', *Language*, 56, 386–412.

Bod, R. (1998), *Beyond Grammar: An Experience-Based Theory of Language*, Stanford, CA: CSLI Publications.

Bod, R. (2001), 'Sentence memory: storage vs. computation of frequent sentences'. Retrieved 19 October 2003 from http://turing.wins.uva.nl/~rens/cuny2001.pdf.

Boesch, C. (1993), 'Aspects of transmission of tool-use in wild chimpanzees', in K. G. Gibson and T. Ingold (eds), *Tools, Language and Cognition in Human Evolution*, Cambridge: Cambridge University Press, pp. 171–83.

Boesch, C. and Boesch-Acherman, H. (2000), *The Chimpanzees of the Tai Forest: Behavioural Ecology and Evolution*, Oxford: Oxford University Press.

Borer, H. and Wexler, K. (1987), 'The maturation of syntax', in T. Roeper and E. Williams (eds), *Parameter-setting and Language Acquisition*, Dordrecht: Reidel, pp. 123–72.

Boudelaa, S. and Gaskell, M. G. (2002), 'A re-examination of the default system for Arabic plurals', *Language and Cognitive Processes*, 17, 321–43.

Bowerman, M. (1976), 'Semantic factors in the acquisition of rules for word use and sentence construction', in D. Morehead and A. Morehead (eds), *Normal and Deficient Child Language*, Baltimore: University Park Press, pp. 99–180.

Bowerman, M. (1993), 'Learning a semantic system: what role do cognitive predispositions play?', in P. Bloom (ed.), *Language Acquisition: Core Readings*, New York: Harverster Wheatsheaf, pp. 329–63.

Bowerman, M. (1996), 'The origins of children's spatial semantic categories: cognitive versus linguistic determinants', in J. Gumperz and S. C. Levinson (eds), *Rethinking Linguistic Relativity*, Cambridge: Cambridge University Press, pp. 145–76.

Braine, M. (1963), 'The ontogeny of English phrase structure', *Language*, 39, 1–14.

Braine, M. (1976), 'Children's first word combinations', *Monographs of the Society for Research in Child Development*, 41 (Serial No. 167), 1–104.

Braze, D., Shankweiler, D., Ni, W. and Palumbo, L. C. (2002), 'Readers' eye movements distinguish anomalies of form and content', *Journal of Psycholinguistic Research*, 31, 25–44.

Briscoe, T. (1994), 'Prospects for practical parsing of unrestricted text: robust statistical parsing techniques', in N. Oostdijk and P. de Haan (eds), *Corpus-Based Research into Language*, Amsterdam: Rodopi, pp. 67–95.

Brooks, P. J. and Tomasello, M. (1999), 'Young children learn to produce passives with nonce verbs', *Developmental Psychology*, 35, 29–44.

Brown, C. M., Hagoort, P. and Kutas, M. (2000), 'Postlexical integration processes in language comprehension: evidence from brain-imaging research', in M. S. Gazzaniga (ed.), *The New Cognitive Neurosciences*, Cambridge, MA: MIT Press, pp. 881–95.

Brown, J. W. (1975), 'On the neural organization of language: thalamic and cortical relationships', *Brain and Language*, 2, 18–30.

Brown, P. (1994), 'The INs and ONs of Tzeltal locative expressions: the semantics of static descriptions of location', *Linguistics*, 32, 743–90.

Brown, P. and Levinson, S. (1993), '"Uphill" and "downhill" in Tzeltal', *Journal of Linguistic Anthropology*, 3, 46–74.

Brown, R. (1968), 'The development of wh-questions in child speech', *Journal of Verbal Learning and Verbal Behavior*, 7, 279–90.

Brown, R. (1973), *A First Language: The Early Stages*, Cambridge, MA: Harvard University Press.

Brown, R. and Hanlon, C. (1970), 'Derivational complexity and order of acquisition in child speech', in J. R. Hayes (ed.), *Cognition and the Development of Language*, New York: Wiley, pp. 11–53.

Brugman, C. (1983), 'The use of body-part terms as locatives in Chalcatongo Mixtec', in A. Schlichter, W. Chafe and L. Hinton (eds), *Studies in Mesoamerican Linguistics*, Berkeley: Survey of California and Other Indian Languages, Report No. 4, pp. 235–90.

Brugman, C. (1988), *The Story of Over: Polysemy, Semantics and the Structure of the Lexicon*, New York: Garland.

Brugman, C. and Macaulay, M. (1986), 'Interacting semantic systems: Mixtec expressions of location', *Proceedings of the Twelfth Annual Meeting of the Berkeley Linguistics Society*, 315–27.

Bull, M. and Aylett, M. (1998), 'An analysis of the timing of turn-taking in a corpus of goal-orientated dialogue', in *Proceedings of ICSLP-98, Sidney, Australia* (Vol. 4), pp. 1175–8.

Bybee, J. L. (1995), 'Regular morphology and the lexicon', *Language and Cognitive Processes*, 10, 425–55.

Bybee, J. L. (2000), 'The phonology of the lexicon: evidence from lexical diffusion', in M. Barlow and S. Kemmer (eds), *Usage-Based Models of Language*, Cambridge: Cambridge University Press, pp. 65–85.

Bybee, J. L. and Scheibman, J. (1999), 'The effect of usage on degrees of constituency: the reduction of don't in English', *Linguistics*, 37, 575–96.

Bybee, J. L. and Slobin, D. I. (1982), 'Rules and schemas in the development and use of the English past tense', *Language*, 58, 265–89.

Cairns, P., Shillcock, R., Chater, N. and Levy, J. (1997), 'Bootstrapping word boundaries: a bottom-up corpus-based approach to speech segmentation', *Cognitive Psychology*, 33, 111–53.

Calvin, W. H. (1983), 'A stone's throw and its launch window: timing precision and its implications for language and hominid brains', *Journal of Theoretical Biology*, 104, 121–35.

Calvin, W. H. (1993), 'The unitary hypothesis: a common neural circuitry for novel manipulations, language, plan-ahead, and throwing?', in K. R. Gibson and T. Ingold (eds), *Tools, Language and Cognition in Human Evolution*, Cambridge: Cambridge University Press, pp. 230–50.

Calvin, W. H. and Bickerton, D. (2000), *Lingua ex Machina: Reconciling Darwin and Chomsky with the Human Brain*, Cambridge, MA: MIT Press.

Calvin, W. H. and Ojemann, G. A. (1994), *Conversations with Neil's Brain: The Neural Nature of Thought and Language*, Reading, MA: Addison-Wesley.

Cameron-Faulkner, T., Lieven, E. and Tomasello, M. (2003), 'A construction-based analysis of child-directed speech', *Cognitive Science*.

Capirci, O., Sabbadini, L. and Volterra, V. (1996), 'Language development in Williams syndrome: a case study', *Cognitive Neuropsychology*, 13, 1017–39, 27, 843–73.

Carey, S. (1978), 'The child as a word learner', in M. Halle, J. Bresnan and G. A. Miller (eds), *Linguistic Theory and Psychological Reality*, Cambridge, MA: MIT Press, pp. 264–93.

Carpenter, M., Akhtar, N. and Tomasello, M. (1998), 'Fourteen through 18-month-old infants differentially imitate intentional and accidental actions', *Infant Behavior and Development*, 21, 315–30.

Casad, E. H. (1977), 'Location and direction in Cora discourse', *Anthropological Linguistics*, 19, 216–41.

Casad, E. H. (1982), 'Cora locationals and structured imagery'. Unpublished PhD dissertation, University of California, San Diego.

Casad, E. H. (1988), 'Conventionalization of Cora locationals', in B. Rudzka-Ostyn (ed.), *Topics in Cognitive Grammar*, Amsterdam and Philadelphia: Benjamins, pp. 593–645.

Casad, E. H. (1996a), 'What good are locationals, anyway?', in M. Pütz and R. Dirven (eds), *The Construal of Space in Language and Thought*, Berlin: Mouton de Gruyter, pp. 249–67.

Casad, E. H. (1996b), *Cognitive Linguistics in the Redwoods: The Expansion of a New Paradigm in Linguistics*, Berlin: Mouton de Gruyter.

Casad, E. H. and Langacker, R. (1985), '"Inside" and "outside" in Cora grammar', *International Journal of American Linguistics*, 51, 247–81.

Casad, E. H. and Palmer, G. B. (eds) (2003), *Cognitive Linguistics and Non-Indo-European Languages*, Berlin: Mouton de Gruyter.

Caselli, C., Casadio, P. and Bates, E. (1999), 'A comparision of the transition from first words to grammar in English and Italian', *Journal of Child Language*, 26, 69–111.

Caselli, M. C., Leonard, L. B., Volterra, V. and Campagnoli, M. G. (1993), 'Towards mastery of Italian morphology: a cross-sectional study', *Journal of Child Language*, 20, 377–93.

Cazden, C. (1968), 'The acquisition of noun and verb inflections', *Child Development*, 39, 433–48.

Celli, M. L., Tomonaga, M., Udono, T., Teramoto, M. and Nagano, K. (2001), 'Learning processes in the acquisition of a tool-using task by captive chimpanzees', *Psychologia*, 44, 70–81.

Chambers English Dictionary (1988), Cambridge: Chambers.

Chiat, S. (1982), 'If I were you and you were me: the analysis of pronouns in a pronoun-reversing child', *Journal of Child Language*, 9, 359–79.

Chiat, S. (1986), 'Personal pronouns', in P. Fletcher and M. Garman (eds), *Language Acquisition*, Cambridge: Cambridge University Press, pp. 339–55.

Chipere, N. (2001), 'Native speaker variations in syntactic competence: implications for first language teaching', *Language Awareness*, 10, 107–24.

Chipere, N. (2003), *Understanding Complex Sentences: Native Speaker Variations in Syntactic Competence*, Basingstoke: Palgrave.

Choi, S. and Bowerman, M. (1991), 'Learning to express motion events in English and Korean: the influence of language-specific lexicalization patterns', *Cognition*, 41, 83–121.

Choi, S., Bowerman, M., Mandler, J. and McDonough, L. (1999), 'Early sensitivity to language-specific spatial categories in English and Korean', *Cognitive Development*, 14, 241–68.

Chomsky, N. (1964), 'Formal discussion of Miller and Ervin', *Monographs of the Society for Research in Child Development*, 29 (Serial No. 92), 35–9.

Chomsky, N. (1975), *Reflections on Language*, New York: Pantheon.

Chomsky, N. (1980a), 'On cognitive structures and their development: a reply to Piaget', in M. Piattelli-Palmarini (ed.), *Language and Learning: The Debate Between Jean Piaget and Noam Chomsky*, London: Routledge and Kegan Paul, pp. 35–52.

Chomsky, N. (1980b), 'Discussion of Putnam's comments', in M. Piattelli-Palmarini (ed.), *Language and Learning: The Debate Between Jean Piaget and Noam Chomsky*, Cambridge, MA: Harvard University Press, pp. 310–24.

Chomsky, N. (1986), *Knowledge of Language: Its Nature, Origin and Use*, New York: Praeger.

Chomsky, N. (1991), 'Linguistics and cognitive science: problems and mysteries', in A. Kasher (ed.), *The Chomskyan Turn*, Cambridge, MA: Blackwell, pp. 26–53.

Chomsky, N. (1999), 'On the nature, use, and acquisition of language', in W. C. Ritchie and T. K. Bhatia (eds), *Handbook of Child Language Acquisition*, San Diego: Academic Press, pp. 33–54.

Chomsky, N. (2000), *New Horizons in the Study of Language and Mind*, Cambridge: Cambridge University Press.

Chouinard, M. M. and Clark, E. V. (2003), 'Adult reformulations of child errors as negative evidence', *Journal of Child Language*, 30, 637–69.

Cienki, A. J., Luka, B. J. and Smith, M. B. (eds) (2001), *Conceptual and Discourse Factors in Linguistic Structure*, Stanford, CA: CSLI Publications.

Clahsen, H. (1999), 'Lexical entries and rules of language: a multidisciplinary study of German inflection', *Behavioral and Brain Sciences*, 22, 991–1060.

Clahsen, H. and Almazan, M. (1998), 'Syntax and morphology in Williams syndrome', *Cognition*, 68, 167–98.

Clahsen, H., Eisenbeiss, S. and Sonnenstuhl-Hennig, I. (1997), 'Morphological structure and the processing of inflected words', *Theoretical Linguistics*, 23, 201–49.

Clahsen, H., Rothweiler, M., Woest, A. and Marcus, G. F. (1992), 'Regular and irregular inflection in the acquisition of German noun plurals', *Cognition*, 45, 225–55.

Clark, E. V. (1973a), 'Non-linguistic strategies and the acquisition of word meaning', *Cognition*, 2, 161–82.

Clark, E. V. (1973b), 'What's in a word? On the child's acquisition of semantics in his first language', in T. Moore (ed.), *Cognitive Development and the Acquisition of Language*, New York: Academic Press, pp. 65–110.

Clark, E. V. (1975), 'Knowledge, context and strategy in the acquisition of meaning', in D. P. Dato (ed.), *Developmental Psycholinguistics: Theory and Applications. Georgetown University Roundatable on Languages and Linguistics 1975*, Washington, DC: Georgetown University Press, pp. 77–98.

Clark, E. V. (1976), 'Universal categories: on the semantics of classifiers and children's early word meanings', in A. Juilland (ed.), *Linguistic Studies Offered to Joseph Greenberg*, Saratoga, CA: Anma Libri, pp. 449–62.

Clark, E. V. (1980), 'Here's the *top*: nonlinguistic strategies in the acquisition of locative terms', *Child Development*, 51, 329–38.

Clark, E. V. (1982), 'The young word maker: a case study of innovation in the child's lexicon', in E. Wanner and L. R. Gleitman (eds), *Language Acquisition: The State of the Art*, Cambridge, MA: Cambridge University Press, pp. 390–425.

Clark, E. V. and Clark, H. (1977), *Psychology and Language*, New York: Harcourt Brace.

Clark, H. (1973), 'Space, time, semantics and the child', in T. Moore (ed.), *Cognitive Development and the Acquisition of Language*, New York: Academic Press, pp. 27–63.

Clark, R. (1974), 'Performing without competence', *Journal of Child Language*, 1, 1–10.

Clark, R. (1977), 'What's the use of imitation?', *Journal of Child Language*, 4, 341–58.

Collins COBUILD English Language Dictonary (1993), London: HarperCollins.

Comrie, B. (1976), *Aspect*, Cambridge: Cambridge University Press.

Conway, C. M. and Christiansen, M. H. (2001), 'Sequential learning in non-human primates', *Trends in Cognitive Sciences*, 5, 539–46.

Corina, D. (1996), 'Sign language and the brain: apes, apraxia and aphasia', *Behavioral and Brain Sciences*, 19, 633–4.

Corina, D. (1998), 'Aphasia in users of signed languages', in P. Coppens, Y. Lebrun and A. Basso (eds), *Aphasia in Atypical Populations*, Mahwah, NJ: Lawrence Erlbaum, pp. 261–309.

Cottrell, G. W. and Plunkett, K. (1994), 'Acquiring the mapping from meanings to sounds', *Connection Science*, 6, 379–412.

Crain, S. (1991), 'Language acquisition in the absence of experience', *Behavioral and Brain Sciences*, 14, 597–650.

Crain, S. and Lillo-Martin, D. (1999), *An Introduction to Linguistic Theory and Language Acquisition*, Malden, MA: Blackwell.

Crain, S. and Thornton, R. (1991), 'Recharting the course of language acquisition: studies in elicited production', in N. A. Krasnegor, D. Rumbargh, M. Studdert-Kennedy and R. Schiefelbusch (eds), *Biological and Behavioral Determinants of Language Development*, Hillsdale, NJ: Lawrence Erlbaum, pp. 321–37.

Croft, W. (2001), *Radical Construction Grammar: Syntactic Theory in Typological Perspective*, Oxford: Oxford University Press.

Crosson, B., Parker, J., Albert, K., Warren, R., Kepes, J. and Tully, R. (1986), 'A case of thalamic aphasia with postmortem verification', *Brain and Language*, 29, 301–14.

Culicover, P. W. (1999), *Syntactic Nuts: Hard Cases, Syntactic Theory and Language Acquisition*, Oxford: Oxford University Press.

Culp, R., Watkins, R., Lawrence, H., Letts, D., Kelly, D. and Rice, M. (1991), 'Maltreated children's language and speech development: abused, neglected and abused and neglected', *First Language*, 11, 377–90.

Curtiss, S. and de Bode, S. (1998), 'Linguistic outcomes for hemispherectomized children', in A. Greenhill, M. Hughes, H. Littlefield and H. Walsh (eds), *Proceedings of the Twenty-Second Boston University Conference on Language Development*, Boston: Cascadilla Press, pp. 121–33.

Curtiss, S. and Tallal, P. (1991), 'On the nature of the impairment in language-impaired children', in J. F. Miller (ed.), *Research on Child Language Disorders: A Decade of Progress*, Austin, TX: Pro-ed, pp. 189–210.

Curtiss, S., Katz, W. and Tallal, P. (1992), 'Delay vs. deviance in the language acquisition of language impaired children', *Journal of Speech and Hearing Research*, 35, 372–83.

Cutler, A. and McQueen, J. M. (1995), 'The recognition of lexical units in speech', in B. de Gelder and J. Morais (eds), *Speech and Reading: A Comparative Approach*, Hove: Lawrence Erlbaum, pp. 33–47.

Dąbrowska, E. (1993), 'O językowej idealizacji świata', *Bulletin de la Société Polonaise de Linguistique*, XLIX, 35–42.

Dąbrowska, E. (1996), 'The linguistic structuring of events: a study of Polish perfectivizing prefixes', in R. Dirven and M. Pütz (eds), *The Construal of Space in Language and Thought*, Berlin: Mouton de Gruyter, pp. 467–90.

Dąbrowska, E. (1997), 'The LAD goes to school: a cautionary tale for nativists', *Linguistics*, 35, 735–66.

Dąbrowska, E. (2000), 'From formula to schema: the acquisition of English questions', *Cognitive Linguistics*, 11, 1–20.

Dąbrowska, E. (2001), 'Learning a morphological system without a default: the Polish genitive', *Journal of Child Language*, 28, 545–74.

Dąbrowska, E. (2004), 'Rules or schemas? Evidence from Polish', *Language and Cognitive Processes*, 19, 225–71.

Dąbrowska, E. and Lieven, E. (2003), 'Learning the linguistic conventions: early Polish and English syntactic combination'. Paper presented at the Biennial Meeting of the Society for Research on Child Development, Tampa, Florida.

Dąbrowska, E. and Lieven, E. (submitted), 'Developing question constructions: lexical specificity and usage-based operations'.

Dąbrowska, E. and Szczerbiński, M. (submitted), 'Polish children's productivity with case marking: the role of regularity, type frequency, and phonological coherence'.

Dale, P. S. and Crain-Thoreson, C. (1993), 'Pronoun reversals: who, when, and why?', *Journal of Child Language*, 20, 573–89.

Daugherty, K. and Seidenberg, M. (1992), 'Rules or connections? The past tense revisited', *Proceedings of the 14th Annual Meeting of the Cognitive Science Society*, Hillsdale, NJ: Lawrence Erlbaum, pp. 259–64.

Dawkins, R. (1986), *The Blind Watchmaker*, Harlow: Longman.

de León, L. (1991), *Strategies in the Acquisition of Spatial Orientation in Tzotzil* (draft paper). Nijmegen: Cognitive Anthropology Research Group, Max Planck Institute for Psycholinguistics.

de León, L. (1994), 'Exploration in the acquisition of geocentric location by Tzotzil children', *Linguistics*, 32, 857–84.

de Villiers, J. and de Villiers, P. (1973), 'A cross-sectional study of the acquisition of gramamtical morphemes in child speech', *Journal of Psycholinguistic Research*, 2, 331–41.

de Villiers, J. G. and de Villiers, P. A. (1985), 'The acquisition of English', in D. I. Slobin (ed.), *The Crosslinguistic Study of Language Acquisition. Volume 1: The Data*, Hillsdale, NJ: Lawrence Erlbaum, pp. 27–140.

Deacon, T. (1997), *The Sympolic Species: The Co-evolution of Language and the Human Brain*, London: Penguin.

Deacon, T. (2000), 'Evolutionary perspectives on language and brain plasticity', *Journal of Communication Disorders*, 33, 273–91.

Deacon, T., Schumacher, J., Dinsmore, J., Thomas, C., Palmer, P., Kott, S., Edge, A., Penney, D., Kassissieh, S., Dempsey, P. and Isacson, O. (1997), 'Histological evidence of fetal pig neural cell survival after transplantation into a patient with Parkinson's disease', *Nature and Medicine*, 3, 350–3.

Deane, P. (1993), *Grammar in Mind and Brain: Explorations in Cognitive Syntax*, Berlin and New York: Mouton de Gruyter.

Della Corte, M., Benedict, H. and Klein, D. (1983), 'The relationship of pragmatic dimensions of mother's speech to the referential–expressive distinction', *Journal of Child Language*, 10, 35–43.

Démonet, J.-F., Wise, R. and Frackowiak, R. (1993), 'Language functions explored in normal subjects by positron emission tomography: a critical review', *Human Brain Mapping*, 1, 39–47.

Démonet, J.-F., Puel, M., Celsis, P. and Cardebat, D. (1991), ' "Subcortical" aphasia: some proposed pathophysiological mechanisms and their rCBF correlates revealed by SPECT', *Journal of Neurolinguistics*, 6, 319–44.

Démonet, J.-F., Viallard, G., Marc-Vergnes, J. P. and Rascol, A. (1992), 'Cerebral blood flow correlates of word monitoring in sentences: influence of semantic incoherence. A SPECT study in normals', *Neuropsychologia*, 30, 1–11.

Dennis, M. (1980), 'Capacity and strategy for syntactic comprehension after left of right hemidecortification', *Brain and Language*, 10, 287–317.

Dennis, M. and Kohn, B. (1975), 'Comprehension of syntax in infantile hemiplegics after cerebral hemidecortification', *Brain and Language*, 2, 475–86.

Dennis, M. and Whitaker, H. (1976), 'Language acquisition following hemidecortication: linguistic superiority of the left over the right hemisphere', *Brain and Language*, 3, 404–33.

Dick, F., Bates, E., Utman, J. A., Wulfeck, B., Dronkers, N. and Gernsbacher, M. A. (2001), 'Language deficits, localization, and grammar: evidence for a distributive model of language breakdown in aphasics and normals', *Psychological Review*, 108, 759–88.

Dickinson, D. D. (1984), 'First impressions: children's knowledge of words gained from a single exposure', *Applied Psycholinguistics*, 5, 359–73.

Diessel, H. and Tomasello, M. (2000), 'The development of relative clauses in spontaneous child speech', *Cognitive Linguistics*, 11, 131–51.

Diessel, H. and Tomasello, M. (2001), 'The acquisition of finite complement clauses in English: a corpus-based analysis', *Cognitive Linguistics*, 12, 97–141.

Dockrell, J. and Campbell, R. (1986), 'Lexical acquisition strategies in the preschool child', in S. Kuczaj and M. Barrett (eds), *The Development of Word Meaning*, New York: Springer-Verlag, pp. 121–54.

Drews, E. (1999), 'Pitfalls in tracking the psychological reality of lexically based and rule-based inflection', *Behavioral and Brain Sciences*, 22, 1022–3.

Dronkers, N. N., Redfern, B. B. and Knight, R. T. (2000), 'The neural architecture of language disorders', in M. S. Gazzaniga (ed.), *The New Cognitive Neurosciences* (2nd edn), Cambridge, MA: MIT Press, pp. 949–58.

Du Bois, J. (1987), 'The discourse basis of ergativity', *Language*, 63, 805–55.

Dunlea, A. (1989), *Vision and the Emergence of Meaning: Blind and Sighted Children's Early Language*, Cambridge: Cambridge University Press.

Eberhard, K. M., Spivey-Knowleton, M. J., Sedivy, J. C. and Tanenhaus, M. K. (1995), 'Eye-movements as a window into real-time spoken language comprehension in natural contexts', *Journal of Psycholinguistic Research*, 24, 409–34.

Ebersberger, I., Metzier, D., Schwarz, C. and Paabo, S. (2002), 'Genome-wide comparison of DNA sequences between humans and chimpanzees', *American Journal of Human Genetics*, 70, 1490–7.

Eeg-Olofsson, M. and Altenberg, B. (1993), 'Discontinuous recurrent word combinations in the London–Lund corpus', in U. Fries, G. Tottie and P. Schneider (eds), *Creating and Using English Language Corpora. Papers from the Fourteenth International Conference on English Language Research on Computerized Corpora, Zürich*, Amsterdam: Rodopi, pp. 63–77.

Ellis, N. C. (2000), 'Frequency effects in language processing: a review with implications for theories of implicit and explicit language acquisition', *Studies in Second Language Acquisition*, 24, 143–88.

Elman, J. L. (1993), 'Learning and development in neural networks: the importance of starting small', *Cognition*, 48, 71–99.

Elman, J. L. (1990), 'Finding structure in time', *Cognitive Science*, 14, 179–211.

Elman, J. L. (1999), 'The emergence of language: a conspiracy theory', in B. MacWhinney (ed.), *The Emergence of Language*, Mahwah, NJ: Lawrence Erlbaum, pp. 1–27.

Elman, J. L., Bates, E., Johnson, M. H., Karmiloff-Smith, A., Parisi, D. and Plunkett, K. (1996), *Rethinking Innateness: A Connectionist Perspective on Development*, Cambridge, MA: MIT Press.

Elstner, W. (1983), 'Abnormalities in the verbal communication of visually-impaired children', in A. E. Mills (ed.), *Language Acquisition in the Blind Child*, London: Croom Helm, pp. 18–41.

Enard, W., Przeworski, M., Fisher, S. E., Lai, C. S. L., Wiebe, V., Kitano, T., Monaco, A. P. and Paabo, S. (2002), 'Molecular evolution of FOXP2, a gene involved in speech and language', *Nature*, 418, 869–72.

Erman, B. and Warren, B. (2000), 'The idiom principle and the open choice principle', *Text*, 20, 29–62.

Ewers, H. (1999), 'Schemata im mentalen Lexikon: Empirische Untersuchungen zum Erwerb der deutschen Pluralbildung', in J. Meibauer and M. Rothweiler (eds), *Das Lexikon im Spracherwerb*, Tübingen: Francke, pp. 106–27.

Farrar, M. J. (1990), 'Discourse and the acquisition of grammatical morphemes', *Journal of Child Language*, 17, 607–24.

Fenson, L., Dale, P. S., Resnick, J. S., Bates, E., Thal, D. and Pethick, S. (1994), 'Variability in early communicative development', *Monographs of the Society for Research in Child Development*, 59 (Serial No. 242).

Ferreira, F. (2003), 'The misinterpretation of noncanonical sentences', *Cognitive Psychology*, 47, 164–203.

Ferreira, F. and Clifton, C., Jr (1986), 'The independence of syntactic processing', *Journal of Memory and Child Language*, 25, 348–68.

Fiez, J. A., Tallal, P., Raichle, M. E., Miezin, F. M., Katz, W. F. and Petersen, S. E. (1995), 'PET studies of auditory and phonological processing: effects of stimulus characteristics and task demands', *Journal of Cognitive Neuroscience*, 7, 357–75.

Fillenbaum, S. (1974), 'Pragmatic normalization: further results for some conjunctive and disjunctive sentences', *Journal of Experimental Psychology*, 102, 574–8.

Fillmore, C. (1978), 'On the organization of semantic information in the lexicon', *Papers from the Parasession on the Lexicon, Chicago Linguistic Society*, 1–11.

Fillmore, C., Kay, P., Michaelis, L. A. and Sag, I. A. (2003), *Construction Grammar*, Stanford, CA: CSLI Publications.

Fillmore, C. J. (1975), 'An alternative to checklist theories of meaning', *Proceedings of the First Annual Meeting of the Berkeley Linguistic Society*, 123–31.

Fillmore, C. J. and Kay, P. (1993), 'Construction grammar'. Unpublished manuscript.

Fisher, S. E., Lai, C. S. L. and Monaco, A. P. (2003), 'Deciphering the genetic basis of speech and language disorders', *Annual Review of Neuroscience*, 26, 57–80.

Fletcher, S., Rowland, C. and Jackson, K. (2003), 'Why modelling does matter: the use of elicitation to study wh-question production in children'. Paper presented at the Child Language Seminar, Newcastle, 9–11 July.

Fodor, J. A. (1970), 'Three reasons for not deriving "kill" from "cause to die"', *Linguistic Inquiry*, 1, 429–38.

Fodor, J. A. (1983), *The Modularity of Mind*, Cambridge, MA: MIT Press.

Fodor, J. D., Fodor, J. A. and Garrett, M. (1975), 'The unreality of semantic representations', *Linguistic Inquiry*, 4, 515–31.

Fodor, J. A., Garrett, M., Walker, E. and Parkes, C. (1980), 'Against definitions', *Cognition*, 8, 263–367.

Foley, W. A. and Van Valin, R. D. (1984), *Functional Syntax and Universal Grammar*, Cambridge: Cambridge University Press.

Foolen, A. and van der Leek, F. (2000), *Constructions in Cognitive Linguistics: Selected Papers from the Fifth International Cognitive Linguistics Conference, Amsterdam 1997*, Amsterdam: John Benjamins.

Fox, P. T., Petersen, S., Posner, M. and Raichle, M. E. (1988), 'Is Broca's area language specific?', *Neurology*, 38 (suppl.), 172.

Fraiberg, S. (1977), 'The acquisition of language', in S. Fraiberg (ed.), *Insights from the Blind*, London: Condor Book Souvenir Press, pp. 221–47.

Frazier, L. (1987), 'Sentence processing: a tutorial review', in M. Coltheart (ed.), *Attention and Performance XII: The Psychology of Reading*, Hove: Lawrence Erlbaum, pp. 559–86.

Friederici, A. D. (1995), 'The time course of syntactic activation during language processing: a model based on neuropsychological and neurophysiological data', *Brain and Language*, 50, 259–81.

Gardner, H. (1974), *The Shattered Mind*, New York: Vintage.

Garnsey, S. M., Pearlmutter, N. J., Myers, E. and Lotocky, M. A. (1997), 'The contribution of verb bias and plausibility to the comprehension of temporarily amgiguous sentences', *Journal of Memory and Language*, 37, 58–93.

Gasser, M. and Smith, L. B. (1998), 'Learning nouns and adjectives: a connectionist account', *Language and Cognitive Processes*, 13, 269–306.

Gathercole, S. E. and Baddeley, A. D. (1990), 'Phonological memory deficits in language disordered children: is there a causal relationship?', *Journal of Memory and Language*, 29, 336–60.

Gawlitzek-Maiwald, I. (1994), 'How do children cope with variation in the input? The case of German plurals and compounding', in R. Tracy and E. Lattey (eds), *How Tolerant is Universal Grammar? Essays on Language Variability and Language Variation*, Tübingen: Niemeyer, pp. 225–66.

Geeraerts, D. (1988), 'Where does prototypicality come from?', in B. Rudzka-Ostyn (ed.), *Topics in Cognitive Linguistics*, Amsterdam: John Benjamins, pp. 207–29.

Gibbs, R. W. (1980), 'Spilling the beans on understanding and memory for idioms in conversation', *Memory and Cognition*, 8, 149–56.

Gibbs, R. W. and Colston, H. L. (1995), 'The cognitive psychological reality of image schemas and their transformations', *Cognitive Linguistics*, 6, 347–78.

Gibbs, R. W., Jr and Gonzales, G. P. (1985), 'Syntactic frozenness in processing and remembering idioms', *Cognition*, 20, 243–59.

Givón, T. (1989), *Mind, Code and Context: Essays in Pragmatics*, Hillsdale, NJ: Lawrence Erlbaum.

Gleitman, L. R. (1981), 'Maturational determinants of language growth', *Cognition*, 10, 103–14.

Gleitman, L. R. (1990), 'The structural sources of verb meanings', *Language Acquisition*, 1, 3–55.

Gleitman, L. R. and Gillette, J. (1995), 'The role of syntax in verb learning', in P. Fletcher and B. MacWhinney (eds), *The Handbook of Child Language*, Oxford: Blackwell, pp. 413–27.

Goldberg, A. E. (1995), *Constructions: A Construction Grammar Approach to Argument Structure*, Chicago: University of Chicago Press.

Goldfield, B. A. and Reznick, J. S. (1990), 'Early lexical acquisition: rate, content and vocabulary spurt', *Journal of Child Language*, 17, 171–84.

Goldman-Eisler, F. (1968), *Psycholinguistics: Experiments in Spontaneous Speech*, London: Academic Press.

Goodall, J. (1986), *The Chimpanzees of Gombe: Patterns of Behavior*, Cambridge, MA: Harvard University Press.

Goodglass, H. (2001), *The Assessment of Aphasia and Related Disorders*, Philadelphia: Lippincott, Williams and Williams.

Goodglass, H. and Kaplan, E. (1972), *The Assessment of Aphasia and Related Disorders*, Philadelphia: Lea and Febiger.

Gordon, P. and Chafetz, J. (1990), 'Verb-based versus class-based accounts of action-ality effects in children's comprehension of passives', *Cognition*, 36, 227–54.

Graham, M. D. (1968), *Multiply Impaired Blind Children: A National Problem*, New York: American Foundation for the Blind.

Grant, J., Valian, V. and Karmiloff-Smith, A. (2002), 'A study of relative clauses in Williams syndrome', *Journal of Child Language*, 29, 403–16.

Grodzinsky, Y. and Finkel, L. (1998), 'The neurology of empty categories', *Journal of Cognitive Neuroscience*, 10, 281–92.

Grosjean, F. (1980), 'Spoken word recognition and the gating paradigm', *Perception and Psychophysics*, 28, 299–310.

Grossman, M. (1980), 'A central processor for hierarchically structured material: evidence from Broca's aphasia', *Neuropsychologia*, 18, 299–309.

Gullo, D. F. (1981), 'Social class differences in preschool children's comprehension of wh-questions', *Child Development*, 52, 736–40.

Haiman, J. (1985), *Iconicity in Syntax*, Cambridge: Cambridge University Press.

Hall, W. S., Nagy, W. E. and Linn, R. (1984), *Spoken Words: Effects of Situation and Social Group on Oral Word Usage and Frequency*, Hillsdale, NJ: Lawrence Erlbaum.

Hampson, J. and Nelson, K. (1993), 'The relation of maternal language to variation in rate and style of language acquisition', *Journal of Child Language*, 20, 313–42.

Hamsher, K. (1998), 'Intelligence and aphasia', in M. T. Sarno (edn), *Acquired Aphasia* (3rd edn), San Diego: Academic Press, pp. 341–73.

Hare, M. and Elman, J. L. (1995), 'Learning and morphological change', *Cognition*, 56, 61–98.

Hare, M., Elman, J. L. and Daugherty, K. G. (1995), 'Default generalization in con-nectionist networks', *Language and Cognitive Processes*, 10, 601–30.

Hart, B. and Risley, R. R. (1995), *Meaningful Differences in the Everyday Experience of Young American Children*, Baltimore: Paul Brooks.

Hart, B. and Risley, R. R. (1999), *The Social World of Children Learning to Talk*, Baltimore: Paul Brookes.

Hauser, M. D., Chomsky, N. and Fitch, W. T. (2002), 'The faculty of language: what is it, who has it, and how did it evolve', *Science*, 298, 1569–79.

Hawkins, J. A. (1994), *A Performance Theory of Order and Constituency*, Cambridge: Cambridge University Press.

Heibeck, T. H. and Markman, E. M. (1987), 'Word learning in children: an examination of fast mapping', *Child Development*, 58, 1021–34.

Heine, B. (1997), *Cognitive Foundations of Grammar*, New York and Oxford: Oxford University Press.

Herskovits, A. (1985), 'Semantics and pragmatics of locative expressions', *Cognitive Science,* 9, 341–78.

Herskovits, A. (1986), *Language and Spatial Cognition,* Cambridge: Cambridge University Press.

Hickey, T. (1993), 'Identifying formulas in first language acquisition', *Journal of Child Language,* 20, 27–41.

Hill, E. L. (2001), 'Non-specific nature of specific language impairment: a review of the literature with regard to concomitant motor impairments', *International Journal of Language & Communication Disorders,* 36, 149–71.

Hirsh-Pasek, K. and Golinkoff, R. M. (1996), *The Origins of Grammar: Evidence from Early Language Comprehension,* Cambridge, MA: MIT Press.

Hjelmslev, L. (1935), *La catégorie des cas,* Copenhagen: Munksgaard.

'How many genes are in the human genome?' (2003). Retrieved 20 September 2003 from Human Genome Project Information website, http://www.ornl.gov/TechResources/Human_Genome/faq/genenumber.html.

Hu, Y.-H., Qiou, Y.-G. and Zhong, G.-Q. (1990), 'Crossed aphasia in Chinese: a clinical survey', *Brain and Language,* 39, 347–56.

Huggins, A. W. F. (1964), 'Distortion of the temporal pattern of speech: interruption and alternation', *Journal of the Acoustical Society of America,* 36, 1055–64.

Huttenlocher, J. (1998), 'Language input and language growth', *Preventive Medicine,* 27, 195–9.

Huttenlocher, J., Smiley, P. and Ratner, H. (1983), 'What do word meanings reveal about conceptual development?', in T. B. Seiler and W. Wannenmacher (eds), *Concept Development and the Development of Word Meaning,* Berlin: Springer Verlag, pp. 210–33.

Huttenlocher, J., Vasilyeva, M., Cymerman, E. and Levine, S. (2002), 'Language input and child syntax', *Cognitive Psychology,* 45, 337–74.

Huttenlocher, J., Haight, W., Bryk, A., Seltzer, M. and Lyons, T. (1991), 'Early vocabulary growth: relation to language input and gender', *Developmental Psychology,* 27, 236–48.

Indefrey, P. (1999), 'Some problems with the lexical status of nondefault inflection', *Behavioral and Brain Sciences,* 22, 1025.

Ingram, D. and Tyack, D. (1979), 'The inversion of subject NP and Aux in children's questions', *Journal of Psycholinguistic Research,* 4, 333–41.

Iwamura, S. G. (1979), '"I don' wanna don't throw": speech formulas in first language acquisition'. Unpublished manuscript, University of Hawaii.

Jackendoff, R. (1983), *Semantics and Cognition,* Cambridge, MA: MIT Press.

Jackendoff, R. (1990), *Semantic Structure,* Cambridge, MA: MIT Press.

Jackendoff, R. (2002), *Foundations of Language: Brain, Meaning, Grammar, Evolution,* Oxford: Oxford University Press.

Jaeger, J. J., Lockwood, A. H., Kemmerer, D. L., Van Valin, R. D. and Murphy, B. W. (1996), 'Positron emission tomographic study of regular and irregular verb morphology in English', *Language,* 72, 451–97.

Jäkel, O. (1995), 'The metaphorical concept of mind: "mental activity is manipulation"', in J. R. Taylor and R. E. MacLaury (eds), *Language and the Cognitive Construal of the World,* Berlin: Mouton de Gruyter, pp. 197–229.

Janda, L. A. (1996), 'Figure, ground and animacy in Slavic declension', *Slavic and East European Journal,* 40, 325–55.

Johnson, M. (1987), *The Body in the Mind: The Bodily Basis of Reason and Imagination*, Chicago: University of Chicago Press.

Johnson, M. H. (1993), 'Constraints on cortical plasticity', in M. H. Johnson (ed.), *Brain Development and Cognition: A Reader*, Cambridge: Blackwell, pp. 703–22.

Johnson, M. H. (1998), 'The neural basis of cognitive development', in D. Kuhn and R. S. Siegler (eds), *Handbook of Child Psychology. Vol. 2: Cognition, Perception and Language*, New York: John Wiley and Sons, pp. 1–50.

Johnston, J. R. (1997), 'Specific language impairment, cognition and the biological basis of language', in M. Gopnik (ed.), *The Inheritance and Innateness of Grammars*, New York: Oxford University Press, pp. 161–80.

Johnston, J. R. and Slobin, D. I. (1979), 'The development of locative expressions in English, Italian, Serbo-Croatian and Turkish', *Journal of Child Language*, 6, 529–45.

Jones, D., von Stienbrugge, W. and Chicralis, K. (1994), 'Underlying deficits in language-disordered children with central auditory processing difficulties', *Applied Psycholinguistics*, 15, 311–28.

Jones, M. J. (1996), 'A longitudinal and methodological investigation of auxiliary verb development'. Unpublished thesis, University of Manchester.

Jones, S. S. and Smith, L. B. (1993), 'The place of perception in children's concepts', *Cognitive Development*, 8, 113–39.

Jou, J. and Harris, R. J. (1991), 'Processing inflections: dynamic processes in sentence comprehension', *Journal of Experimental Psychology: Learning Memory and Cognition*, 17, 1082–94.

Kaplan, J. (1998), Message posted to Funknet, *Funknet Archive, 13 October 1998*. Retrieved 8 December 2003 from https://mailman.rice.edu/pipermail/funknet/1998-October.txt.

Karmiloff-Smith, A. (1998), 'Is atypical development necessarily a window on the normal mind/brain? The case of Williams syndrome', *Developmental Science*, 1, 273–7.

Karmiloff-Smith, A., Grant, J., Bethoud, I., Davies, M., Howlin, P. and Udwin, O. (1997), 'Language and Williams syndrome: how intact is "intact"?', *Child Development*, 68, 246–62.

Karmiloff-Smith, A., Tyler, L. K., Voice, K., Sims, K., Udwin, O., Howlins, P. and Davies, M. (1998), 'Linguistic dissociations in Williams syndrome: evaluating receptive syntax in on-line and off-line tasks', *Neuropsychologia*, 36, 343–51.

Katz, J. (1972), *Semantic Theory*, New York: Harper and Row.

Katz, J. (1987), 'Common sense in semantics', in E. Lepore (ed.), *New Directions in Semantics*, London: Academic Press, pp. 157–234.

Katz, J. J. and Fodor, J. A. (1963), 'The structure of semantic theory', *Language*, 39, 170–210.

Kegl, J., Senghas, A. and Coppola, M. (1999), 'Creation through contact: sign language emergence and sign language change in Nicaragua', in M. DeGraf (ed.), *Language Creation and Language Change: Creolization, Diachrony and Development*, Cambridge, MA: MIT Press, pp. 179–238.

Keil, K. and Kaszniak, A. W. (2002), 'Examining executive function in individuals with brain injury: a review', *Aphasiology*, 16, 305–35.

Kertesz, A. and Osmán-Sági, J. (2001), 'Manifestations of aphasic symptoms in Hungarian', *Journal of Neurolinguistics*, 14, 313–19.

Kidd, E., Bavin, E. L. and Rhodes, B. (2001), 'Two-year-olds' knowledge of verbs and argument structure', in M. Almgren, A. Barreña, M.-J. Ezeizabarrena, I. Idiazabal and B. MacWhinney (eds), *Research on Child Language Acquisition. Proceedings of the 8th Conference of the International Association for the Study of Child Language*, Somerville: Cascadilla Press, pp. 1368–82.

Kim, J. J., Pinker, S., Prince, A. S. and Prasada, S. (1991), 'Why no mere mortal has ever flown out to center field', *Cognitive Science*, 15, 173–218.

Kim, J. J., Marcus, G. F., Pinker, S., Hollander, M. and Coppola, M. (1994), 'Sensitivity of children's inflections to grammatical structure', *Journal of Child Language*, 21, 173–209.

Kimura, D. (1993), *Neuromotor Mechanisms in Human Communication*, Oxford: Oxford University Press.

Kiparsky, P. (1985), 'Some consequences of lexical phonology', *Phonology Yearbook*, 2, 85–138.

Kirby, S. (1998), 'Fitness and the selective adaptation of language', in J. R. Hurford, M. Studdert-Kennedy and C. Knight (eds), *Approaches to the Evolution of Language: Social and Cognitive Bases*, Cambridge: Cambridge University Press, pp. 359–83.

Klima, E. S. and Bellugi, U. (1966), 'Syntactic regularities in the speech of children', in J. Lyons and R. J. Wales (eds), *Psycholinguistics Papers. Proceedings of the 1966 Edinburgh Conference*, Edinburgh: Edinburgh University Press, pp. 183–208.

Kluender, K., Diehl, R. and Killeen, P. (1987), 'Japanese quail can learn phonetic categories', *Science*, 237, 1195–7.

Kluender, R. (1998), 'On the distinction between strong and weak islands: a processing perspective', in P. W. Culicover and L. McNally (eds), *Syntax and Semantics 29: The Limits of Syntax*, San Diego: Academic Press, pp. 241–79.

Kluender, R. and Kutas, M. (1993), 'Subjacency as a processing phenomenon', *Language and Cognitive Processes*, 8, 573–633.

Köpcke, K.-M. (1988), 'Schemas in German plural formation', *Lingua*, 74, 303–35.

Köpcke, K.-M. (1998), 'The acquisition of plural marking in English and German revisited: schemata versus rules', *Journal of Child Language*, 25, 293–319.

Kottum, S. E. (1981), 'The genitive singular form of masculine nouns in Polish', *Scando-Slavica*, 27, 179–86.

Kövecses, Z. (1986), *Metaphors of Anger, Pride and Love*, Amsterdam: Benjamins.

Krashen, S. D. and Scarcella, R. (1978), 'On routines and patterns in language acquisition and performance', *Language Learning*, 28, 283–300.

Kuczaj, S. and Brannick, N. (1979), 'Children's use of the wh-question modal auxiliary placement rule', *Journal of Experimental Child Psychology*, 28, 43–67.

Kuczaj, S. A. (1976), '-*ing*, -*s* and -*ed*: a study of the acquisition of certain verb inflections'. Unpublished PhD dissertation, University of Minnesota.

Kuczaj, S. A. and Maratsos, M. P. (1983), 'Initial verbs in yes-no questions: a different kind of general grammatical category?', *Developmental Psychology*, 19, 440–4.

Kuhl, P. K. (1981), 'Discrimination of speech by nonhuman animals: basic auditory sensitivities conducive to the perception of speech-sound categories', *Journal of the Acoustical Society of America*, 70, 340–9.

Kuiper, K. (1996), *Smooth Talkers: The Linguistic Performance of Auctioneers and Sportscasters*, Mahwah, NJ: Lawrence Erlbaum.

Kurcz, I., Lewicki, A., Sambor, J., Szafran, K. and Woronczak, J. (1990), *Słownik frekwencyjny polszczyzny współczesnej*, Kraków: Polska Akademia Nauk.

Kutas, M. and King, J. W. (1995), 'The potentials for basic sentence processing: differentiating integrative processes', in T. Inui and J. L. McClelland (eds), *Attention and Performance XVI: Information Integration in Perception and Communication*, Cambridge, MA: MIT Press, pp. 501–46.

Labov, W. and Labov, T. (1978), 'Learning the syntax of questions', in R. N. Campbell and P. T. Smith (eds), *Recent Advances in the Psychology of Langauge* (Vol. 4B), New York: Plenum Press, pp. 1–44.

Lachter, J. and Bever, T. (1988), 'The relation between linguistic structure and associative theories of language learning: a constructive critique of some connectionist learning models', *Cognition*, 28, 195–247.

Lai, C. S. L., Fisher, S. E., Hurst, J. A., Vargha-Khadem, F. and Monaco, A. P. (2001), 'A forkhead-domain gene is mutated in a severe speech and language disorder', *Nature*, 413, 519–23.

Lakoff, G. (1987), *Women, Fire and Dangerous Things: What Categories Reveal about the Mind*, Chicago: Chicago University Press.

Lakoff, G. and Johnson, M. (1980), *Metaphors We Live By*, Chicago: Chicago University Press.

Landau, B. and Gleitman, L. R. (1985), *Language and Experience: Evidence from the Blind Child*, Cambridge, MA: Harvard University Press.

Langacker, R. W. (1987), *Foundations of Cognitive Grammar. Vol. 1: Theoretical Prerequisites*, Stanford, CA: Stanford University Press.

Langacker, R. W. (1991a), *Foundations of Cognitive Grammar. Vol. 2: Descriptive Application*, Stanford, CA: Stanford University Press.

Langacker, R. W. (1991b), *Concept, Image and Symbol: The Cognitive Basis of Grammar*, Berlin: Mouton de Gruyter.

Langacker, R. W. (1995), 'Raising and transparency', *Language*, 71, 1–62.

Langacker, R. W. (2000), 'A dynamic usage-based model', in M. Barlow and S. Kemmer (eds), *Usage-Based Models of Language*, Stanford, CA: CSLI Publications, pp. 1–63.

Lebrun, Y. and Hoops, R. (1974), *Intelligence and Aphasia*, Amsterdam: Swets and Zeitlinger B.V.

Levine, S. C. and Carey, S. (1982), 'Up front: the acquisition of a concept and a word', *Journal of Child Language*, 9, 645–57.

Levinson, S. C. (1994), 'Vision, shape and linguistic description: Tzeltal body-part terminology and object description', *Linguistics*, 94, 791–855.

Lieberman, P. (1991), *Uniquely Human: The Evolution of Speech, Thought, and Selfless Behavior*, Cambridge, MA: Harvard University Press.

Lieberman, P. (1998), *Eve Spoke: Human Language and Human Evolution*, London: Picador.

Lieberman, P. (2002), 'On the nature and evolution of the neural bases of human language', *Yearbook of Physical Anthropology*, 45, 36–62.

Lieberman, P., Friedman, J. and Feldman, L. S. (1990), 'Syntax comprehension deficits in Parkinson's disease', *Journal of Nervous and Mental Disease*, 178, 360–5.

Lieberman, P., Kako, E. T., Friedman, J., Tajchman, G., Feldman, L. S. and Jiminez, E. B. (1992), 'Speech production, syntax comprehension, and cognitive deficits in Parkinson's disease', *Brain and Language*, 43, 169–89.

Lieven, E. V. (1994), 'Crosslinguistic and crosscultural aspects of language addressed to children', in C. Gallaway and B. J. Richards (eds), *Input and Interaction in Language Acquisition*, Cambridge: Cambridge University Press, pp. 56–73.

Lieven, E. V. (1997), 'Variation in a crosslinguistic context', in D. I. Slobin (ed.), *The Crosslinguistic Study of Language Acquisition. Vol. 5: Expanding the Contexts*, Mahwah, NJ: Lawrence Erlbaum, pp. 199–263.

Lieven, E. V. (2003), 'Memory, productivity and constructions in early English multi-word utterances'. Paper presented at the Biennial Meeting of the Society for Research on Child Development, Tampa, Florida.

Lieven, E. V., Pine, J. M. and Baldwin, G. (1997), 'Lexically-based learning and early grammatical development', *Journal of Child Language*, 24, 187–219.

Lieven, E. V., Pine, J. M. and Barnes, H. D. (1992), 'Individual differences in early vocabulary development: redefining the referential–expressive distinction', *Journal of Child Language*, 19, 287–310.

Lightfoot, D. (1989), 'The child's trigger experience: degree-0 learnability', *Behavioral and Brain Sciences*, 12, 321–75.

Linebarger, M. C. (1989), 'Neuropsychological evidence for linguistic modularity', in G. N. Carlson and M. K. Tanenhaus (eds), *Linguistic Structure in Language Processing*, Dordrecht: Kluwer Academic, pp. 197–238.

Linebarger, M. C. (1990), 'Neuropsychology of sentence parsing', in A. Caramazza (ed.), *Cognitive Neuropsychology and Neurolinguistics*, Hillsdale, NJ: Lawrence Erlbaum, pp. 55–122.

Linebarger, M. C., Schwartz, M. F. and Saffran, E. M. (1983), 'Sensitivity to grammatical structure in so-called agrammatic aphasics', *Cognition*, 13, 361–92.

Lock, A. and Colombo, M. (1996), 'Cognitive abilities in a comparative perspective', in A. Lock and C. R. Peters (eds), *Handbook of Human Symbolic Evolution*, Oxford: Clarendon Press, pp. 596–643.

Lock, A. and Peters, C. R. (1996), 'Editorial appendix II: evolution of the human vocal apparatus', in A. Lock and C. R. Peters (eds), *Handbook of Human Symbolic Evolution*, Oxford: Clarendon Press, pp. 116–25.

Locke, A. and Ginsborg, J. (submitted), 'Spoken language in the early years: the cognitive and linguistic developemnt of three- to five-year-old children from socio-economically deprived backgrounds'.

Locke, A., Ginsborg, J. and Peers, I. (2002), 'Development and disadvantage: implications for the early years and beyond', *International Journal of Language and Communication Disorders*, 37, 3–15.

Logan, G. D. (1988), 'Toward an instance theory of automatization', *Psychological Review*, 95, 492–527.

MacDonald, M. C. (1994), 'Probabilistic constraints and syntactic ambiguity resolution', *Language and Cognitive Processes*, 9, 157–201.

MacDonald, M. C. (1999), 'Distributional information in language comprehension, production and acquisition: three puzzles and a moral', in B. MacWhinney (ed.), *The Emergence of Language*, Mahwah, NJ: Lawrence Erlbaum, pp. 177–96.

Maclay, H. and Osgood, C. E. (1959), 'Hesitation phenomena in spontaneous English speech', *Word*, 15, 19–44.

MacWhinney, B. (1985), 'Hungarian language acquisition as an exemplification of a general model of grammatical development', in D. I. Slobin (ed.), *The Crosslinguistic Study of Language Acquisition. Vol. 2: Theoretical Issues*, Hillsdale, NJ: Lawrence Erlbaum, pp. 1069–155.

MacWhinney, B. (1995), *The CHILDES Project: Tools for Analyzing Talk*, Hillsdale, NJ: Lawrence Erlbaum.

MacWhinney, B. and Leinbach, J. (1991), 'Implementations are not conceptualizations: revising the verb learning model', *Cognition*, 29, 121–57.

MacWhinney, B., Osmán-Sági, J. and Slobin, D. I. (1991), 'Sentence comprehension in aphasia in two clear case-marking languages', *Brain and Language*, 41, 234–49.

Major, D. (1974), *The Acquisition of Modal Auxiliaries in the Language of Children*, The Hague: Mouton.

Mandler, J. M. (1992), 'How to build a baby II: Conceptual primitives', *Psychological Review*, 99, 587–604.

Maratsos, M. (2000), 'More overregularizations after all: new data and discussion on Marcus, Pinker, Ullmann, Hollander, Rosen & Xu', *Journal of Child Language*, 27, 183–212.

Marchman, V. A. (1993), 'Constraints on plasticity in a connectionist model of the English past tense', *Journal of Cognitive Neuroscience*, 5, 215–34.

Marcus, G. F. (1998), 'Can connectionism save constructivism?', *Cognition*, 66, 153–82.

Marcus, G. F. and Fisher, S. E. (2003), 'FOXP2 in focus: what can genes tell us about speech and language?', *Trends in Cognitive Science*, 7, 257–62.

Marcus, G. F., Brinkmann, U., Clahsen, H., Wiese, R. and Pinker, S. (1995), 'German inflection: the exception that proves the rule', *Cognitive Psychology*, 29, 189–256.

Marcus, G. F., Pinker, S., Ullman, M., Hollander, M., Rosen, T. J. and Xu, F. (1992), 'Overregularization in language acquisition', *Monographs of the Society for Research in Child Development*, 57 (Serial No. 22), 1–180.

Markman, E. M. (1987), 'How children constrain the possible meanings of words', in U. Neisser (ed.), *Concepts and Conceptual Development: Ecological and Intellectual Factors in Categorization*, Cambridge: Cambridge University Press, pp. 255–87.

Markman, E. M. (1990), 'Constraints children place on word meanings', *Cognitive Science*, 14, 57–77.

Markson, L. and Bloom, P. (1997), 'Evidence against a dedicated system for word learning in children', *Nature*, 385, 813–15.

Marshall, J. C. (1986), 'The description and interpretation of aphasic language disorder', *Neuropsychologia*, 24, 5–24.

Marslen-Wilson, W. and Tyler, L. K. (1987), 'Against modularity', in J. L. Garfield (ed.), *Modularity in Knowledge Representation and Natural-Language Processing*, Cambridge, MA: MIT Press, pp. 37–62.

Marslen-Wilson, W. D. (1973), 'Linguistic structure and speech shadowing at very short latencies', *Nature*, 244, 522–3.

Marslen-Wilson, W. D. (1987), 'Functional parallelism in spoken word-recognition', *Cognition*, 25, 71–102.

Marslen-Wilson, W. D. and Tyler, L. K. (1997), 'Dissociating types of mental computation', *Nature*, 387, 592–4.

Marslen-Wilson, W. D. and Tyler, L. K. (1998), 'Rules, representations, and the English past tense', *Trends in Cognitive Science*, 2, 428–35.

Martin, W. K., Church, K. and Patil, R. (1987), 'Preliminary analysis of a breadth-first parsing algorithm: theoretical and experimental results', in L. Bolc (ed.), *Natural Language Parsing Systems*, Berlin: Springer Verlag, pp. 267–328.

Martins, I. P. and Ferro, J. M. (1992), 'Recovery of acquired aphasia in children', *Aphasiology*, 6, 431–8.

Martins, I. P. and Ferro, J. M. (1993), 'Acquired childhood aphasia: a clinicoradiological study of 11 stroke patients', *Aphasiology*, 7, 489–95.

Massaro, D. W. (1994), 'Psychological aspects of speech perception: implications for research and theory', in M. A. Gernsbacher (ed.), *Handbook of Psycholinguistics*, San Diego: Academic Press, pp. 219–63.

Matsuki, K. (1995), 'Metaphors of anger in Japanese', in J. R. Taylor and R. E. MacLaury (eds), *Language and the Cognitive Construal of the World*, Berlin: Mouton de Gruyter, pp. 137–51.

Mattys, S. L., Jusczyk, P. W., Luce, P. A. and Morgan, J. L. (1999), 'Phonotactic and prosodic effects on word segmentation in infants', *Cognitive Psychology*, 38, 465–94.

Mazziotta, J. C. and Metter, J. E. (1988), 'Brain cerebral metabolic mapping of normal and abnormal language and its acquisition during development', in F. Plum (ed.), *Language, Communication and the Brain*, New York: Raven, pp. 245–66.

Mazziota, J. C., Phelps, M. E., Carson, R. E. and Kuhl, D. E. (1982), 'Tomographic mapping of human cerebral metabolism: auditory stimulation', *Neurology*, 32, 921–37.

Meltzoff, A. (1995), 'Understanding the intentions of others: re-enactment of intended acts by 18-month-old children', *Developmental Psychology*, 24, 470–6.

Menn, L. and Obler, L. K. (eds) (1990), *Agrammatic Aphasia: A Cross-Language Narrative Sourcebook*, Amsterdam: Benjamins.

Merzenich, M. M., Jenkins, W. M., Johnston, P., Schreiner, C., Miller, S. L. and Tallal, P. (1996), 'Temporal processing deficits in language-learning impaired children ameliorated by training', *Science*, 271, 77–81.

Miller, G. A. (1986), 'Dictionaries in the mind', *Language and Cognitive Processes*, 1, 171–85.

Miller, G. A. and Gildea, P. M. (1987), 'How children learn words', *Scientific American*, 257, 86–9.

Miller, G. A. and Johnson-Laird, P. N. (1976), *Language and Perception*, Cambridge: Cambridge University Press.

Miller, J. E. (1972), 'Towards a generative semantic account of aspect in Russian', *Journal of Linguistics*, 8, 217–36.

Miller, J. E. (1974), 'A localist account of the dative case in Russian', in R. D. Brecht and C. V. Chvany (eds), *Slavic Transformational Syntax*, Ann Arbor: University of Michigan, pp. 244–61.

Miller, J. L. and Jusczyk, P. W. (1989), 'Seeking the neurobiological bases of speech perception', *Cognition*, 33, 111–37.

Mills, A. (1985), 'The acquisition of German', in D. I. Slobin (ed.), *The Cross-Linguistic Study of Language Acquisition. Vol. 1: The Data*, Hillsdale, NJ: Lawrence Erlbaum, pp. 141–254.

Mitchell, D. C. (1994), 'Sentence parsing', in M. A. Gernsbacher (ed.), *Handbook of Psycholinguistics*, New York: Academic Press, pp. 357–409.

Miyake, A., Carpenter, P. A. and Just, M. A. (1994), 'A capacity approach to syntactic comprehension disorders: making normal adults perform like aphasic patients', *Cognitive Neuropsychology*, 11, 671–717.

Mogford, K. (1993), 'Language development in twins', in K. Mogford and D. Bishop (eds), *Language Development in Exceptional Circumstances*, Hove: Lawrence Erlbaum, pp. 80–95.

Montgomery, J. (1995), 'Examination of phonological working memory in specifically language-impaired children', *Applied Psycholinguistics*, 16, 355–78.

Moon, R. (1998), 'Frequencies and forms of phrasal lexemes in English', in A. P. Cowie (ed.), *Phraseology: Theory, Analysis and Applications*, Oxford: Clarendon Press, pp. 79–100.

Mueller, R. A. G. and Gibbs, R. W. (1987), 'Processing idioms with multiple meanings', *Journal of Psycholinguistic Research*, 16, 63–81.

Mühlhäusler, P. (1986), *Pidgin and Creole Linguistics*, Oxford: Blackwell.

Mulford, R. (1988), 'First words of the blind', in M. D. Smith and J. L. Locke (eds), *The Emergent Lexicon: The Child's Development of a Linguistic Vocabulary*, New York: Academic Press, pp. 293–338.

Müller, R.-A. (1992), 'Modularism, holism, connectionism: old conflicts and new perspectives in aphasiology and neuropsychology', *Aphasiology*, 6, 443–75.

Müller, R.-A. (1996), 'Innateness, autonomy, universality? Neurobiological approaches to langauge', *Behavioral and Brain Sciences*, 19, 611–75.

Murray, A. D., Johnson, J. and Peters, J. (1990), 'Fine-tuning of utterance length to preverbal infants: effects on later language development', *Journal of Child Language*, 17, 511–25.

Nagell, K., Olguin, K. and Tomasello, M. (1993), 'Processes of social learning in the tool use of chimpanzees (*Pan troglodytes*) and human children (*Homo sapiens*)', *Journal of Comparative Psychology*, 107, 174–86.

Nagórko, A. (1998), *Zarys gramatyki polskiej (ze słowotwórstwem)*, Warsaw: PWN.

Naigles, L. R. (1990), 'Children use syntax to learn verb meaning', *Journal of Child Language*, 17, 357–74.

Nelson, K. (1973), 'Structure and strategy in learning to talk', *Monographs of the Society for Research in Child Development*, 38 (Serial No. 149), 1–135.

Nelson, K. (1981), 'Individual differences in language development: implications for development and language', *Developmental Psychology*, 17, 170–87.

Neville, H. J. and Bavelier, D. (2000), 'Specificity and plasticity in neurocognitive development in humans', in M. S. Gazzaniga (ed.), *The New Cognitive Neurosciences*, Cambridge, MA: MIT Press, pp. 83–98.

Neville, H. J., Mills, D. L. and Bellugi, U. (1993), 'Effects of altered auditory sensitivity and age of language acquisition on the development of language-relevant neural systems: preliminary studies of Williams syndrome', in S. Broman and J. Grafman (eds), *Cognitive Deficits in Developmental Disorders: Implications for Brain Function*, Hillsdale, NJ: Lawrence Erlbaum, pp. 67–83.

New, H. (1972), 'Ranking of constraints on /t, d/ deletion in American English: a statistical analysis', in W. Labov (ed.), *Locating Language in Time and Space*, New York: Academic Press, pp. 37–54.

Ni, W., Crain, S. and Shankweiler, D. (1996), 'Sidestepping garden paths: assessing the contributions of syntax, semantics, and plausibility in resolving ambiguities', *Language and Cognitive Processes*, 11, 283–334.

Obler, L. K. and Gjerlow, K. (1999), *Language and the Brain*, Cambridge: Cambridge University Press.

Ogden, J. A. (1988), 'Language and memory functions after long recovery periods in left hemispherectomised subjects', *Neuropsychologia*, 26, 645–59.

Osterhout, L. and Nicol, J. (1999), 'On the distinctiveness, independence and time course of the brain responses to syntactic and semantic anomalies', *Language and Cognitive Processes*, 14, 283–317.

Paivio, A. (1986), *Mental Representations: A Dual Coding Approach*, New York: Oxford University Press.

Paradis, M. (1977), 'Bilingualism and aphasia', in H. Whitaker (ed.), *Studies in Neurolinguistics* (Vol. 3), New York: Academic Press, pp. 65–121.

Paradis, M. (1998), 'Acquired aphasia in bilingual speakers', in M. T. Sarno (ed.), *Acquired Aphasia* (3rd edn), San Diego: Academic Press, pp. 531–49.

Paradis, M., Goldblum, M. C. and Abidi, R. (1982), 'Alternate antagonism with paradoxical translation in two bilingual aphasic patients', *Brain and Language*, 15, 55–69.

Park, T. Z. (1978), 'Plurals in child speech', *Journal of Child Language*, 5, 237–50.

Paterson, S. J., Brown, J. H., Gsödl, M. H., Johnson, M. H. and Karmiloff-Smith, A. (1999), 'Cognitive modularity and genetic disorders', *Science*, 286, 2355–8.

Pawley, A. and Syder, F. H. (1983), 'Two puzzles for linguistic theory: nativelike selection and nativelike fluency', in J. C. Richards and R. W. Schmidt (eds), *Language and Communication*, London: Longman, pp. 191–226.

Pérez-Pereira, M. (1994), 'Imitations, repetitions, routines and the child's analysis of language: insights from the blind', *Journal of Child Language*, 21, 317–37.

Pérez-Pereira, M. and Castro, J. (1997), 'Language acquisition and the compensation of visual deficit: new comparative data on a controversial topic', *British Journal of Developmental Psychology*, 15, 439–59.

Pérez-Pereira, M. and Conti-Ramsden, G. (1999), *Language Development and Social Interaction in Blind Children*, Hove: Psychology Press.

Peters, A. M. (1977), 'Language learning strategies: does the whole equal the sum of the parts?', *Language*, 53, 560–73.

Peters, A. M. (1983), *The Units of Language Acquisition*, Cambridge: Cambridge University Press.

Peters, A. M. (1985), 'Language segmentation: operating principles for the perception and analysis of language', in D. I. Slobin (ed.), *The Cross-Linguistic Study of Language Accquisition. Vol. 2: Theoretical Issues*, Hillsdale, NJ: Lawrence Erlbaum, pp. 1029–67.

Peters, A. M. (1995), 'Strategies in the acquisition of syntax', in P. Fletcher and B. MacWhinney (eds), *The Handbook of Child Language*, Oxford: Blackwell, pp. 462–82.

Peters, A. M. (2001), 'Filler syllables: what is their status in emerging grammar?', *Journal of Child Language*, 28, 229–42.

Peters, A. M. and Menn, L. (1993), 'False starts and filler syllables: ways to learn grammatical morphemes', *Language*, 69, 742–77.

Peterson, R. and Burgess, C. (1993), 'Syntactic and semantic processing during idiom comprehension: neurolinguistic and psycholinguistic dissociations', in C. Cacciari and P. Tabossi (eds), *Idioms: Processing, Structure and Interpretation*, Hillsdale, NJ: Lawrence Erlbaum, pp. 201–25.

Petitto, L. A. (1987), 'On the autonomy of language and gesture: evidence from the acquisition of personal pronouns in American Sign Language', *Cognition*, 27, 1–52.

Piattelli-Palmarini, M. (1989), 'Evolution, selection and cognition: from "learning" to parameter setting in biology and the study of language', *Cognition*, 31, 1–44.

Pick, A. (1973) [1913], *Aphasia*, trans. and ed. J. Brown, Springfield, IL: Charles C. Thomas.

Pine, J. (1994), 'The language of primary caregivers', in C. Gallaway and B. J. Richards (eds), *Input and Interaction in Language Acquisition*, Cambridge: Cambridge University Press, pp. 15–37.

Pine, J. M. and Lieven, E. V. (1993), 'Reanalysing rote-learned phrases: individual differences in the transition to multi-word speech', *Journal of Child Language*, 20, 551–71.

Pinker, S. (1984), *Language Learnability and Language Development*, Cambridge, MA: Harvard University Press.

Pinker, S. (1987), 'The bootstrapping problem in language acquisition', in B. MacWhinney (ed.), *Mechanisms of Language Acquisition*, Hillsdale, NJ: Lawrence Erlbaum, pp. 399–441.

Pinker, S. (1991), 'Rules of language', *Science*, 253, 530–5.

Pinker, S. (1995), 'Facts about human language relevant to its evolution', in J.-P. Changeux and J. Chavaillon (eds), *Origins of the Human Brain*, Oxford: Clarendon Press, pp. 262–83.

Pinker, S. (1998), 'Words and rules', *Lingua*, 106, 219–42.

Pinker, S. (1999), *Words and Rules: The Ingredients of Language*, London: Weidenfeld and Nicolson.

Pinker, S. and Bloom, P. (1990), 'Natural language and natural selection', *Behavioral and Brain Sciences*, 13, 707–84.

Pinker, S. and Prince, A. (1988), 'On language and connectionism: analysis of a parallel distributed processing model of language acquisition', *Cognition*, 28, 73–193.

Pinker, S. and Prince, A. (1992), 'Regular and irregular morphology and the psychological status of rules of grammar', *Berkeley Linguistics Society*, 17, 230–51.

Pizzuto, E. and Caselli, M. C. (1992), 'The acquisition of Italian morphology: implications for models of language development', *Journal of Child Language*, 19, 491–557.

Plunkett, K. and Marchman, V. (1991), 'U-shaped learning and frequency effects in a multi-layered perceptron: implications for child langauge acquisition', *Cognition*, 38, 43–102.

Plunkett, K. and Marchman, V. (1993), 'From rote learning to system building: acquiring verb morphology in children and connectionist nets', *Cognition*, 48, 21–69.

Plunkett, K. and Nakisa, R. C. (1997), 'A connectionist model of the Arabic plural system', *Language and Cognitive Processes*, 12, 807–36.

Pollack, I. and Pickett, J. M. (1964), 'Intelligibility of excerpts from fluent speech: auditory vs. structural context', *Journal of Verbal Learning and Verbal Behavior*, 3, 79–84.

Posner, M. I., Petersen, S., Fox, P. and Raichle, M. (1988), 'Localization of cognitive operations in the human brain', *Science*, 240, 1627–31.

Prasada, S. and Pinker, S. (1993), 'Generalization of regular and irregular morphological patterns', *Language and Cognitive Processes*, 8, 1–56.

Premack, D. (1980), 'Representational capacity and the accessibility of knowledge: the case of chimpanzees', in M. Piattelli-Palmarini (ed.), *Language and Learning: The Debate Between Jean Piaget and Noam Chomsky*, London: Routledge and Kegan Paul, pp. 203–21.

Preuss, T. M. (2000), 'What's human about the human brain?', in M. S. Gazzaniga (ed.), *The New Cognitive Neurosciences*, Cambridge, MA: MIT Press, pp. 1219–34.

Pullum, G. K. and Scholz, B. C. (2002), 'Empirical assessment of stimulus poverty arguments', *Linguistic Review*, 19, 9–50.

Pulvermüller, F. (1998), 'On the matter of rules: past-tense formation and its significance for cognitive neuroscience', *Network*, 9, R1–R52.

Putnam, H. (1988), *Representation and Reality*, Cambridge, MA: MIT Press.

Quirk, R., Greenbaum, S., Leech, G. and Svartnik, J. (1985), *A Comprehensive Grammar of the English Language*, London: Longman.

Radford, A. (1990), *Syntactic Theory and the Acquisition of English Syntax: The Nature of Early Child Grammars of English*, Oxford: Blackwell.

Ramscar, M. (2002), 'The role of meaning in inflection: why the past tense does not require a rule', *Cognitive Psychology*, 45, 45–94.

Rayner, K., Carlson, M. and Frazier, L. (1983), 'The interaction of syntax and semantics during sentence processing', *Journal of Verbal Learning and Verbal Behavior*, 22, 358–74.

Redington, M. and Chater, N. (1998), 'Connectionist and statistical approaches to language acquisition: a distributional perspective', *Language and Cognitive Processes*, 13, 129–92.

Regier, T. (1996), *The Human Semantic Potential: Spatial Language and Constrained Connectionism*, Cambridge, MA: MIT Press.

Richards, B. J. (1990), *Language Development and Individual Differences: A Study of Auxiliary Verb Learning*, Cambridge: Cambridge University Press.

Richards, M. (1979), 'Adjective ordering in the language of young children: an experimental investigation', *Journal of Child Language*, 6, 253–78.

Rosch, E. (1975), 'Cognitive reference points', *Cognitive Psychology*, 7, 532–47.

Rosch, E. (1977), 'Human categorization', in N. Warren (ed.), *Studies in Cross-Cultural Psychology* (Vol. 1), London: Academic Press, pp. 1–49.

Rowland, C. F. and Pine, J. M. (2000), 'Subject-auxiliary inversion errors and wh-question acquisition: "what children do know?"', *Journal of Child Language*, 27, 157–81.

Rubino, R. B. and Pine, J. M. (1998), 'Subject–verb agreement in Brazilian Portuguese: what low error rates hide', *Journal of Child Language*, 25, 35–59.

Rudzka-Ostyn, B. (1985), 'Metaphoric processes in word formation: the case of prefixed verbs', in W. Paprotté and R. Dirven (eds), *The Ubiquity of Metaphor. Metaphor in Language and Thought*, Amsterdam: John Benjamins, pp. 209–41.

Rudzka-Ostyn, B. (ed.) (1988), *Topics in Cognitive Linguistics*, Amsterdam: John Benjamins.

Rumelhart, D. E. and McClelland, J. L. (1986), 'On learning the past tenses of English verbs', in D. E. Rumelhart and J. L. McClelland (eds), *Parallel Distributed Processing: Explorations in the Microstructure of Cognition. Vol. 2: Psychological and Biological Models*, Cambridge, MA: MIT Press, pp. 216–71.

Sachs, J. (1983), 'Talking about the there and then: the emergence of displaced reference in parent–child discourse', in K. E. Nelson (ed.), *Children's Language* (Vol. 4), Hillsdale, NJ: Lawrence Erlbaum, pp. 1–28.

Sachs, J., Bard, B. and Johnson, M. L. (1981), 'Language learning with restricted input: case studies of two hearing children of deaf parents', *Applied Psycholinguistics*, 2, 33–54.

Samuel, A. G. (1986), 'The role of the lexicon in speech perception', in E. B. Schwab and H. C. Nusbaum (eds), *Pattern Recognition by Humans and Machines. Vol. 1: Speech Perception*, Orlando: Academic Press, pp. 89–111.

Savage, C., Lieven, E., Theakston, A. and Tomasello, M. (submitted), 'Testing the abstractness of children's linguistic representations: lexical and structural priming of syntactic constructions in young children'.

Schneider, W. and Bjorklund, D. F. (1998), 'Memory', in D. Kuhn and R. S. Siegler (eds), *The Handbook of Child Psychology. Vol. 2: Cognition, Perception and Language*, New York: John Wiley and Sons, pp. 467–522.

Schreuder, R., de Jong, N., Krott, A. and Baayen, H. (1999), 'Rules and rote: beyond the linguistic either-or fallacy', *Behavioral and Brain Sciences*, 22, 1038–9.

Seidenberg, M. S. and Hoeffner, J. H. (1998), 'Evaluating behavioral and neuroimaging data on past tense processing', *Language*, 74, 104–22.

Seidenberg, M. S., Tanenhaus, M. K., Leiman, J. M. and Bienkowski, M. (1982), 'Automatic access of the meanings of ambiguous words in context: some limitations of knowledge-based processing', *Cognitive Psychology*, 14, 489–537.

Senghas, A. and Coppola, M. (2001), 'Children creating language: how Nicaraguan Sign Language acquired a spatial grammar', *Psychological Science*, 12, 323–8.

Sereno, J., Zwitserlood, P. and Jongman, A. (1999), 'Entries and operations: the great divide and the pitfalls of form frequency', *Behavioral and Brain Sciences*, 22, 1039.

Sereno, J. A. and Jongman, A. (1997), 'Processing of English inflectional morphology', *Memory and Cognition*, 25, 425–37.

Silverberg, R. and Gordon, H. W. (1979), 'Differential aphasia in two bilingual individuals', *Neurology*, 29, 51–5.

Simpson, G. B. (1994), 'Context and the processing of ambiguous words', in M. A. Gernsbacher (ed.), *Handbook of Psycholinguistics*, San Diego: Academic Press, pp. 359–74.

Sinclair, J. (1987), 'Introduction', in J. Sinclair (ed.), *Collins COBUILD English Language Dictionary*, London: HarperCollins, pp. xv–xxi.

Sinha, C. and Kuteva, T. (1995), 'Distributed spatial semantics', *Nordic Journal of Linguistics*, 18, 167–99.

Sinha, C., Thorseng, L. A., Hayashi, M. and Plunkett, K. (1994), 'Comparative spatial semantics and language acquisition: evidence from Danish, English, and Japanese', *Journal of Semantics*, 11, 253–87.

Slobin, D. I. (1973), 'Cognitive prerequisites for the development of grammar', in C. A. Ferguson and D. I. Slobin (eds), *Studies in Child Language Development*, New York: Holt, Rinehart and Winston, pp. 175–208.

Slobin, D. I. (1991), 'Aphasia in Turkish: speech production in Broca's and Wernicke's patients', *Brain and Language*, 41, 149–64.

Smith, L. B., Jones, S. S. and Landau, B. (1992), 'Count nouns, adjectives and perceptual properties in children's novel word interpretation', *Developmental Psychology*, 28, 273–86.

Smith, N. and Tsimpli, I. M. (1991), 'Linguistic modularity? A case study of a "savant" linguist', *Lingua*, 84, 315–51.

Smith, N. and Tsimpli, I. M. (1995), *The Mind of a Savant: Language Learning and Modularity*, Oxford: Blackwell.

Smoczyńska, M. (1985), 'The acquisition of Polish', in D. I. Slobin (ed.), *The Crosslinguistic Study of Language Acquisition. Vol. 1: The Data*, Hillsdale, NJ: Lawrence Erlbaum, pp. 595–683.

Smoczyńska, M. (1998), 'Krakowskie dane językowe dzieci w systemie CHILDES', in M. Smoczyńska (ed.), *Studia z psychologii rozwojowej i psycholingwistyki*, Kraków: Universitas, pp. 283–96.

Snow, C. (1986), 'Conversations with children', in P. Fletcher and M. Garman (eds), *Language Acquisition* (2nd edn), Cambridge: Cambridge University Press, pp. 69–89.

Snow, C. E. (1981), 'The uses of imitation', *Journal of Child Language*, 8, 205–12.

Snow, C. E. (1983), 'Saying it again: the role of expanded and deferred imitations in language acquisition', in K. E. Nelson (ed.), *Children's Language* (Vol. 4), Hillsdale, NJ: Lawrence Erlbaum, pp. 29–58.

Snow, C. E. (1995), 'Issues in the study of input: finetuning, universality, individual and developmental differences, and necessary causes', in P. Fletcher and B. MacWhinney (eds), *The Handbook of Child Language*, Oxford: Blackwell, pp. 180–93.

Sonnenstuhl, I., Eisenbeiss, S. and Clahsen, H. (1999), 'Morphological priming in the German lexicon', *Cognition*, 72, 203–36.

Spivey, M. J., Tanenhaus, M. K., Eberhard, K. M. and Sedivy, J. C. (2002), 'Eye movements and spoken language comprehension: effects of visual context on syntactic ambiguity resolution', *Cognitive Psychology*, 45, 447–81.

Springer, S. (1979), 'Speech perception and the biology of language', in M. Gazzaniga (ed.), *Handbook of Behavioral Neurobiology. Vol. 2: Neuropsychology*, New York: Plenum Press, pp. 153–77.

Stemberger, J. P. and MacWhinney, B. (1986), 'Frequency and the lexical storage of regularly inflected forms', *Memory and Cognition*, 14, 17–26.

Stemberger, J. P. and MacWhinney, B. (1988), 'Are lexical forms stored in the lexicon?', in M. Hammond and M. Noonan (eds), *Theoretical Morphology: Approaches in Modern Linguistics*, London: Academic Press, pp. 101–16.

Stojanovik, V., Perkins, M. and Howard, S. (in press), 'Williams syndrome and specific language impairment do not support claims for developmental double dissociations', *Journal of Neurolinguistics*.

Stromswold, K. (1995), 'The acquisition of subject and object wh-questions', *Language Acquisition*, 4, 5–48.

Stromswold, K. (1996), 'Genes, specificity, and the lexical/functional distinction in language acquisition', *Behavioral and Brain Sciences*, 19, 648–9.

Stromswold, K. (2000), 'The cognitive neuroscience of language acquisition', in M. S. Gazzaniga (ed.), *The New Cognitive Neurosciences*, Cambridge, MA: MIT Press, pp. 909–32.

Stromswold, K. (2001), 'The heritability of language: a review and metaanalysis of twin, adoption and linkage studies', *Language*, 77, 647–723.

Sutton-Spence, R. and Woll, B. (1999), *The Linguistics of British Sign Language: An Introduction*, Cambridge: Cambridge University Press.

Svorou, S. (1994), *The Grammar of Space*, Amsterdam: John Benjamins.

Tager-Flusberg, H. (1986), 'Constraints on the representation of word meaning: evidence from autistic and mentally retarded children', in S. A. Kuczaj and M. Barrett (eds), *The Development of Word Meaning*, New York: Springer-Verlag, pp. 69–81.

Talmy, L. (1983), 'How language structures space', in H. Pick and L. Acredolo (eds), *Spatial Orientation: Theory, Research and Application*, New York: Plenum Press, pp. 225–82.

Talmy, L. (1985), 'Force dynamics in language and thought', *Parasession on Causatives and Agentivity, 21st Regional Meeting, Chicago Linguistic Society*, 293–337.

Tanenhaus, M. K., Leiman, J. M. and Seidenberg, M. S. (1979), 'Evidence for multiple stages in the processing of ambiguous words in syntactic contexts', *Journal of Verbal Learning and Verbal Behavior*, 18, 427–40.

Taylor, J. R. (1989), *Linguistic Categorization: Prototypes in Linguistic Theory*, Oxford: Clarendon Press.

Taylor, J. R. (2002), *Cognitive Grammar*, Oxford: Oxford University Press.

Tesak, J. (1994), 'Cognitive load and the processing of grammatical items', *Neurolinguistics*, 8, 43–8.

Thal, D., Bates, E. and Bellugi, U. (1989), 'Language and cognition in two children with Williams syndrome', *Journal of Speech and Hearing Research*, 32, 489–500.

Thal, D. J., Bates, E., Zappia, M. J. and Oroz, M. (1996), 'Ties between lexical and grammatical development: evidence from early talkers', *Journal of Child Language*, 23, 349–68.

Theakston, A., Lieven, E., Pine, J. and Rowland, C. (2000), 'The role of performance limitations in the acquisition of "mixed" verb-argument structure at stage 1', in M. Perkins and S. Howard (eds), *New Directions in Language Development and Disorders*, New York: Plenum Press, pp. 119–28.

Thomas, M. S. C., Grant, J., Barham, Z., Gsödl, M., Laing, E., Lakusta, L., Tyler, K., Grice, S., Paterson, S. and Karmiloff-Smith, A. (2001), 'Past tense formation in Williams syndrome', *Language and Cognitive Processes*, 16, 143–76.

Thornton, R. and Crain, S. (1994), 'Successful cyclic movement', in T. Hoekstra and B. D. Schwartz (eds), *Language Acquisition Studies in Generative Grammar*, Amsterdam: John Benjamins, pp. 215–52.

Todd, P. (1982), 'Tagging after red herrings: evidence against the processing capacity explanation in child language', *Journal of Child Language*, 9, 99–114.

Todd, P. and Aitchison, J. (1980), 'Learning language the hard way', *First Language*, 1, 122–40.

Tomasello, M. (1987), 'Learning to use prepositions: a case study', *Journal of Child Language*, 14, 79–98.

Tomasello, M. (1992), *First Verbs: A Case Study of Early Grammatical Development*, Cambridge: Cambridge University Press.

Tomasello, M. (1995), 'Language is not an instinct', *Cognitive Development*, 10, 131–56.

Tomasello, M. (1999), *The Cultural Origins of Human Cognition*, Cambridge, MA: Harvard University Press.

Tomasello, M. (2000), 'Do young children have adult syntactic competence?', *Cognition*, 74, 209–53.

Tomasello, M. (2003), *Constructing a Language: A Usage-Based Theory of Child Language Acquisition*, Cambridge, MA: Harvard University Press.

Tomasello, M. and Abbot-Smith, K. (2002), 'A tale of two theories: response to Fisher', *Cognition*, 83, 207–14.

Tomasello, M. and Todd, J. (1983), 'Joint attention and lexical acquisition style', *First Language*, 4, 197–212.

Tomasello, M., Akhtar, N., Dodson, K. and Rekau, L. (1997), 'Differential productivity in young children's use of nouns and verbs', *Journal of Child Language*, 24, 373–87.

Tomblin, J. B. and Buckwalter, P. R. (1998), 'Heritability of poor language achievement among twins', *Journal of Speech Language and Hearing Research*, 41, 188–99.

Traugott, E. C. (1978), 'On the expression of spatio-temporal relations in language', in J. Greenberg, C. Ferguson and E. Moravcsik (eds), *Universals of Human Language* (Vol. 3), Stanford, CA: Stanford University Press, pp. 369–400.

Trueswell, J. C. (1996), 'The role of lexical frequency in syntactic ambiguity resolution', *Journal of Memory and Language*, 35, 566–85.

Trueswell, J. C., Tanenhaus, M. K. and Garnsey, S. M. (1994), 'Semantic influences on parsing: use of thematic role information in syntactic ambiguity resolution', *Journal of Memory and Language*, 33, 285–318.

Trueswell, J. C., Tanenhaus, M. K. and Kello, C. (1993), 'Verb-specific constraints in sentence-processing: separating effects of lexical preference from garden-paths', *Journal of Experimental Psychology: Learning Memory and Cognition*, 19, 528–53.

Ulatowska, H. K., Sadowska, M. and Kądzielowa, D. (2001), 'A longitudinal study of agrammatism in Polish: a case study', *Journal of Neurolinguistics*, 14, 321–36.

Ullman, M., Bergida, R. and O'Craven, K. M. (1997), 'Distinct fMRI activation patterns for regular and irregular past tense', *NeuroImage*, 5, S549.

Ullman, M. T. (1999), 'Acceptability ratings of regular and irregular past tense forms: evidence for a dual-system model of language from word frequency and phonological neighborhood effects', *Language and Cognitive Processes*, 14, 47–67.

Ullman, M. T., Corkin, S., Coppola, M., Hickok, G., Growdon, J. H., Koroshetz, W. J. and Pinker, S. (1997), 'A neural dissociation within language: evidence that the mental dictionary is part of declarative memory, and that grammatical rules are processed by the procedural system', *Journal of Cognitive Neuroscience*, 9, 2–27.

Urwin, C. (1984), 'Communication in infancy and the emergence of language in blind children', in R. L. Schiefelbusch and J. Pickar (eds), *The Acquisition of Communicative Competence*, Baltimore: University Park Press, pp. 479–524.

van Hoek, K. (1997), *Anaphora and Conceptual Structure*, Chicago: Chicago University Press.

van Hout, A. (1991), 'Outcome of acquired aphasia in childhood: prognosis factors', in I. Pavão Martins, A. Castro-Caldas, H. R. van Dongen and A. van Hout (eds), *Acquired Aphasia in Children: Acquisition and Breakdown of Language in the Developing Brain*, Dordrecht: Kluwer, pp. 163–9.

van Mourik, M., Verschaeve, M., Boon, P., Paquier, P. and Vanharskamp, F. (1992), 'Cognition in global aphasia: indicators for therapy', *Aphasiology*, 6, 491–9.

Van Petten, C., Coulson, S., Rubin, S., Plante, E. and Parks, M. (1999), 'Time course of word identification and semantic integration in spoken language', *Journal of Experimental Psychology: Learning Memory and Cognition*, 25, 394–417.

Vargha-Khadem, F. and Polkey, C. E. (1992), 'A review of cognitive outcome after hemidecortication in humans', in F. D. Rose and D. A. Johnson (eds), *Recovery from Brain Damage: Reflections and Directions*, New York: Plenum Press, pp. 137–51.

Vargha-Khadem, F., Watkins, K., Alcock, K., Fletcher, P. and Passingham, R. (1995), 'Praxic and nonverbal cognitive deficits in a large family with a genetically transmitted speech and langauge disorder', *Proceedings of the National Academy of Sciences of the United States of America*, 92, 930–3.

Verhagen, A. (forthcoming), *Constructions of Intersubjectivity*, Oxford: Oxford University Press.

Volterra, V., Caparci, O., Pezzini, G., Sabbadini, L. and Vicari, S. (1996), 'Linguistic abilities in Italian children with Williams syndrome', *Cortex*, 32, 663–77.

Warburton, E., Wise, R. J. S., Price, C. J., Weiller, C., Hadar, U., Ramsay, S. and Frackowiak, R. S. J. (1996), 'Noun and verb retrieval by normal subjects: studies with PET', *Brain*, 119, 159–79.

Wason, P. C. and Reich, S. S. (1979), 'A verbal illusion', *Quarterly Journal of Experimental Psychology*, 31, 591–7.

Wayland, S. C., Berndt, R. S. and Sandson, J. R. (1996), 'Aphasic patients' sensitivity to structural and meaning violations when monitoring for nouns and verbs in sentences', *Neuropsychology*, 10, 504–16.

Wegener, H. (1994), 'Variation in the acquisition of German plural morphology by second language learners', in R. Tracy and E. Lattey (eds), *How Tolerant is Universal Grammar? Essays on Language Variability and Language Variation*, Tübingen: Niemeyer, pp. 267–94.

Wegener, H. (1999), 'Die Pluralbildung im Deutschen: ein Versuch im Rahmen der Optimalitätstheorie', *Linguistik online*, 4, http://viadrina.euv-frankfurt-o.de/~wjournal/3{I99/wegener.html.

Wells, C. G. (1979), 'Learning and using the auxiliary verb in English', in V. Lee (ed.), *Language Development*, London: Croom Helm, pp. 250–70.

Wells, G. (1985), *Language Development in the Preschool Years*, Cambridge: Cambridge University Press.

Westfal, S. (1956), *A Study in Polish Morphology: The Genitive Singular Masculine*, The Hague: Mouton.

Whiten, A., Custance, D. M., Gomez, J. C., Teixidor, P. and Bard, K. A. (1996), 'Imitative learning of artificial fruit processing in children (*Homo sapiens*) and chimpanzees (*Pan troglodytes*)', *Journal of Comparative Psychology*, 110, 3–14.

Wilson, B. and Peters, A. M. (1988), 'What are you cookin' on a hot? A three-year-old blind child's violation of universal constraints on constituent movement', *Language*, 64, 249–73.

Wise, R. J. S., Chollet, F., Hadar, U., Friston, K., Hoffner, E. and Frackowiak, R. (1991), 'Distribution of cortical networks in word comprehension and word retrieval', *Brain*, 114, 1803–17.

Worden, R. (1998), 'The evolution of language from social intelligence', in J. R. Hurford, M. Studdert-Kennedy and C. Knight (eds), *Approaches to the Evolution of Language: Social and Cognitive Bases*, Cambridge: Cambridge University Press, pp. 148–66.

Wulfeck, B. and Bates, E. (1991), 'Differential sensitivity to errors of agreement and word order in Broca's aphasia', *Journal of Cognitive Neuroscience*, 3, 258–72.

Wulfeck, B., Bates, E. and Capasso, R. (1991), 'A crosslinguistic study of grammaticality judgments in Broca's aphasia', *Brain and Language*, 41, 311–36.

Yamada, J. E. (1990), *Laura: A Case for Modularity of Language*, Cambridge, MA: MIT Press.

Zattore, R., Evans, A. C., Meyer, E. and Gjedde, A. (1992), 'Lateralization of phonetic and pitch discrimination in speech processing', *Science*, 256, 846–9.

Index